MW01044503

THE COMPREHENSIVE
NCLEX-RN® REVIEW

Complete Source of Vital NCLEX® Exam Information

FOURTEENTH EDITION

PATRICIA A. HOEFLER, MSN, RN

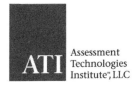

ATI Assessment
Technologies
Institute™, LLC

7500 W. 160TH ST.
STILWELL, KS 66085
WWW.ATITESTING.COM

THE COMPREHENSIVE NCLEX-RN® REVIEW

CONTRIBUTING AUTHOR

Karyn Plante, MSN, RN
Associate Professor

CONTRIBUTING REVIEWERS

Tracey Bousquet, MSN, RN
Consultant

Jennifer Burks, MSN, RN
Consultant

Janet Gysi, MSN, RN
Associate Professor

Carol Jernigan, MSN, RN
Clinical Nurse Specialist

Lynn Jordan, MSN, RN
Professor of Nursing

Elizabeth Kassel, MSN, RN
Associate Professor

Teresa LaFave, NP, MS, RN
Nurse Practitioner, Consultant

Marian Kovatchitch, MSN, RN
Associate Professor

Laura McQueen, PhD, RN, CS
Ph.D. Candidate
Clinical Specialist

Michele Michael, PhD, RN
Professor of Nursing

Cherralene Peer, MSN, RN
Associate Professor

May Phillips, PhD, RN
Professor

Margaret Poole, MSN, RN
Associate Professor

Sandra Schuler, MSN, RN
Professor

Donna Snelson, MSN, RN
Associate Professor

Eleanor Walker, PhD, RN
Professor

Lois Walker, PhD, RN
Psychotherapist

TABLE OF CONTENTS

TABLE OF CONTENTS

LIST OF TABLES & GRAPHICS

AN INTRODUCTION TO

THE COMPREHENSIVE NCLEX-RN® REVIEW

Complete Source of Vital NCLEX® Exam Information
Fourteenth Edition

Welcome to ATI's *COMPREHENSIVE NCLEX-RN® REVIEW!* ATI is a professional organization directed by nurse educators and dedicated to excellence in nursing education.

If you are now beginning an ATI review - in live or online format - you are in good company! ATI is the leader in NCLEX-RN® exam reviews.

This fourteenth edition features:

- ✓ Thoroughly revised and updated content throughout
- ✓ New Community Health unit
- ✓ Updated unit on the NCLEX® Exam Alternate Test Item Formats
- ✓ An outline of ATI's unique test-taking strategies
- ✓ Easy-to-understand charts and graphs
- ✓ Expanded appendices
- ✓ An easy-to-use Pharmacology Guide

We hope this outline will facilitate your review of nursing information for the NCLEX® exam. You have our best wishes for success on the exam and for success and fulfillment in your career as a professional nurse.

For more information about ATI products, contact ATI at (800) 667-7531 or visit our Web site at www.atitesting.com. We always are pleased to assist you.

INTRODUCTION

REVIEW OF TEST-TAKING STRATEGIES FOR THE NCLEX-RN® EXAM

UNIT CONTENT

SYMBOLS

 Key Points

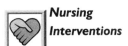 Nursing Interventions

 Points to Remember

PREPARING FOR THE EXAM

A. What You Should Know About the NCLEX-RN® Exam

1. General information
   a. The first integrated exam was given in July 1982
   b. The purpose of the exam is to determine that a candidate is prepared to practice entry-level nursing safely
   c. The exam is designed to test essential knowledge of nursing and a candidate's ability to apply that knowledge to clinical situations
   d. The purpose of the new test plan is to bring the exam in line with current nursing behaviors (the nursing process and decision making)
   e. Exam is "pass/fail," and no other score is given
2. Computerized Adaptive Testing
   a. Computer program continuously scores answers and selects questions suitable for each candidate's competency level for a more precise measurement of competency
   b. A higher weight is assigned to difficult questions, so a passing score can be obtained by answering a lot of easier questions or, a smaller number of more difficult questions
   c. Special screen design is used (see SCREEN DESIGN below)
   d. Use the mouse to move the cursor on the screen to the desired location. Single-click your mouse to select an option as your answer.
   e. A drop-down calculator is also featured. Double-click your mouse on the calculator icon, and the drop-down calculator will appear.
   f. After you have confirmed your selection, click on "next" to input your answer and proceed to the next screen
   g. After you proceed to the next screen, you CANNOT go back to a previous question to change your answer.
3. Exam schedule
   a. Given year-round
   b. Retake policy: The exam can only be repeated every 45 days
4. Number of questions and time allowed
   a. No minimum amount of time; however, a candidate must answer a minimum of 75 test questions
   b. Maximum time is 6 hr, with a maximum of 265 test questions
   c. About one out of three candidates completes the exam in less than 2 hr; one in three will use the complete 6 hr
   d. The computer will automatically stop as soon as one of the following occurs:
      1) Candidate's measure of competency is determined to be above or below the passing standard
      2) Candidate has answered all 265 test questions
      3) Maximum amount of time (6 hr) has expired

Case Scenario and Stem

SCREEN DESIGN

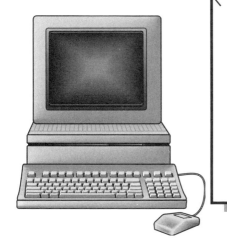

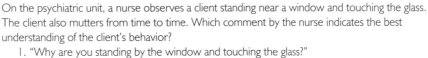

> On the psychiatric unit, a nurse observes a client standing near a window and touching the glass. The client also mutters from time to time. Which comment by the nurse indicates the best understanding of the client's behavior?
>
> 1. "Why are you standing by the window and touching the glass?"
>
> 2. "There you are. I came to see if you wanted to see the video we are showing on the unit?"
>
> 3. "What are you looking at through the window?"
>
> 4. "Are you hearing voices or seeing things?"

Choices 1, 2, 3, and 4

5. A candidate will pass by either:
   a. Answering 75 to 265 questions above the passing standard (the required weighted score) for all questions answered, within the time allowed; or
   b. Answering at least 75 questions within the time allowed and achieving the passing standard for the last 60 questions answered
6. Types of questions
   a. The majority of questions are standard multiple choice
      1) Standard multiple choice questions have four choices
      2) The best option is the only correct answer
   b. Exam includes 15 unmarked questions that do not impact your score.
   c. A small percentage of the questions are alternative format questions, including:
      1) Fill-in-the-blank (calculation) items
      2) Drag-and-drop (sequencing) items
      3) Multiple response items
      4) Hot spot (point and click) items
      5) Items with graphs, tables, or charts
7. Exam procedure:
   a. Look for the BEST answer to each question
   b. It is not possible to skip questions or return to previous questions
   c. Mandatory 10-min break after first 2 hr and after another 1 and ½ hr
   d. Paper or erase board provided for calculations to be returned at end of exam
8. Structure of the test plan
   a. Safe, Effective Care Environment
      1) Management of Care   13-19%
      2) Safety and Infection Control   8-14%
   b. Health Promotion and Maintenance   6-12%
   c. Psychosocial Integrity   6-12%
   d. Physiological Integrity
      1) Basic Care and Comfort   6-12%
      2) Pharmacological and Parenteral Therapies   13-19%
      3) Reduction of Risk Potential   13-19%
      4) Physiological Adaptation   11-17%
      Information courtesy of the National Council of State Boards of Nursing, Inc., Test Plan April 2007.

B. Schedule Your Study Time

1. The minimum time for preparation is 2 hr a day for 6 to 8 weeks
   a. Spend ⅓ of your time reviewing content
   b. Spend ⅔ of your time answering test questions
2. For content review, use an NCLEX-RN® exam review book such as this one, which outlines content

3. Begin with areas that are most difficult for you, or the areas that are least familiar.
4. For more detailed information on your difficult or less familiar areas, use a good nursing reference manual.
5. Review medical-surgical, child health, women's health, and mental health nursing, as well as nursing management and alternate test item formats.
6. Use a body systems approach for medical-surgical and child health nursing areas.
7. When studying body systems and the associated diseases, remember to:
   a. Define the disease in terms of the pathophysiological process that is occurring.
   b. Identify the client's early and late manifestations.
   c. Identify the most important or life-threatening complications.
   d. Define the medical treatment.
   e. Identify and prioritize the nursing. interventions associated with early and late manifestations.
   f. Identify what the nurse teaches the client/family to prevent or adapt to disease.
8. To schedule your study time:
   a. List the areas you need to review.
   b. Count the number of days you have available to study.
   c. Estimate the amount of time needed for each area.
   d. On your calendar, write the area to review, the number of questions to answer, and the amount of time needed for each study day.

C. Answer Many Questions

1. Answering questions will develop your test-taking skills.
2. Use questions similar to those on the NCLEX® exam.
3. Answer a minimum of 3,000 test questions
4. Include answering test questions in your study plan. For example, answer 100 questions each day for a month.
5. If you are at high risk, answer 5,000 test questions.
6. Use at least three different question-and-answer books.
7. Use a variety of books that provide more comprehensive preparation.
8. Use an online question-and-answer program that mimics the NCLEX® exam. This will give you a more realistic experience with answering alternative-item format questions.

D. Assess Your Progress

1. Each time you answer questions, check the number of questions you answered correctly.
   a. If you answer less than 65% correctly, this is a warning signal. Spend lots of time reviewing content and answering more questions in this area of nursing.
   b. If you answer 65 to 75% correctly, your performance is average. Success in this area is uncertain. Continue working with this content until your score is above 75%. Work on building your confidence by answering more questions in this area.
   c. If you answer 75 to 85% correctly, your performance is very good. Only return to this area after you have at least 75% in all other areas. Feel confident.
   d. If you answer 85 to 95% correctly, your performance is superior. Don't waste time on this. Feel very confident.
2. For each wrong answer, identify why you answered wrong
   a. You may have answered a question wrong because you did not know the facts or got confused about the information.
      1) Identify this as a content weakness.
      2) Review the content again.
   b. You may have answered a question wrong because you misread the question, did not understand what it was asking, or did not know how to select the best answer.
      1) Identify this as a test-taking deficiency.
      2) Seek assistance using other ATI products.
3. Check the number of questions that you identified as difficult and went back to answer later. See how many of them you answered correctly.

SECTION II

ANSWERING QUESTIONS

A. Identify the Critical Elements in the Question

1. Identify the issue in the question.
   a. The issue is the problem about which the question is asking.
   b. The issue may be a:
      1) Medication: for example, digoxin (*Lanoxin*), furosemide (*Lasix*)
      2) Nursing problem: for example, alteration in comfort, potential for infection
      3) Behavior: for example, restlessness, agitation
      4) Disorder: for example, diabetes mellitus, ulcerative colitis
      5) Procedure: for example, glucose tolerance test, cardiac catheterization

2. Identify the client in the question.
   a. The client in the question is usually the person with the health problem.
   b. The client in a test question may also be a relative or significant other or another member of the health care team with whom the nurse is interacting.
   c. The correct answer to the question must relate to the client in the question.
3. Look for the key words.
   a. Key words focus attention on what is important.
   b. Key words may appear in bold print.
   c. Examples:
      1) During the early period, which of the following nursing procedures would be **best**?
      2) The nurse would expect to find which of the following characteristics in an **adult** diabetic?
      3) Which of the following nursing actions is **vital**?
      4) Which of the following nursing actions would be best **initially**?
4. Identify what the stem is asking and determine whether the question has a true response stem, a false response stem, or a priority stem.
   a. Be clear about what the stem is asking before you look at the options.
   b. If the question is not clear to you, rephrase it using your own words.
   c. Determine whether the question has a true response stem, a false response stem, or a priority stem.
      1) True response stem
         a) Definition: A true response stem requires an answer that is a true statement
         b) Examples:
            (1) The nurse would assign the nursing assistant to:
            (2) Which manifestation would the nurse expect to assess?
            (3) The therapeutic response by the nurse would be:
            (4) The nurse evaluates that the client has a positive response to the medication when the client has:
      2) False response stem
         a) Definition: A false response stem requires an answer that is a false statement

b) Examples:
(1) Which of the following nursing actions would be inappropriate?
(2) Which of the following statements by the client would indicate a need for further instruction?
(3) Which of the following describes incorrect placement of the hands during CPR?
(4) Which of the following actions would place the client at risk?

3) Priority response stem
a) Definition: A priority response stem requires the candidate to select the best answer from four plausible responses
b) Examples:
(1) Which client would the nurse assess first?
(2) The nurse's initial action would be to:
(3) The nurse should give immediate consideration to which of the following findings?
(4) The task that the nurse has the nursing assistant complete first would be:

B. Use a Selection Procedure to Eliminate Incorrect Options

1. Most NCLEX® questions are standard multiple choice questions that have four options. The correct answer is the BEST answer. The other three options are "distractors."
2. Distractors are options made to look like correct answers. They are intended to distract you from answering correctly.
3. As you read each of the four options, make a decision about it.
   a. This option is true (+)
   b. This option is false (−)
   c. I am not sure about this option (?)
4. If the stem is a true response stem:
   a. An option that is true (+) might be the correct answer
   b. An option that is false (−) is a distractor. Eliminate this option.
   c. An option that you are not sure about (?) is possibly the correct answer.
5. If the stem is a false response stem:
   a. An option that is true (+) is a distractor. Eliminate this option.
   b. An option that is false (−) may be the correct answer.

c. An option that you are not sure about (?) is possibly the correct answer.
6. Do not return to options you have eliminated.
7. If you are left with one option, that is your answer.
8. If you are left with one (+) option and one (?) option, select the (+) option as your answer.
9. If you are left with two (+) options, use strategies to select the best answer.

C. Use Test-Taking Strategies When You Are Unable to Select the Best Option

1. The Global Response Strategy
   a. A global response is a general statement that may include ideas of other options within it.
   b. Look for a global response when more than one option appears to be correct.
   c. The global response option will probably be the correct answer.
2. The Similar Distractors Strategy
   a. Similar distractors say basically the same thing using different words.
   b. Since there is only one correct answer in a question, similar distractors must be wrong.
   c. Eliminate similar distractors. Select for your answer an option that is different.
3. The Similar Word or Phrase Strategy
   a. When more than one option appears to be correct, look for a similar word or phrase in the stem of the question and in one of the four options.
   b. The option that contains the similar word or phrase may be the correct answer.
   c. Use this strategy after you have tried to identify a global response option and eliminated similar distractors.
4. The Absolute Word Strategy
   a. Absolute words include words such as "only", "every", "always", and "never."
   b. When a response includes an absolute word it is unlikely to be the correct answer.

D. Answering Communication Questions

1. The NCLEX® exam includes many communication questions because the ability to communicate therapeutically is essential for safe practice.
2. Identify the critical elements as in all questions. Pay particular attention to identification of the client in the question. Remember that the answer must relate to the client.
3. Learn to identify communication tools that enhance communication.
   a. Being silent: Nonverbal communication
   b. Offering self: "Let me sit with you."
   c. Showing empathy: "You are upset."
   d. Focusing: "You say that . . ."
   e. Restatement: "You feel anxious?"

f. Validation/clarification: "What you are saying is . . .?"
g. Giving information: "Your room is 423."

4. Learn to identify nontherapeutic communication blocks.
   a. Giving advice: "If I were you, I would . . ."
   b. Showing approval/disapproval: "You did the right thing."
   c. Using clichés and false reassurances: "Don't worry. It will be all right."
   d. Requesting an explanation: "Why did you do that?"
   e. Belittling feelings: "Everyone feels that way."
   f. Being defensive: "Every nurse on this unit is exceptional."
   g. Focusing on inappropriate issues or persons: "Have I said something wrong?"
   h. Placing the client's issues "on hold": "Talk to your doctor about that."

5. When answering communication questions, select an option that illustrates a therapeutic communication tool. Eliminate options that illustrate nontherapeutic communication blocks.

E. Answering Questions that Focus on Setting Priorities

1. Priority-setting questions ask the test taker to identify either what comes first, is most important, or gets the highest priority.

2. Examples:
   a. What is the nurse's initial response?
   b. The nurse should give immediate consideration to which of the following?
   c. Which nursing action receives the highest priority?
   d. What should the nurse do first?

3. Use guidelines to help you to answer priority setting questions
   a. Maslow's Hierarchy of Needs indicates that physiological needs come first.
   b. Maslow's Hierarchy of Needs indicates that when no physiological need is identified, safety needs come first.
   c. Nursing Process indicates that assessment comes first.
   d. Communication Theory indicates focusing on feelings first.
   e. Teaching/Learning Theory indicates focusing on motivation first.

A. Plan for Everything

1. Assemble everything you will need for the exam the night before:
   a. Identification: two IDs with signatures, including one with recent photograph
   b. Watch
   c. Several sharpened pencils (with erasers) for calculations

2. Plan to arrive at the test site early:
   a. Know the route to the exam site.
   b. Know how long it will take to get there.
   c. Know where you will park and if you will need coins for a parking meter.

3. Pay close attention to your own physiological needs:
   a. Dress in layers.
   b. Get a good night's sleep the night before the exam.
   c. Eat a good breakfast.
   d. Avoid stimulants and depressants.
   e. Use the bathroom just before the exam.

4. During the exam:
   a. Listen to the instructions.
   b. Pace yourself; don't spend too long on any one question.
   c. Don't let yourself become distracted. Focus your attention on answering the questions.
   d. Go with your first choice. Use test-taking strategies only when you cannot decide between close options.
   e. Keep your thoughts positive.

B. Manage Your Anxiety Level

1. Moderate levels of anxiety increase your effectiveness.
2. Don't cram the night before the exam.
3. Do something enjoyable and relaxing the night before the exam.
4. Learn and practice measures to manage your anxiety level during the exam as needed.
   a. Take a few deep breaths.
   b. Tense and relax muscles.
   c. Tell yourself positive affirmations.
   d. Visualize a peaceful scene.
   e. Visualize your success.

C. Test-Taking Tips

1. Prepare comprehensively and be sure to be well rested for the exam.

2. Read each question carefully, identifying the critical elements. Each question must be answered in sequence, and you may not skip or go back to change your answers to any questions.

3. Don't panic if the computer stops after a short time. It does not mean that you failed. The computer stops when the exam is able to determine with at least 95% certainty that you have demonstrated the ability, or inability, to practice safely at the minimal level of nursing competency.

4. It is helpful to know that most students pass by answering a maximum of 119 questions. However, you can still pass the exam even if you answered all 265 questions.

5. If you are having difficulty choosing between the best two options, use the test taking strategies you have learned in this review.

MEDICAL- SURGICAL NURSING

UNIT CONTENT

SYMBOLS

 Key Points   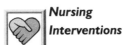 Nursing Interventions   Points to Remember

SECTION I

REVIEW OF FLUIDS AND ELECTROLYTES, ACID-BASE BALANCE

Fluids and Electrolytes

A. Body Fluids
1. Adults
   a. Women: 50 to 55% body weight is water
   b. Men: 60 to 70% body weight is water
   c. Older adults: 47% body weight is water
2. Infants: 75 to 80% body weight is water
3. Intracellular: 80% of total body water
4. Extracellular: 20% of total body water
   a. Interstitial
   b. Intravascular (plasma)
   c. Other: cerebrospinal fluid, intraocular fluid, bone water, gastrointestinal secretions

B. Electrolytes (normal values may vary slightly between institutions and laboratories)
1. Extracellular
   a. Na^+ 135 to145 mEq/L
   b. Ca^{++} 8.5 to 10 mg/dL
   c. Cl^- 85 to 115 mEq/L
   d. HCO_3^- 22 to 26 mEq/L
2. Intracellular
   a. K^+ 3.5 to 5.0 mEq/L
   b. PO_4 2.5 to 4.5 mg/dL
   c. Mg^+ 1.8 to 3.0 mEq/L
3. Function
   a. Promote neuromuscular excitability.
   b. Maintain fluid volume.
   c. Distribute water between fluid compartments.
   d. Regulate acid-base balance.

C. Movement of Fluids and Electrolytes
1. Diffusion: molecules move from an area of higher concentration to an area of lower concentration
2. Osmosis: water moves from an area of lower concentration of particles to an area of higher concentration
3. Filtration: water and dissolved substances move from an area of greater hydrostatic pressure to an area of lower hydrostatic pressure
4. Types of solution
   a. Isotonic 0.9% sodium chloride
      1) Same osmolarity as plasma
      2) Example: D_5W: To replace fluid volume or increase antidiuretic hormone (ADH) activity
   b. Hypertonic 3.0% sodium chloride
   c. Hypotonic 0.45% sodium chloride

5. Types of pressures
   a. Osmotic
   b. Hydrostatic

D. Mechanisms of Fluid Balance
1. Kidneys: regulate fluids and electrolytes, secrete renin
2. Lungs: regulate CO_2 levels, water vapor
3. Skin: regulate fluid losses (sweat)
4. Hormonal control
   a. Antidiuretic Hormone (ADH)
   b. Aldosterone

E. Assessment of Fluid and Electrolyte Balance/Imbalance
1. Fluid-volume deficit: water and electrolytes lost in same proportion (blood and urine become concentrated)
   a. Causes
      1) Fever
      2) Vomiting
      3) Diarrhea or ostomy losses
      4) Increased urine output
      5) Increased respirations
      6) Use of diuretics
      7) Insufficient IV fluid replacement
      8) Draining fistulas
      9) Third spacing (burns, ascites)
   b. Manifestations
      1) Weight loss
      2) Poor skin turgor
      3) Urine: decrease in volume, dark, odorous, increased specific gravity
      4) Increased respirations
      5) Dry, mucous membrane
      6) Increased heart rate
      7) Increased Hct (hemoconcentration)
      8) Decreased central venous pressure
    c. **NURSING INTERVENTIONS**
      1) Weigh client daily.
      2) Monitor I&O.
      3) Replace fluid - by mouth or IV (lactated Ringer's, 0.9% NS) per order.
      4) Assess urine specific gravity; normal range 1.010 to 1.025.
      5) Correct underlying cause.
2. Fluid volume excess
   a. Causes
      1) Excessive IV fluids
      2) Decreased kidney function, heart failure, cirrhosis
      3) Excessive intake of sodium
   b. Manifestations (same as heart failure)
      1) Cough, dyspnea, crackles, tachypnea
      2) Increased blood pressure, pulse
      3) Decreased Hct (hemodilution)
      4) Headache
      5) Weight gain (1 L of water = 1 kg of weight gain)

MEDICAL-SURGICAL NURSING - **UNIT ONE** ❖ **11**

6) Increased central venous pressure
7) Flushed skin
8) Late signs
   a) Bilateral jugular vein distention, tachycardia
   c) Pitting edema

 c. **NURSING INTERVENTIONS**
   1) Administer diuretics - furosemide (*Lasix*) as per order.
   2) Restrict fluids, monitor I&O.
   3) Weigh client daily.
   4) Provide skin care.
   5) Use semi-Fowler's position.
   6) Maintain low-sodium diet.
3. Electrolyte imbalances: (See Table I-1 Major Electrolytes: Imbalance/Interventions.)

POINTS TO REMEMBER

 1. Clients with low sodium will present with acute onset of confusion (increased risk of falls in older adult clients)
2. Never give potassium to a client who is not voiding (no "P," no "K")
3. When a client has a high calcium level, phosphorus levels will be low and vice versa; there is an inverse relationship

F. Regulation of Body pH
1. Normal value is 7.35 to 7.45
2. Mechanisms regulating pH
   a. Chemical buffers: protein molecules, phosphate
   b. Lungs: control carbon dioxide levels
   c. Kidneys: sodium bicarbonate

Metabolic/Respiratory Imbalance-Acidosis/Alkalosis

A. Acid-Base Imbalance
1. Metabolic acidosis
   a. Definition: base bicarbonate deficit; increase in hydrogen ion concentration
   b. Causes
      1) Diarrhea
      2) Renal failure
      3) Systemic infections
      4) Diabetic acidosis
      5) Starvation, malnutrition, ketogenic (high-fat) diet
      6) Excessive exercise
   c. Manifestations
      1) Headache
      2) Confusion, stupor
      3) Loss of consciousness
      4) pH below 7.35
      5) HCO_3^- below 22

6) Tachypnea (increased respirations) or Kussmaul breathing
 d. **NURSING INTERVENTIONS**
   1) Promote good air exchange.
   2) Monitor potassium level.
   3) Give sodium bicarbonate as prescribed.
2. Metabolic alkalosis
   a. Definition: base bicarbonate excess; decrease in hydrogen ion concentration
   b. Causes
      1) Vomiting (excessive loss of chloride)
      2) Gastric suction
      3) Alkali ingestion (excessive bicarbonate)
      4) Long-term diuretic therapy
   c. Manifestations
      1) CNS symptoms: confusion, irritability, agitation, coma
      2) Shallow respirations
      3) Tetany
      4) pH above 7.45
      5) HCO_3^- above 26
 d. **NURSING INTERVENTIONS**
   1) Restore fluid volume.
   2) Prevent metabolic alkalosis.
      a) Monitor potassium level.
      b) Evaluate need for IV potassium replacement for clients on gastric suction.
      c) Promote intake of potassium-rich foods or oral replacement for clients on long-term diuretic therapy.
3. Respiratory acidosis
   a. Definition: excess carbonic acid; increase in hydrogen ion concentration
   b. Causes
      1) Acute: respiratory suppression or obstruction due to pulmonary edema, over-sedation, pneumonia
      2) Chronic: chronic airflow limitation or COPD
   c. Manifestations
      1) Acute
         a) Confusion
         b) Restlessness
         c) Weakness
         d) Headache
         e) Coma
         f) pH below 7.35
         g) pCO_2 above 45 mm Hg
      2) Chronic (These symptoms are classic signs of COPD)
         a) pCO_2 above 45 mm Hg
         b) Tachypnea
         c) Dyspnea
         d) Weight loss

TABLE I-1
MAJOR ELECTROLYTES: IMBALANCE/INTERVENTIONS

ELECTROLYTE	NORM VALUE	SOURCES	LOW CAUSES	MANIFESTA-TIONS	NURSING INTERVEN.	EXCESS CAUSES	MANIFES-TATIONS	NURSING INVERVEN.
1. Potassium: (K+)	3.5 to 5.0 mEq/L	Fruits: bananas, peaches, melons, raisins, dried fruits, black licorice Juices: tomato, orange, grape Nuts Vegetables	Hypokalemia associated with renal loss, diuretics, burns, massive trauma, colitis, uncontrolled diabetes mellitus, diarrhea, excessive perspiration, decreased intake, vomiting, gastric suction	Muscle cramping, muscle weakness, weak pulse, dyspnea, mental changes, loquacious, hallucinations, depression, ECG changes (sensitivity to digitalis), respiratory arrest	- Keep I&O - Observe for ECG changes - Potassium supplements: Never give bolus injection IV or by mouth - Check renal function before giving - Dilute and mix well before adm. Not greater than 40 mEq/L	Hyperkalemia, renal failure, cell damage, Addison's disease, acidosis	CNS stimulation, listlessness, weakness, flaccid paralysis, abdominal cramps, arrhythmias, muscle weakness	- Monitor IV glucose and insulin (promote entry of K into cells), - Give fluids to increase urinary output, Kayexalate exchanges Na+ for K+ ion
2. Sodium: (Na+)	135 to 145 mEq/L	Table salt, processed foods, baking soda, MSG	Hyponatremia, increased perspiration, drinking water, gastrointestinal suction, irrigation of tube with plain water, adrenal insufficiency, potent diuretics	Lethargy, hypotension, cramps, vomiting, oliguria, apprehension, muscular weakness, headache, convulsions	- Use NS (not distilled water) for irrigation - Avoid tap water enemas - Drink juices and bouillon	Hypernatremia, decreased water intake, diarrhea, impaired renal function, acute tracheo bronchitis, unconsciousness, base bicarbonate deficit	Edema, hypertonicity, dry sticky mucous membranes, elevated temperature, flushed skin, thirst	- D$_5$W - Give water between tube feedings - Older adult clients to drink up to 10 glasses - Check humidifier water level
3. Calcium: (Ca++)	8.5 to 10 mg/dL	Milk, cheese, sardines, salmon, tofu, soy nuts, yogurt	Hypocalcemia, massive infection, burns, administration of citrated blood, hypoparathyroidism, surgical removal of parathyroids	Tetany cramps, tingling, numbness, hyperactive reflexes, cardiac arrhythmias Chvostek's sign and Trousseau's sign	- Teach proper use of antacids/laxatives, Importance of adequate milk intake - Keep 10% calcium gluconate on hand for use, start after thyroid surgery	Hypercalcemia, excessive vitamin D milk ingestion, hyperparathyroid, multiple myeloma, prolonged bed rest, renal disease	Renal calculi, nausea, anorexia, weight loss, deep bone pain, flank pain, lethargy, anorexia, muscle weakness, pathological fractures	- Increase mobility - Avoid large doses of vitamin D supplementation - Adequate hydration
4. Magnesium: (mg++)	1.8 to 3.0 mEq/L	Fruit, peas, beans, nuts, pumpkin seeds, sunflower seeds, spinach, salmon, halibut, black beans, navy beans	Hypomagnesemia, vomiting, diarrhea, chronic alcoholism, impaired GI absorption, enterostomy drainage. Use of diuretics	Disorientation, convulsion, hyperactive deep reflexes, tremors, arrhythmias, headaches, increased blood pressure	Encourage tap water and foods high in Mg++; bananas, seafood, dark, green vegetables, nuts, grains, oranges, chocolate. Monitor respiratory/cardiac systems.	- Hypermagnesemia, hypotension, respiratory, paralysis - Associated with renal failure, DM, dehydration	Contraindicated to administer antacids containing magnesium to clients with renal failure.	

d. **NURSING INTERVENTIONS**
   1) Administer sodium bicarbonate per order.
   2) Promote good respiratory exchange.
   3) Administer bronchodilators per order.
   4) Monitor ABGs.
4. Respiratory alkalosis
   a. Definition: carbonic acid deficit; decrease in hydrogen ion concentration
   b. Causes
      1) Hyperventilation - secondary to pain, anxiety, thyroid toxicosis
      2) Decreased O_2 (pneumonia, pulmonary edema)
      3) Elevated body temperature
      4) Salicylate intoxication
   c. Manifestations
      1) Unconsciousness
      2) Circumoral numbness
      3) pCO_2 below 35 mm Hg

   d. **NURSING INTERVENTIONS**
      1) Have client breathe into paper bag
      2) Have client breathe into cupped hands
      3) Provide oxygen if hypoxic

B. Blood Gases
1. ABGs
   a. Most accurate means of assessing respiratory function
   b. Must be sterile, anaerobic
   c. Drawn into heparinized syringe
   d. Keep on ice and transport to laboratory immediately
   e. Document amount of oxygen delivered
   f. Document client's body temperature
   g. Apply pressure to site for 5 to 10 min
2. Components
   a. pH
      1) Measure of acidity or alkalinity of blood
      2) Normal is between 7.35 and 7.45
         a) Acidosis: pH less than 7.35
         b) Alkalosis: pH greater than 7.45
   b. pCO_2
      1) Partial pressure of carbon dioxide
      2) Respiratory parameter influenced by lungs only
         a) Hyperventilation results in hypocapnia, or too little CO_2
         b) Hypoventilation results in hypercapnia, or too much CO_2
      3) Normal is between 35 and 45 mm Hg
   c. pO_2
      1) Partial pressure of oxygen
      2) Measure of amount of oxygen delivered to the lungs
      3) Normal is between 80 and 100 mm Hg

d. HCO_3^-
   1) Bicarbonate
   2) Metabolic parameter influenced only by metabolic factors, primarily the kidneys
   3) Normal is between 22 and 26 mEq/L

POINTS TO REMEMBER:

1. If acid/base imbalance has a respiratory origin, the pCO_2 is inversely related to the pH
   a. Respiratory acidosis: elevated pCO_2 and lowered pH
   b. Respiratory alkalosis: lowered pCO_2 and elevated pH
2. If acid/base imbalance has a metabolic origin, the HCO_3^- is directly related to the pH
   a. Metabolic alkalosis: elevated HCO_3^- and elevated pH
   b. Metabolic acidosis: lowered HCO_3^- and lowered pH
3. Normal values
   a. pH: 7.35 to 7.45
   b. pCO_2: 35 to 45 mm Hg
   c. HCO_3^-: 22 to 26 mEq/L
4. In relation to pH, apply ROME: Respiratory Opposite, Metabolic Equal

TABLE I-2
ACID-BASE IMBALANCE

	pH	pCO_2	HCO_3^-
Respiratory Acidosis	↓	↑	Normal or ↓
Respiratory Alkalosis	↑	↓	Normal or ↑
Metabolic Acidosis	↓	↓	↓
Metabolic Alkalosis	↑	↑	↑

SECTION II

REVIEW OF RESPIRATORY SYSTEM DISORDERS

Anatomy and Physiology

A. Function of the Lungs
1. Respiration: overall process by which exchange takes place between the atmosphere and the cells of the body; Normal adult respiratory rate is 12 to 20/min
2. Ventilation: movement of air in and out of the airways, intermittently replenishing the oxygen and removing the carbon dioxide from the lungs
3. Dead space: the 150 mL area where there is no air exchange; anatomically from the nose and mouth to the alveoli; therefore, 150 mL of the tidal volume is not used in any air exchange

B. Thoracic Cavity-Lined by Visceral and Parietal Pleura
1. Right pulmonary space
2. Left pulmonary space
3. Pericardial space
4. Mediastinal space contains the esophagus, trachea, great vessels, and heart

C. Subdivisions of the Lungs
1. Right: 3 lobes, 10 segments
2. Left: 2 lobes, 8 segments
3. Alveoli: tiny distal air sacs where gas exchange takes place; produce surfactant, a phospholipid secretion of the alveoli (Type II cells) that reduces the surface tension of fluid lining the alveoli allowing expansion to take place; Without surfactant, the lungs would collapse; oxygen is required for surfactant production
4. Diffusion: exchange of gases (oxygen and carbon dioxide) at the alveolar/capillary membrane

D. Factors Affecting Airflow
1. Normally, airways are open, moist, intact, and not inflamed. Cilia clear foreign substances.
2. Objective of care is to keep the airways healthy by the nursing interventions:
   a. Promote adequate fluid intake.
   b. Prevent exposure to infections.
   c. Decrease exposure to tobacco smoke.
   d. Decrease environmental pollutants.
   e. Avoid triggers that cause inflammation of airways, such as allergens.
3. If airways are affected, the diameter of the airways narrows causing an increase in airway resistance.

E. General Causes of Airway Illnesses
1. Infections that cause mucus and swelling
2. Allergens that cause swelling and bronchospasm
3. Foreign bodies that cause obstruction
4. Obstructive disorders: COPD, bronchiectasis
5. Restrictive disorders: kyphoscoliosis, abdominal distension, edema
6. Trauma: stab wound, surgery

Diagnostic Tests

A. Chest x-ray (CXR): noninvasive procedure with no special preparation; use a lead shield for women who are of child-bearing age

B. Mantoux Test: positive result indicates exposure to tuberculosis (TB). The test does not diagnose active TB. Diagnosis confirmed with acid-fast bacillus (AFB) sputum culture.

1. Administration method
   a. Given in the upper 1/3 inner surface of the forearm
   b. Needle is inserted bevel up
   c. 0.1 mL of purified protein derivative inserted intradermally
2. Evaluation method
   a. Must be read in 48 to 72 hr for accuracy
   b. Induration (area of elevation) is measured: if 10 mm or greater, it is a positive reading; for HIV or clients who are immunosuppressed, a reaction of 5 mm or greater may be considered positive

C. Sputum Examination
1. Obtain a first morning specimen is preferable, approximately 15 mL required.
2. Always attempt to obtain sputum sample prior to initiating antibiotics.
3. Instruct client to rinse mouth before collecting specimen to decrease oral flora and improve accuracy of results.

D. Thoracentesis: aspiration of pleural fluid and/or air from the pleural space
1. Preparation
   a. Ensure that informed consent has been obtained.
   b. Explain procedure to client; obtain baseline, and preprocedure vital signs.
   c. Position client sitting on side of bed with feet on chair, leaning over bedside table.
2. Postprocedure
   a. Apply pressure to puncture site, assess for bleeding, crepitus.
   b. Use semi-Fowler's position or puncture site up.
   c. Monitor for complications: shock, pneumothorax, respiratory arrest, subcutaneous emphysema.
   d. Assess breath sounds.

E. Bronchoscopy: direct examination of tracheobronchial tree using a bronchoscope
1. Preparation
   a. Ensure that informed consent has been obtained.
   b. Client must be NPO after midnight.
   c. Explain procedure to client; obtain baseline, preprocedure vital signs, and ABGs.
2. Postprocedure
   a. Keep client NPO until return of gag reflex returns.
   b. Monitor vital signs until stable.
   c. Assess for respiratory distress.

d. Notify provider if client experiences fever, and/or difficulty breathing.
e. Use semi-Fowler's position.
f. Give water as first fluid.
g. Inform client that it is possible to expectorate some blood-tinged mucus secretions, especially when a biopsy was performed.

Management of Clients with Respiratory System Disorders

A. COPD; Also Called Chronic Airflow Limitation (CAL)

1. Definition: a group of chronic lung diseases including pulmonary emphysema, chronic bronchitis, and bronchial asthma
2. Major diseases
   a. Pulmonary emphysema ("pink puffer")
      1) Definition: destruction of alveoli, narrowing of small airways (bronchioles), and the trapping of air resulting in loss of lung elasticity
      2) Etiology: cigarette smoking (#1 preventable cause of respiratory problems), deficiency of alpha antitrypsin (enzyme that blocks the action of proteolytic enzymes that are destructive to elastin and other substances in the alveolar walls)
      3) Manifestations
         a) Shortness of breath
         b) Difficult exhalation
         c) Pursed-lip breathing
         d) Wheezing, crackles
         e) Shallow, rapid respirations
         f) Hypoxia
         g) Productive cough
         h) Respiratory acidosis
         i) Barrel chest
         j) Anorexia, weight loss
         k) Finger clubbing
       4) **NURSING INTERVENTIONS**
         a) Position client sitting up, leaning forward.
         b) Provide pulmonary toilet.
            (1) Bronchodilator medications via nebulization as ordered
            (2) Chest physiotherapy/pulmonary drainage (CPT/PD)
            (3) Evaluate if treatment regimen is effective by checking the breath sounds and the pulse oximetry on a routine basis
         c) Encourage frequent rest periods.
         d) Use intermittent positive pressure breathing.

         e) Administer oxygen at low flow rate limited to 1 L, but may go no higher than a maximum 3 L or less): to prevent CO_2 narcosis.
         f) Encourage fluids of 3,000 mL per day if not contraindicated.
         g) Administer prophylactic antibiotics as prescribed.
         h) Provide appropriate nutrition and decrease carbohydrates to decrease carbon dioxide. Increase calories and protein to meet increased energy requirements. Lower intake of gas-forming foods to decrease dyspnea.
         i) Promote deep breathing exercises.
         j) Promote energy conservation exercises to enhance rest.
         k) Provide emotional support to decrease anxiety.
         l) Address sexual concerns.
         m) Provide teaching
            (1) No crowds
            (2) Diaphragmatic breathing
            (3) Pursed-lip breathing
            (4) Report first sign of upper respiratory infection
            (5) Avoid allergens (e.g., dust, odors, dander)
   b. Chronic bronchitis ("blue bloater")
      1) Definition: excessive mucus secretions within the airways and recurrent cough
      2) Etiology: heavy cigarette smoking, pollution, infection
      3) Manifestations
         a) Cough (copious sputum)
         b) Dyspnea on exertion, later at rest
         c) Hypoxemia resulting in polycythemia: ruddy look to skin, compensation
         d) Crackles, rhonchi
         e) Pulmonary hypertension leading to cor pulmonale and signs of right heart failure such as peripheral dependent edema
       4) **NURSING INTERVENTIONS**
         a) Prevent exposure to irritants.
         b) Increase humidity to 70%.
         c) Relieve bronchospasm through deep breathing and medications.
         d) Provide chest physiotherapy/pulmonary drainage.
         e) Promote breathing techniques.
   c. Asthma
      1) Definition: condition of abnormal bronchial hyper-reactivity to certain substances ("triggers")

2) Etiology
   a) Extrinsic: antigen-antibody reaction triggered by food, medications, or inhaled particles
   b) Intrinsic: pathophysiological conditions within the respiratory tract, nonallergic form
3) Manifestations: acute attack
   a) Severe, sudden dyspnea
   b) Use of accessory muscles; for adults neck muscles; children will get retractions
   c) Sitting up
   d) Diaphoresis
   e) Anxiety, apprehension
   f) Wheezing
   g) Cyanosis: very late sign
   h) An improvement in wheezing with no improvement in the client's condition may actually indicate worsening of the condition and tightening of airways to the point where air flow is diminishing.
   i) Decrease in tidal volume is measured by a spirometer.

 4) **NURSING INTERVENTIONS**
   a) Remain with client who is experiencing acute shortness of breath.
   b) Use high-Fowler's position.
   c) Provide emotional support.
   d) Monitor respiratory status: ABGs, lung sounds, and pulse oximetry.
   e) Promote hydration with fluids.
   f) Administer epinephrine hydrochloride (*Adrenalin*) subcutaneously and monitor its effectiveness.
   g) Administer aminophylline (*Theophylline*) IV or by mouth.
      (1) Monitor for side effects such as gastrointestinal upset (nausea and vomiting) and seizures.
      (2) Monitor aminophylline level to assure therapeutic action and prevent toxic effects. Therapeutic serum level is 10 to 20 mcg/mL.
   h) Provide bronchodilators via nebulization and metered-dose inhalers.
   i) Monitor oxygen therapy.
   j) Administer corticosteroids to decrease airway inflammation and open airways.

5) Status asthmaticus: severe life-threatening episode of airway obstruction that does not respond to common therapy; medical emergency
   a) Use high-Fowler's position.
   b) Monitor client for signs of hypoxia and administer continuous pulse oximetry.
   c) Monitor respiratory status.
   d) Administer potent systemic bronchodilators, steroids, epinephrine.
   e) Administer oxygen.
   f) Provide emotional support.
   g) Be prepared for emergency intubation.

B. Complications of COPD/CAL
1. Cor pulmonale (form of heart failure)
   a. Definition: right ventricular hypertrophy or failure secondary to disease of the lungs, pulmonary vessels or chest wall
   b. Etiology: causes increased pressure and pulmonary hypertension
      1) Decrease in the size of the pulmonary vascular bed from destruction of the pulmonary capillary
      2) Increased resistance of pulmonary capillary bed
      3) Shunting of unaerated blood across the collapsed alveoli
   c. Manifestations: signs of heart failure; initially the right side of the heart fails, then the left, because of decreased cardiac output
      1) Right-sided heart failure
         a) Peripheral edema (dependent)
         b) Jugular vein distension
      2) Left-sided heart failure
         a) Dyspnea
         b) Cyanosis
         c) Cough
         d) Substernal pain
         e) Syncope on exertion
         f) Paroxysmal nocturnal dyspnea and orthopnea
    d. **NURSING INTERVENTIONS**
      1) Promote bed rest.
      2) Monitor oxygen therapy.
      3) Maintain low-sodium diet.
      4) Monitor for signs of Lanoxin (*Digoxin*) toxicity.
2. Carbon dioxide narcosis/oxygen toxicity
   a. Definition: near comatose state secondary to increased CO_2 due to chronic retention
   b. Etiology: carbon dioxide retention secondary to excessive oxygen delivery

c. Manifestations: signs of hypoxia
   1) Drowsiness
   2) Irritability
   3) Hallucinations
   4) Coma
   5) Paralysis
   6) Convulsions
   7) Tachycardia
   8) Arrhythmias
   9) Poor ventilation

 d. **NURSING INTERVENTIONS**
   1) Avoid high concentrations of oxygen. Keep below 4 L/min (no more than 70% oxygen delivered). Make sure you know the approximate concentration delivered by the oxygen delivery method you are using. (cannula: 40%; mask: 60%; rebreather mask: 100%)
   2) Monitor response to oxygen therapy, blood gases, and continuous oximetry. If the client's pCO_2 is above normal, his oxygen saturation or PaO_2 should be at a normal level. This will shut off the hypoxic drive, which is triggered by a low O_2 level, and may cause the client to go into respiratory arrest.

3. Pneumothorax
   a. Definition: collection of air or fluid in the pleural space; can come from outside chest wall or inside the lung
   b. Etiology
      1) Trauma: gunshot, stabbing
      2) Thoracic surgery: open thoracotomy
      3) Positive pressure ventilation: causes segment of the lung to rip open, exposing pleural space
      4) Iatrogenic, as a complication of:
         a) Thoracentesis
         b) Central venous catheter insertion
         c) Surgery
   c. Types
      1) Spontaneous
      2) Tension: due to build up of pressure; causes mediastinal shift, a shift of the major organs and vessels in the chest cavity
      3) Open: from trauma such as a gunshot or stab wound to the chest cavity
   d. Manifestations: depend on severity, type
      1) Spontaneous
         a) Sudden, sharp chest pain
         b) Sudden shortness of breath with violent attempts to breathe
         c) Hypotension
         d) Tachycardia
         e) Hyper-resonance and decreased breath sounds over the affected lung

         f) Anxiety, diaphoresis, restlessness
      2) Tension
         a) Subcutaneous emphysema (crepitus), dyspnea
         b) Cyanosis
         c) Acute chest pain
         d) Tympany on percussion
         e) Mediastinal shift: contents of mediastinum pushed toward the unaffected side
            (1) Tracheal deviation – away from affected side
            (2) Cardiovascular compromise: may have signs and symptoms depending on degree of deviation

 e. **NURSING INTERVENTIONS**
   1) Remain with client and remain calm.
   2) Position in high-Fowler's.
   3) Assess vital signs, continuous oximetry, and breath sounds.
   4) Provide oxygen therapy as ordered.
   5) Prepare for chest x-ray.
   6) Provide thoracentesis tray to reestablish negative pressure or relieve pressure of tension pneumothorax.
      a) Assist with insertion of chest tube(s).
      b) Use upper chest tube for evacuation of air.
      c) Use lower chest tube for evacuation of fluid.
         (1) At the bedside or in operating room by provider
         (2) Aseptic technique
         (3) Local anesthetic, stab wound
         (4) Occlusive dressing
         (5) Chest x-ray immediately following insertion
   7) Monitor ABGs.
   8) Monitor for shock.

C. Closed-Chest Drainage
1. Purposes
   a. Remove fluid and/or air from the pleural space.
   b. Re-establish normal negative pressure in the pleural space.
   c. Promote re-expansion of the lung.
   d. Prevent reflux of air/fluid into pleural space from the drainage apparatus.
   e. This procedure is commonly used after thoracic surgery or as a treatment of pneumothorax.
2. General principles the nurse must consider when confronted with any chest drainage system:
   a. Water seal: Where is it? How can it be maintained?

b. Suction control: What controls the suction in the system, gravity or negative pressure? What is the setting?
c. Drainage: Where does the drainage collect? How is the patency of the system maintained? How is it measured?

3. Usage: the most commonly used systems today are disposable chest tube systems (*Pleur-Evac, Thora-seal*)
   a. Considered a "three-chamber system," these are made of molded plastic to form three chambers
      1) Suction control chamber (closest to suction): when on, should be continuously bubbling at a "gentle roll"; amount of suction is usually determined by the prescribed water level in the suction control chamber; make sure evaporation does not change the amount of suction by lowering the water level
      2) Water seal chamber is middle seal; intermittent bubbling occurs if there is air in the chest; tidaling, the rise and fall of fluid in the water seal chamber, may be observed with respirations
      3) Drainage collection chamber should not having bubbling. Amount of drainage noted each shift; decreases over time.

   b. Note: newer systems are waterless and amount of suction is controlled by dial on device

4. **NURSING INTERVENTIONS**
   a. Observe for gentle bubbling in suction control chamber (if applicable).
   b. Observe for tidaling in the water seal chamber.
   c. Assess respiratory status, continuous oximetry.
   d. Turn client, ask to cough, and then deep breathe.
   e. Calculate and demarcate amount of drainage at the end of each shift.
   f. Note character of drainage.
   g. Be sure tubing is without kinks or dependant loops, keep coiled on the bed.
   h. Keep closed-chest drainage system below level of client's heart.
   i. Maintain water seal.
   j. Maintain dry, sterile, occlusive dressing.
   k. Do not strip or milk chest tubes.
   l. Obtain daily chest x-ray, as ordered.

5. Removal of chest tubes: done by provider
   a. Provide equipment: suture removal kit, sterile gauze, petroleum gauze, occlusive tape.
   b. Use semi or high-Fowler's position.
   c. Instruct client that removal of tubes will be done during expiration or at the end of full inspiration.
   d. Apply occlusive dressing immediately after removal.

   e. Obtain chest x-ray immediately following removal.
   f. Assess for complications: subcutaneous emphysema, respiratory distress, reaccumulation of pneumothorax.

POINTS TO REMEMBER:

1. Problem: Continuous, rapid bubbling in water-seal bottle/chamber
   Solution: Locate leak in the system; repair or replace. Start at the chest and move down the tubing to see where the leak is.

2. Problem: No fluctuation in water-seal chamber with respirations
   Solution: Check for kinks in the tubing. Listen for breath sounds. Assess for respiratory distress. Lungs may have completely re-expanded.

3. Problem: No bubbling in suction-control bottle/chamber (if not waterless system)
   Solution: Turn up suction until gentle continuous bubbling is noted; check fluid level to ensure that it is filled to prescribed amount.

4. Problem: Damaged system or chest tube disconnected from water seal
   Solution: Insert end of chest tube into sterile water until the system can be replaced.

5. Problem: Tube accidentally pulled out (e.g., by client who is agitated or confused)
   Solution: Cover wound site with an occlusive sterile dressing and call the provider immediately.

D. Infectious Pulmonary Diseases
1. Tuberculosis (TB)
   a. Reportable, communicable, infectious, inflammatory disease that can occur in any part of the body
   b. Etiology: mycobacterium tuberculosis (nonmotile, aerobic, killed by heat and ultraviolet light); droplet nuclei spread by laughing, sneezing, coughing; can spread to other areas of the body and is called miliary TB; causes caseation in the lungs and Ghon tubercles, which can stay with the client for years, lay dormant, and then open again and reinfect the client

c. Risk factors
   1) Overcrowded, poor living conditions
   2) Poor nutritional status
   3) Previous infection
   4) Inadequate treatment of primary infection leads to multi-medication resistant organisms
   5) Close contact with infected person
   6) Immune dysfunction; HIV infection
   7) Long-term care facilities; prisons
   8) Older adults
   9) Substance abuse
d. Manifestations: same as other pulmonary inflammations and infections
   1) Productive cough
   2) Night sweats, low-grade fever
   3) Hemoptysis
   4) Dyspnea
   5) Malaise
   6) Weight loss
   7) Anorexia, vomiting, indigestion
   8) Pallor
e. Diagnostic tests
   1) Mantoux test
   2) Sputum for acid-fast bacillus, specimen obtained each morning for 3 days
   3) Chest x-ray
   4) History and physical exam
f. Multicombination medication therapy - common adverse reactions include GI, hepatic, and/or peripheral nerves
   1) Antituberculin medications
      a) Ethambutol (*Myambutol*): contraindicated in children due to optic neuritis
      b) Rifampin (*Rifampicin*): GI distress, shock, acute renal failure, thrombocytopenia, discoloration of body fluids
      c) Isoniazid (*INH*): peripheral neuritis (vitamin B_6), increases liver enzymes, increases seizures in clients with seizure disorder
      d) Streptomycin sulfate: aminoglycoside used in combination antitubercular therapy; monitor for ototoxicity and nephrotoxicity
      e) Pyrazinamide: major side effects: hepatoxicity, hyperuricemia; must monitor hepatic function and uric acid levels routinely

 2) **NURSING INTERVENTIONS**
   a) Teaching plan
      (1) Initiate infection control measures.
      (2) Medications must be taken in combination to avoid bacterial resistance.
      (3) Medications should be taken either once each day or 2 to 3 times per week, but always at the same time of day and on an empty stomach.
      (4) Medications must be taken for 6 to 12 months (as prescribed).
      (5) Maintain adequate nutritional status.
      (6) Promote yearly checkups
      (7) Make sure the client knows to have liver function tests.
      (8) Teach client to avoid tyramine-containing foods, because they may cause reaction with some antitubular agents.
      (9) Instruct client to notify provider if signs of hepatitis and hepatoxicity, neurotoxicity, and visual changes occur.
   b) Hospital care
      (1) Teaching: handwashing; Cover nose and mouth when sneezing, coughing.
      (2) Wear special particulate respirator mask when in the client's room.
      (3) Isolation room should be ventilated to outside (negative-pressure room). This is required for airborne precautions. Precautions discontinued when client no longer considered infectious.
      (4) Psychological support: Reinforce the need to take medications. Many clients, once discharged, stop taking medications.

POINTS TO REMEMBER:

 2. Pneumonia
   a. Definition: inflammation of the lung parenchyma caused by infectious agents
   b. Etiology: classified as community acquired or hospital acquired (nosocomial)
      1) Community acquired
         a) *Streptococcus pneumoniae* or pneumococcal
         b) Haemophilus influenzae

c) Legionella pneumonia
d) Atypical pneumonia: most commonly seen in children; usual organism is mycoplasma pneumoniae; differs from the others in that minimal mucus is produced
2) Hospital acquired
   a) *Staphylococcus aureus*
   b) Klebsiella pneumoniae
   c) Pseudomonas pneumoniae
   d) Fungi (various types, i.e., histoplasmosis;
c. Clients at increased risk
1) Older adults
2) Infants
3) Substance abusers
4) Cigarette smokers
5) Postoperative clients or those on prolonged bed rest
6) Clients with chronic illnesses such as COPD/CAL
7) Clients with AIDS (increased risk for *Pneumocystis carinii* pneumonia)
8) Clients who are immunosuppressed
d. Common manifestations
1) Sudden onset of chills, fever
2) Cough: dry and painful at first, later produces rusty-colored sputum
3) Dyspnea
4) Flushed cheeks
5) Pallor, cyanosis
6) Pleuritic pain that increases with respiration
7) Tachypnea, tachycardia

e. **NURSING INTERVENTIONS**
1) Administer medication therapy as prescribed.
   a) Cough suppressants (be careful giving to children and clients who have chest congestion; generally only given to them for sleep), expectorants
   b) Bronchodilators; teach use of metered-dose inhaler.
   c) Give antibiotics as prescribed.
   d) Give mild analgesic as needed to decrease pain and enable client to deep breathe.
2) Encourage ambulation as tolerated.
3) Provide pulmonary toilet.
4) Assess for sputum thickness and color.
5) Administer oxygen to maintain oxygen saturations > 95%.
6) Provide small, frequent meals and increase fluid intake.
7) Maintain fluid and electrolyte balance.
8) Isolate as indicated.
9) Provide oral hygiene.

1. Tuberculous
  a. Obtain sputum specimens before medication therapy is initiated.
  b. Multiple medication therapy is necessary to prevent the development of resistant organisms.
  c. Give medications in a single daily dose.
  d. Medication therapy must be continued for 6 to 12 months even if the x-ray, sputum specimens, and manifestations are within normal limits.
  e. Clients who are hospitalized must be on airborne precautions until noninfectious.
  f. Client is generally considered noninfectious after 2 to 3 weeks of continuous medication therapy.
  g. Client should avoid use of alcohol during medication therapy to reduce risk of hepatotoxicity.
2. Pneumonia
  a. Most pneumonias have a sudden onset.
  b. Penicillin remains the medication of choice for pneumococcal pneumonias (unless client is allergic).
  c. Antibiotics must be given on time to maintain blood levels.
  d. Watch for side effects of penicillin therapy, especially allergies.

E. Cancer of the Lung (See also page 77.)
1. Definition: primary or secondary (metastatic from a primary site) malignant tumor located in the lung or bronchi
2. Etiology: cigarette smoking and exposure to asbestos and other carcinogens (coal dust, uranium, nickel)
3. Manifestations:
  a. Asymptomatic in the early stages
  b. Later stages:
    1) Coughing
    2) Dyspnea
    3) Hemoptysis
    4) Anorexia and weight loss
    5) Hoarseness
    6) Chest pain, weakness

  c. **NURSING INTERVENTIONS**
    1) Support cessation of smoking.
    2) Postoperative care for lung excision
      a) Pneumonectomy (removal of entire lung)
        (1) Position client dorsal recumbent or semi-Fowler's position, slightly toward affected side.
        (2) Encourage range of motion to affected shoulder.

(3) No closed-chest drainage is required since goal is to allow serum fluid to accumulate in empty thoracic cavity, consolidate and therefore, prevent shift of mediastinum, heart, and remaining lung.

    b) Lobectomy (removal of a lobe): chest tube(s) will be required postoperatively

    c) Segmentectomy (removal of a portion of a lobe): chest tube(s) will be required postoperatively

    d) Wedge resection (removal of a small portion of lung tissue): chest tube(s) will be required postoperatively

3) Encourage client to turn, cough, and deep breathe.

4) Administer oxygen.

5) Provide pain interventions so that the client will be able to move and deep breathe.

6) Promote fluids to maintain thin respiratory tract secretions.

7) Instruct client to splint chest incision when coughing.

8) Teach client exercises for arm on affected side to prevent frozen shoulder.

9) Place needed articles on side of surgery so client will move arm to get them.

10) Assess wound for infection.

F. Disorders of the Pleural Space

1. Pleural effusion (secondary to other disorders)
   a. Definition: accumulation of nonpurulent fluid in the pleural cavity
   b. Etiology
      1) Blood vessels exudate
      2) Tissue surfaces transudate, associated with leukemia, lymphomas, pneumonia, pulmonary edema, cirrhosis of the liver, following cardiac (coronary artery bypass graft) and pulmonary surgery

2. Empyema
   a. Definition: accumulation of pus in the pleural cavity
   b. Etiology: spread of infection from lungs, chest wall; complication of pneumonia, TB, abscess, bronchiectasis
   c. Treatment: antibiotics, possible chest tube
   d. Interventions
      1) Follow care of a client with a chest tube. Drainage will depend on what is present in the pleural space. If only a limited amount of effusion or pus is present, may be able to remove with a thoracentesis.

2) Assess respiratory status.

3) Maintain infection control measures.

Pulmonary Therapies

A. Chest Physiotherapy (CPT) (using cupped hands)

1. Definition: percussion and vibration over the thorax to loosen secretions in the affected areas of the lung

2. Procedure
   a. Keep a layer of material (gown or pajamas) between your hands and the client's skin.
   b. Stop if pain occurs.
   c. Perform procedure in the morning upon rising, 1 hr before meals or 2 to 3 hr after meals.
   d. Client must be instructed to deep breathe and cough during the procedure.
   e. Procedure should be followed with oral hygiene.

3. Contraindications
   a. When bronchospasm is increased by its use
   b. History of pathological fractures, rib fractures, or osteoporosis
   c. Obesity
   d. New incisions in the chest area or upper abdominal area
   e. Pain in the chest

B. Postural Drainage (PD)

1. Definition: use of gravity to drain secretions from segments of the lung; may be combined with chest physiotherapy

 2. **NURSING INTERVENTIONS**
   a. Provide for proper positioning (lung segment to be drained is uppermost).
   b. Stop if cyanosis or exhaustion occurs.
   c. Provide mouth care after procedure; best time is in the morning upon rising, 1 hr before meals, or 2 to 3 hr after meals.
   d. Maintain position 5 to 20 min, or as tolerated.

3. Contraindications
   a. Unstable vital signs
   b. Increased intracranial pressure

C. Pulmonary Toilet

1. Turn, cough, deep breathe
2. Chest physiotherapy
3. Incentive spirometry
4. Ambulation

D. Intermittent Positive Pressure Breathing

1. Definition: delivery of aerosolized medications to the bronchial tree by positive pressure
2. Adverse effects
   a. Dizziness
   b. Headache

c. Anxiety
d. Cardiac arrhythmias
e. Pneumothorax

E. Inhalers and Nebulizer Treatments

1. Inhaler Therapy:
   a. Doses may vary per order; generally, two puffs are standard for metered-dose inhalers, with no more than 12 puffs administered in 24 hr.
   b. For maximum effectiveness, administer ordered bronchodilators and nebulizer treatments prior to CPT
   c. Types of inhalers
      1) Bronchodilators
         a) Relax airways and open diameter, thereby decreasing airway resistance
         b) Common side effects
            (1) Tachycardia, palpitations
            (2) Cardiac dysrhythmias
            (3) Restlessness, tremors, nervousness
            (4) Anorexia, nausea, and vomiting
            (5) Hyperglycemia (use with caution in clients who have diabetes mellitus)
            (6) Mouth dryness
            (7) Headaches and dizziness
            (8) May decrease clotting time
         c) Type:
            (1) Albuterol (*Proventil*)
            (2) Ipratropium bromide (*Atrovent, Combivent*)
            (3) Terbutaline (*Brethine*)
            (4) Salmeterol xinafoate (*Serevent*)
               a) Used for long-term maintenance therapy of asthma
               (b) Prevents bronchospasm
               (c) Cannot be used to treat acute symptoms
      2) Steroids
         a) Decrease inflammation and open airways, thereby decreasing airway resistance
         b) May cause oral superinfection; therefore, always follow with oral hygiene
         c) May mask the signs of infection
         d) When administering inhalers, always give the steroid last
         e) Type:
            (1) Triamcinolone acetonide (*Azmacort*)
            (2) Fluticasone propionate (*Flovent*)
      3) Inhaled nonsteroidal antiallergy agents: mast-cell stabilizers (cromolyn sodium [*Intal*])
         a) Antiasthmatic and antiallergic; inhibit mast-cell release after exposure to antigens
         b) Can cause cough or bronchospasm following inhalation
         c) Do not discontinue abruptly as rebound attack can occur
      4) Leukotriene modifiers: montelukast (*Singulair*)
         a) Used in prophylaxis and treatment of chronic asthma
         b) Instruct client not to discontinue even during symptom-free periods.
2. Teach client how to correctly use metered-dose inhalers.
   a. Remove cap and shake inhaler.
   b. Tilt head back slightly and exhale.
   c. Hold inhaler open mouth or create seal by closing mouth.
   d. Press down inhaler to release medication and inhale slowly.
   e. Hold breath for 10 to 15 seconds.
   f. Repeat as directed. Wait 1 min between puffs of same medication; 2 to 5 min of second medication.
3. Use of spacer devices
   a. Used to deliver inhalant medications
   b. Increase the amount of medication delivered to the lungs significantly over standard inhalers and should be used whenever possible.

F. Suctioning

1. Indications: client is unable to raise secretions after coughing or chest physiotherapy; to obtain a sputum sample; airway filled with secretions
2. Can be oral or via endotracheal tube/tracheostomy
   a. Oral is not sterile
   b. Endotracheal tube/tracheostomy is sterile
3. Tracheostomy
   a. Prelubricate catheter before insertion with NS.
   b. Preoxygenate client.
   c. Advance catheter during inspiration without suction.
   d. Pull catheter back 2 to 3 cm after reaching the bronchial bifurcation.
   e. Withdraw catheter while applying intermittent suction and rotating catheter between thumb and index finger for a maximum of 10 to 15 seconds.
   f. Give client oxygen.
   g. Rinse catheter and discard with gloves.
   h. Document client response and character and volume of sputum.

i. Maintain standard precautions including mask, goggles, and gloves.
j. Listen to breath sounds to determine effectiveness of intervention.
4. Adverse effects
   a. Hypoxia
   b. Cardiac dysrhythmia
   c. Bronchospasm/bronchoconstriction
   d. Infection

SECTION III

REVIEW OF GENERAL PREOPERATIVE AND POSTOPERATIVE CARE

Preoperative Care

A. Purposes
1. Ensure the client is in the best physical and psychological condition for surgery.
2. Eliminate or reduce postoperative discomfort and complications.
3. Preoperative teaching
   a. Enhances client participation
   b. Decreases anxiety
   c. Helps to ensure good postoperative recovery

B. General Preoperative Care
1. Psychological support: stress experience, consider the effects
2. Client teaching specific to scheduled procedure
   a. Pulmonary toilet measures
   b. Incentive spirometry
   c. Leg exercises
   d. Turning, positioning, and ambulation
   e. Analgesics and pain control: discuss the option of PCA
   f. Recovery room procedures
   g. Other postoperative expectations: type of dressing, NG tube drains, IV
3. Informed consent: nurse only witnesses permit, surgeon must explain procedure to client
4. Latex allergies: assess for and identify clients at risk (multiple invasive procedures or spina bifida)
5. Preoperative checklist must be complete
6. Physical care
   a. Baseline vital signs: client must be afebrile
   b. Nutritional support for wound healing
   c. Skin preparation as indicated
   d. Oral hygiene: check loose teeth
   e. Prophylactic antibiotic as indicated
7. Preoperative medications
   a. Purpose
      1) Reduce anxiety
      2) Decrease secretions
      3) Reduce amount of general anesthesia required
      4) Control nausea and vomiting
   b. Preoperative medications
      1) Meperidine (*Demerol*) - morphine sulfate
      2) Antihistamines - hydroxyzine (*Vistaril*)
      3) Antiemetic - odansetron HCL (Zofran)
      4) Anticholinergics - atropine sulfate
      5) Benzodiazepines - lorazepam (Ativan), diazepam (Valium)
      6) Barbituates - pentobarbital sodium (Nembutal), secobarbital sodium (Seconal)
      7) Sedatives - midazolam (Versed)
      8) Prophylactic antibiotics - specific to type of surgery

C. Anesthetics
1. General: Causes the most effects postoperatively
   a. Inhalation
   b. IV
2. Local
   a. Topical
   b. Spinal
      1) Side effects: hypotension, nausea, vomiting, headache
       2) **NURSING INTERVENTIONS**
         a) Increase fluids per order.
         b) Increase caffeine per order.
         c) Have client lie flat for 6 to 8 hr postoperative.
         d) Monitor vital signs and respiratory system

General Postoperative Care

A. Immediate "Head-to-Toe" Assessment
1. Pulmonary
   a. Airway (check gag reflex)
   b. Bilateral breath sounds
   c. Encourage coughing, deep breathing
2. Neurological
   a. Level of consciousness
   b. Reflexes/pattern of movement
3. Circulatory
   a. Vital signs
   b. Peripheral perfusion
4. Gastrointestinal
   a. Bowel sounds
   b. Distention
5. Genitourinary
   a. Urinary output
   b. I&O

TABLE I-3
COMMON POSTOPERATIVE COMPLICATIONS

COMPLICATION	PREVENTION	COMMON CAUSES	OCCURRENCE	MANIFESTATIONS
Atelectasis	Cough and deep breathe	Shallow respirations	First 48 hr	Fever, increased pulse and respiration
Hypostatic pneumonia	Cough and deep breathe	Shallow respirations	After 48 hr	- Fever, increased pulse and respiration - Crackles and rhonchi
Hypoxia	- Cough and deep breathe - Ambulation and turning	Anesthesia causing depressed respirations	48 hr	Confusion, increased BP and pulse, SOB
Nausea	Slowly progress with diet	Reaction to anesthesia or narcotics	48 hr	Nausea
Shock	- Assess routinely for signs of shock - Identify populations at risk - Monitor for bleeding	- Loss of fluids and electrolytes - Bleeding from wound or surgical site	48 hr	-Decreased BP, pulse, urinary output -Cold, clammy, pale skin -Change in level of consciousness
Urinary retention	- Upright to void (male) - Monitor I&O	- Medications (narcotic) - Local edema	2 to 3 days or later	Inability to void, restlessness, bladder distention
Wound hemorrhage	Monitor site for healing	Slipping of suture, wound evisceration	Immediately or later	- Signs of shock - Bleeding (sanguinous drainage) from tubes or site of surgery
Thrombophlebitis	- Leg exercises, elastic stockings, pneumatic stockings - Identify at-risk populations for intervention	Venous stasis, IV irritation, pressure to legs	7 to 14 days	Redness, warmth, pain and swelling at the site
Wound infection	- Maintain nutritional status - Maintain aseptic technique with manipulations of dressings	Poor aseptic technique, debilitated, to obesity	3 to 5 days	Wound area red and edematous, increased pain in incisional area, increase in the amount and/or change in the character of the drainage: common for drainage to be purulent
Wound dehiscence and evisceration	- Identify those at risk - Maintain nutritional status in high-risk populations	Debilitated, obese, older adults	4 to 15 days	Wound opens and contents may come out onto abdominal area; intervention: place sterile saline-soaked gauze over site and place in recumbent position
Urinary tract infection	- Maintain sterility of catheter, increase fluids - Remove catheter as soon as possible	Indwelling urinary catheter, urinary retention post anesthesia	5 to 8 days	Dysuria, hematuria, urgency, frequency

6. Equipment
   a. IV
   b. Dressings: expect mostly serosanguineous drainage
   c. Drainage tubes: expect some sanguineous drainage postoperative, but monitor amount and evaluate in light of vital signs
   d. NG tube: evaluate need for potassium chloride in IV to prevent metabolic alkalosis

B. NURSING INTERVENTIONS

 1. Assess for complications
   a. Take vital signs routinely according to policy.
   b. Remain NPO until alert and gag reflex returns.
   c. Suction oral cavity PRN.
   d. Monitor I&O.
2. Pain Interventions
   a. Pharmacologic interventions
      1) PRN scheduling: pain medication is given, as prescribed, to the client on a demand basis when pain occurs; is least effective strategy
      2) Fixed scheduling: pain medication is given around the clock (usually every 4 hr); not only treats, but prevents pain.
      3) PCA: pain medication is self administered by client via an infusion system; client must be able to participate in this intervention
      4) Most pharmacologic interventions use narcotic medications; therefore, client must be carefully assessed for the complication of respiratory depression.
   b. Nonpharmacologic interventions
      1) Distraction
      2) Relaxation techniques
      3) Back rubs
      4) Acupuncture, acupressure
3. Positioning
   a. Head to side, chin forward if unconscious
   b. Lateral Sims', semiprone
   c. Turn and position the client; have the client cough and deep breathe

SECTION IV

REVIEW OF GASTROINTESTINAL, HEPATIC, AND PANCREATIC DISORDERS

Nursing Assessment

A. Assessment/Health History
1. Description of present illness or chief report

a. Onset, course, and duration
b. Location
c. Alleviating or precipitating factors
d. Risk factors
   1) Low-fiber diet
   2) Cigarette smoking
   3) Alcohol consumption
   4) Inactivity
   5) Stress
   6) Familial predisposition to gastrointestinal disorders
2. Assessment of gastrointestinal system
   a. Pain
      1) Location, quality of pain/discomfort (stabbing, crampy), and duration
         a) Abdominal, epigastric
         b) Indigestion
      2) Timing (before or after medications)
      3) Measures which alleviate pain
         a) Positional changes
         b) Use of over-the-counter medications
         c) Use of home remedies
   b. Examination of abdomen
      1) Inspection: color, contour, distention, previous scars
      2) Auscultation: bowel sounds
      3) Percussion: tympany or dullness
      4) Palpation: tenderness or masses
   c. Elimination pattern
      1) Constipation
      2) Diarrhea
      3) Rectal bleeding
      4) Laxative use
   d. Nutritional issues
      1) Loss of appetite
      2) Anorexia
      3) I&O
      4) Difficulty swallowing
      5) Nausea and vomiting
   e. Other associated manifestations or reports
      1) Flatus
      2) Eructation (belching)
      3) Heartburn
      4) Dark urine
      5) Jaundice
      6) Excessive weight loss or gain

Diagnostic Procedures

A. Barium Swallow Series
1. Upper gastrointestinal tract examination under fluoroscopy after ingesting barium sulfate (radiopaque) to detect anatomical or functional abnormalities of the esophagus, stomach, and/or small intestines

2. **NURSING INTERVENTIONS**
   a. Preparation
      1) Keep client NPO after midnight the day before the test.
      2) Tell client to avoid smoking, chewing, or eating before the procedure.
   b. Postprocedure
      1) Instruct client to increase fluids to assist in passage of barium.
      2) Laxative may be prescribed after procedure; monitor stools for chalky-white appearance as barium is eliminated.

B. Barium Enema Study
   1. Lower gastrointestinal study done by x-ray and fluoroscopic examination of the large intestine after rectal insertion of a barium (radiopaque) enema

   2. **NURSING INTERVENTIONS**
      a. Preparation
         1) Give clear liquid diet and laxative the day before the procedure.
         2) Tell client to remain NPO after midnight the day before the procedure.
         3) Give cleansing enema the morning of the test.
      b. Postprocedure
         1) Instruct client to increase fluids to assist in passage of barium.
         2) Laxative may be prescribed after procedure. Monitor stools for chalky-white appearance, as barium is eliminated.
         3) Notify provider if no bowel movement in 48 hr.

C. Endoscopic Studies
   1. Lower gastrointestinal tract
      a. Colonoscopy: Fiberoptic endoscopic visualization of the lining of the large intestine; biopsies and polypectomies can be done
      b. Sigmoidoscopy/Proctoscopy: use of a flexible scope to examine rectum and sigmoid colon; biopsies and polypectomies can be done
      c. Anoscopy: rigid scope to examine anal canal

   2. **NURSING INTERVENTIONS**
      a. Preparation: for endoscopic examinations of the lower gastrointestinal tract
         1) Evacuation and cleansing of colon is necessary for visualization; specifics of cleansing regimen may depend on provider preference, but in general will include:
            a) Clear liquid diet the day before the test

         b) Administration of an osmotic laxative (*Fleet Phospho-Soda*) or polyethylene glycol and electrolyte solution (*GoLYTELY*) the day before the test
      2) Tell the client to remain NPO after midnight on day before the test.
      3) Administer IV midazolam (Versed) for conscious sedation.
   b. During examination
      1) Monitor cardiac and respiratory functions.
      2) Position client on left side with knees drawn up to chest. Position may be changed to facilitate passage of scope.
   c. Postprocedure
      1) Remain on bedrest until alert.
      2) Monitor for manifestations of perforation, bleeding.
   3. Upper gastrointestinal tract: Esophagogastroduodenoscopy
      a. Endoscope is passed down the esophagus to visualize the gastric wall, sphincters, duodenum
      b. Tissue biopsies can be obtained

   4. **NURSING INTERVENTIONS**
      a. Preparation: for endoscopic examinations of the upper gastrointestinal tract
         1) Tell the client to remain NPO after midnight on day before the test
         2) Administer IV midazolam (Versed) for conscious sedation.
      b. During examination
         1) Monitor cardiac and respiratory functions.
         2) Position client on left side; position may be changed to facilitate passage of scope.
      c. Postprocedure
         1) Remain on bedrest until alert.
         2) Monitor for manifestations of perforation.
         3) Keep client NPO until gag reflex returns; observe for dysphagia.

D. Analysis of Gastrointestinal Secretions
   1. Stool analysis: laboratory test to inspect stool specimen
      a. Assessment for fecal urobilinogen, nitrates, bacteria, parasites

      b. **NURSING INTERVENTIONS**
         1) Inspect sample for color, consistency, and occult blood (guaiac).
         2) Do not refrigerate.
         3) Send specimen promptly to the laboratory.
   2. Gastric analysis: passage of NG tube into the stomach to aspirate gastric contents; measures the amount of acid secreted by the stomach in baseline conditions

a. Common diagnostic reasons
    1) Pernicious anemia: deficiency of vitamin B_{12} as a result of a lack of stomach acid
    2) Zollinger-Ellison syndrome: increased levels of gastrin are produced, causing the stomach to produce excess hydrochloric acid
    3) Pre- and postacid suppressing therapy (to evaluate adequacy of medication dose)

b. **NURSING INTERVENTIONS**
    1) Have client remain NPO after midnight the day of the test.
    2) Antacids and H2-receptor antagonists should not be given to the client for 24 to 48 hr prior to procedure.
    3) Instruct client to avoid smoking and/or chewing tobacco for 6 hr before the test.

E. Evaluation of the Gallbladder and Liver
1. Cholecystogram (gallbladder series): x-ray imaging procedure that examines the gallbladder to diagnose disorders of the liver and gallbladder, including gallstones and tumors

    a. **NURSING INTERVENTIONS**
        1) Check for allergy to x-ray contrast material.
        2) On the day prior to the procedure, the client is instructed to adhere to the following diet: at 1200 consume high-fat meal; at 1700 consume a low fat meal.
        3) Twelve hours before the procedure, instruct client to take tablets that contain the contrast medium.
        4) After taking the tablets, instruct the client to remain NPO until after the test.
2. Percutaneous transhepatic cholangiogram (PTCA): x-ray of the bile ducts inside and outside the liver taken after the contrast medium is injected into a liver bile duct; PTCA can assist in identification of a blockage causing jaundice and pancreatitis
    a. Procedure: long, thick flexible needle is inserted through right-upper quadrant of the abdomen into the liver; under fluoroscopy, the bile duct is located and contrast medium is injected, allowing for visualization of ducts

    b. **NURSING INTERVENTIONS**
        1) Prior to procedure: check for allergy to x-ray contrast material
        2) Postprocedure: Monitor client for manifestations of complications such as bleeding, infection (sepsis or peritonitis), inflammation of the bile ducts.

F. Abdominal x-ray (KUB or flat plate): abdominal x-ray to identify suspected problems in the urinary system or a blockage in the intestine; may also assist in diagnosing abdominal pain, distention, or unexplained nausea

G. Liver Biopsy: a needle is inserted through the rib cage or abdominal wall and into the liver to obtain a sample for biopsy or microscopic examination
1. Procedure: client is placed in supine or left-lateral position; performed under fluoroscopy

2. **NURSING INTERVENTIONS**
    a. Preparation
        1) Ensure that informed consent is obtained
        2) Assess PT, aPTT, INR, and platelet count laboratory levels.
        3) Have the client remain NPO after midnight the day before the procedure.
    b. Postprocedure
        1) Position client on right side for 1 to 2 hr.
        2) Monitor for manifestations of complications: bleeding, pneumothorax, infection.

H. Paracentesis: removal of abdominal fluid accumulated in the peritoneum for evaluation of clients with ascites
1. Indications
    a. New onset ascites or ascites of unknown origin
    b. Clients with ascites who develop fever, painful abdominal distention, peritoneal irritation, hypotension, encephalopathy or sepsis, difficulty breathing
    c. Suspected malignant ascites
    d. Peritoneal dialysis clients with suspected peritonitis (fever, abdominal pain, or sepsis)
2. Procedure
    a. Client is positioned supine with head elevated 20 to 30°
    b. Local anesthetic is administered to the abdominal wall, followed by insertion of paracentesis needle
    c. Gradual removal of up to 4 L of fluid
    d. If fluid is greater than 5 L, IV serum albumin may be given to prevent hypotension

3. **NURSING INTERVENTIONS**
    a. Preparation
        1) Ensure that informed consent is obtained.
        2) Have client void before procedure.
        3) Measure weight and abdominal girth.
    b. Postprocedure
        1) Measure weight and abdominal girth.
        2) Client must remain supine 2 to 4 hr.
        3) Observe for manifestations of complications: hypovolemia, shock, infection.

I. Liver Function Tests
1. Alkaline phosphatase: nonspecific indicator of liver or bone disease or hypoparathyroidism; tumor marker for malignancy of liver or bone disease

2. Prothrombin time: value is prolonged with liver damage (PT normal at 1.5 to 2.5 times control value)
3. Blood ammonia: assess liver's ability to deaminate protein by products (normal ammonia level 35 to 65 mcg/dL)
4. Serum transaminase studies
   a. ALT/SGPT normal range 10 to 25 units/L
   b. AST/SGOT normal range 8 to 38 units/L
5. Cholesterol
   a. Total normal < 200 mg/dL
   b. LDL normal < 140 mg/dL
   c. HDL normal > 40 to 70 mg/dL
   d. Triglycerides normal < 150 mg/dL
6. Bilirubin
   a. Total normal 0 to 1.5 mg/dL adults; 1 to 12 mg/dL infants
   b. Direct normal 0.1 to 0.3 mg/dL
   c. Indirect: subtract direct value from total value to determine degree of liver failure

Gastrointestinal Intubation

A. Types
1. NG tube: decompression of stomach
2. Salem sump: for continuous or intermittent suction, prevents trauma to stomach lining
3. Miller-Abbot/Anderson: intestinal suction – Reposition client hourly for insertion of the tube and movement into the intestines.
4. Ewald: removal of secretions through the mouth
5. Sengstaken-Blakemore: for treatment of esophageal varices, requires intensive care; not used much because of the trauma and potential complications it causes for the client; major complications are rebleeding, pneumonia and respiratory obstruction

B. NG Tube Feeding/Suction

1. **NURSING INTERVENTIONS**
   a. Feeding
      1) Assess placement before each feeding and every 4 hr with continuous feeding.
      2) Place in semi-Fowler's position.
      3) Check for residual: always refeed unless amount exceeds 100 mL.
      4) Provide nose and mouth care.
   b. Suction
      1) Drain stomach contents.
      2) Overtime, should see a decrease in volume of drainage.

C. Gastrostomy Tube/Jejunostomy Tube
1. Tube is sutured in place; skin care is important
2. Primarily placed for long term feeding needs

D. Percutaneous Endoscopic Gastrostomy (PEG)
1. No need to check placement
2. Primarily placed for long-term feeding needs

3. Preferred over gastrostomy tube because of ease of insertion and care

Total Parenteral Nutrition (TPN)

A. Definition: IV administration of a hyperosmotic (3 to 6 times the osmolarity of blood) solution of glucose, nitrogen, lipids, electrolytes, and other nutrients in the client whose nutritional requirements cannot be achieved via the enteral route; must be administered by a central line for rapid dilution and blood flow

B. Indications for Use
1. Gastrointestinal motility disorders
2. Inability to achieve or maintain enteral nutrition to meet body requirements
3. Disorders that impair the absorption of nutrients
4. Gastrointestinal tract dysfunction

C. NURSING INTERVENTIONS

1. Perform chest x-ray immediately after central line insertion for proper placement.
2. Assess weight, baseline electrolytes, blood glucose, and albumin level (normal 3.8 to 5.0 g/dL).
3. Maintain aseptic (sterile) technique during dressing changes.
4. Maintain infusion rate, do not increase or decrease rate without order; may cause hyper or hypoglycemia.
5. Assess weight daily: should maintain or increase weight while receiving TPN.
6. Change all tubing and filter every 24 hr.
7. Monitor for complications.
   a. Infection-filters and tubing changed with every bottle
   b. Hypoglycemia/hyperglycemia: check fingerstick blood glucose every 4 hr; if behind in administration rate, do NOT attempt to catch up in administration of TPN
   c. Air embolism: never open subclavian central line to air; chance of air embolism is decreased with multiple lumen set-ups and peripherally inserted central catheters (PICC lines); when central line is inserted or opened, have client perform Valsalva maneuver and place in Trendelenburg position.
   d. Pneumothorax, especially during insertion of subclavian central line
   e. Fluid overload. be careful rate does not increase quickly
   f. Hyperglycemic, hyperosmolar nonketotic coma
   g. Monitor for hyper and hyponatremia.
8. Continually evaluate effectiveness of therapy. Seek consultation if it is not effective.
9. Follow protocol for discontinuing TPN.

10. Turn off TPN for 1 full min before drawing all laboratories.
11. Ensure safe medication administration with regard to compatibility.

Gastroesophageal Reflux Disease

A. Definition: a condition in which the lower esophageal sphincter does not close properly and stomach contents reflux into the esophagus

B. Risk Factors
1. Hiatal hernia
2. Alcohol use
3. Obesity
4. Pregnancy
5. Smoking

C. Manifestations
1. Persistent heartburn
2. Chest pain
3. Hoarseness in the morning
4. Dysphagia
5. Dry cough
6. Halitosis

D. Diagnostic Tests
1. Barium swallow
2. Upper endoscopy
3. pH study

E. NURSING INTERVENTIONS

1. Teach client
   a. Avoid smoking.
   b. Avoid alcohol.
   c. Maintain ideal body weight.
   d. Avoid foods that may contribute to manifestations: citrus fruits, chocolate, caffeine, fried foods, garlic, onions, tomato-based foods, foods that are fatty or spicy.
   e. Eat small meals and avoid lying down for 3 hr after a meal.
   f. Wear loose-fitting clothes.
2. Administer medications:
   a. Antacids
   b. H$_2$ blockers: cimetidine (*Tagamet*), famotidine (*Pepcid*), ranitidine (*Zantac*), nizatidine (*Axid*)
   c. Proton-pump inhibitors (*PPI*): omeprazole (*Prilosec*), lansoprazole (*Prevacid*), pantoprazole (*Protonix*), esomeprazole (*Nexium*), rabeprazole (*AcipHex*)

F. Complications
1. Bleeding/ulcers of the esophagus
2. Barrett's esophagus
3. Aggravation of asthma, chronic cough, and pulmonary fibrosis

G. Surgical Treatment
1. Reserved for severe cases
2. Fundoplication: upper portion of the stomach is wrapped around the lower esophageal sphincter to strengthen the sphincter and prevent acid reflux

Hiatal Hernia

A. Definition: portion of the stomach is herniated through the esophageal hiatus of the diaphragm

B. Manifestations
1. Heartburn
2. Dysphagia
3. Chest pain
4. Reflux

C. NURSING INTERVENTIONS

1. Provide client small, frequent meals.
2. Position client upright during and after meals.
3. Elevate head of bed.
4. Administer antacids.
5. Avoid anticholinergic medications.
6. Avoid coughing.
7. Reduce intra-abdominal pressure by avoiding lifting and tight clothes around waist area.
8. Reduce spicy food intake.

Duodenal and Gastric Ulcer

A. Types of Ulcers
1. Chronic duodenal and gastric ulcers (See Table I-4.)
2. Stress ulcers
   a. May be caused by physical as well as psychological stress
   b. Burns cause Curling's ulcer
   c. Steroid therapy
      1) Usually occurs at least 1 to 2 weeks after stress
      2) No pain
      3) May be diagnosed due to gastric bleeding and resulting low Hgb and Hct

B. NURSING INTERVENTIONS

1. Major goal is to prevent complications and allow ulcer to heal
   a. Rest: physical and mental; lower stress
   b. Eliminate stimulants: caffeine, alcohol, spicy foods, cigarette smoking
   c. Diet has no therapeutic effect; milk may be used but is not recommended
   d. Antacid: aluminum hydroxide (*Amphojel*); magnesium carbonate (*Maalox*)
   e. Cimetidine (*Tagamet*): decreases acid production

TABLE I-4
COMPARISON OF CHRONIC DUODENAL AND CHRONIC GASTRIC ULCERS

	CHRONIC DUODENAL	CHRONIC GASTRIC
Age:	Usually 25 to 50 years	Usually 50 years or more
Sex:	M:F–3:1	M:F–2:1
Incidence:	80%	20%
General nourishment:	Well-nourished	Malnourished
Etiology factors:	Most result from *Helicobacter pylori* infection, smoking, 0 blood type	Excessive ingestion of salicylates, smoking
Acid production in stomach:	Hypersecretion	Normal to hyposecretion
Location:	Within 3 cm of pylorus	Lesser curvature
Pain:	2 to 3 hr after meal; night, early morning; ingestion of food relieves pain; pain is a gnawing sensation sharply localized in mid-epigastrium or in back	1/2 to 1 hour after meal; rarely at night; relieved by vomiting; ingestion of food does not help; sometimes causes pain
Vomiting:	Uncommon	Common: caused by pyloric obstruction either by muscular spasm of pylorus or by mechanical obstruction from scarring
Hemorrhage:	Melena more common than hematemesis	Hematemesis more common than melena
Malignancy possibility:	None	Usually less than 10%

f. Ranitidine (*Zantac*): decreases acid production
g. Sucralfate (*Carafate*): protects lining of stomach
h. Omeprazole (*Prilosec*): heals ulcer
i. For *Helicobacter pylori* ulcers: antibiotic therapy and symptomatic relief

C. Gastric Resection
1. Types
   a. Billroth I (gastroduodenostomy)
   b. Billroth II (gastrojejunostomy)
   c. Total gastrectomy: will cause pernicious anemia

2. **NURSING INTERVENTIONS**
   a. Do not move NG tube, as it may stimulate bleeding at surgical site.
   b. Evaluate need for KCL in IV to prevent metabolic alkalosis.

c. Keep client NPO until suture line is totally healed.
d. Assess drainage. Will initially be sanguinous, but should change to greenish in 2 to 3 days.
3. Complications
   a. Hemorrhage
   b. Pulmonary
   c. "Dumping syndrome": due to rapid entry of ingested food into the jejunum without proper mixing and normal digestive process of the duodenum
      1) Early: 5 to 30 min after eating, vertigo, sweating, diarrhea, nausea; due to fluid shifts
      2) Late: 2 to 3 hr after meals, hypoglycemia occurs due to excess insulin secretion

3) Intervention: avoid salty, high-carbohydrate meals; eat small, frequent meals; avoid liquids with meals; lie down after meals (30 to 60 min); avoid antispasmodics; eat high-protein, high-fat, low-carbohydrate meals; no fluids for 1 hr before, with, or 2 hr after meals

    d. Major complication: Peritonitis

Diverticulitis and Diverticulosis

A. Definition:
1. Outpouching of colon is diverticulosis
2. When the outpouching becomes infected, it is called diverticulitis

3. Problem: the pouch gets filled with feces, becomes inflamed, can obstruct and perforate leading to peritonitis

B. NURSING INTERVENTIONS

1. Encourage client to eat low-residue diet to heal, and high-fiber diet to prevent.
2. Avoid all seeds.
3. Prevent constipation by using bulk agents and increasing water intake.

Inflammatory Bowel Disease

A. Inflammatory bowel disease is a group of conditions of the large intestine (and in some cases the small intestine). It should not be confused with irritable bowel syndrome, which is less severe.

TABLE I-5
COMPARISON OF CROHN'S DISEASE AND ULCERATIVE COLITIS

	CROHN'S DISEASE Small Bowel	ULCERATIVE COLITIS Large Bowel
Pathology:	Transmural: primarily involving ileum and right colon	Mucosal ulceration of lower colon and rectum
Age:	20 to 30, 40 to 50	20 to 40
Etiology factors:	Unknown genetic, Jewish	Unknown familial, Jewish
Bleeding:	Usually not	Common, severe
Perianal involvement:	Common	Rare, mild
Fistulas:	Common	Rare
Pain:	Colicky	Varies from mild to severe
Rectal involvement:	20%	100%
Diarrhea:	Presenting manifestation	Severe
Abdominal pain after eating:	Yes	Yes
Weight loss:	Yes	Yes
Medical treatment:	Steroids: anti-inflammatories such as sulfasalazine (*Azulfidine*); immune modulators such as infliximab (*Remicade*); hyperalimentation	Steroids: anti-inflammatories such as sulfasalazine (*Azulfidine*); immune modulators such as infliximab (*Remicade*)
Surgical treatment:	Even a complete removal of the diseased portion of bowel is only a temporary "cure" as disease will tend to reoccur	Ileostomy: complete colon removal is only "cure"; newer surgery allows either continent ileostomy or ileo-anal anastomosis

B. The major forms of inflammatory bowel disease are Crohn's disease and ulcerative colitis (See Table I-5 for comparison.)

Irritable Bowel Syndrome

A. Definition: irritable bowel syndrome is a disorder characterized by a colon that is sensitive to certain foods and stress; the specific etiology remains unknown but may include the immune system

B. Manifestations: there is not a specific diagnostic test for irritable bowel syndrome, although testing (x-ray, colonoscopy, stool sample) may be done to rule out other conditions; if the results are negative, irritable bowel syndrome may be diagnosed on the basis of the manifestations
  1. Crampy abdominal pain, which is typically relieved by having a bowel movement
  2. Abdominal distension
  3. Bowel pattern disturbance
     a. Constipation, diarrhea
     b. Constipation alternating with diarrhea
  4. Manifestations may subside and return, or may progressively worsen

C. NURSING INTERVENTIONS

  1. Teach client
     a. Avoid eating large meals.
     b. Avoid foods known to aggravate the condition: wheat, rye, barley, chocolate, milk products.
     c. Avoid alcohol and caffeine.
     d. Avoid stress or emotional upset.
     e. Include adequate fluids and fiber in the diet.
  2. Anticholinergic medications relieve spasms and cramps of small intestines. Dicyclomine hydrochloride (Bentyl) taken 30 min before meals.

Hernia

A. Definition:
  1. Protrusion of bowel through the muscles of the abdominal cavity
  2. Serious complication: strangulation and gangrene of the bowel (surgical emergency)

B. Types
  1. Umbilical
  2. Ventral
  3. Inguinal

C. NURSING INTERVENTIONS

  1. Wear abdominal binder for support of herniated area.
  2. Prevent constipation.

  3. Arrange for surgical repair with open or laparoscopic surgery.
  4. Avoid lifting objects greater than 10 lb for 4 to 6 weeks after surgical repair.

Intestinal Obstruction

A. Etiology: a condition in which the normal peristaltic action of the colon does not take place due to scar tissue, adhesions from prior surgery, malignant lesions, inflammation and edema of the gastrointestinal tract, decreased gastrointestinal motility, or incarcerated hernia

B. Manifestations:
  1. Intermittent abdominal cramping and pain
  2. Nausea and vomiting
  3. Abdominal distention
  4. Abdominal tenderness
  5. Constipation
  6. Fecal vomiting

C. NURSING INTERVENTIONS

  1. Insert NG tube to low wall suction.
  2. Ambulate.
  3. Treat cause and relieve.
  4. Arrange for possible surgery if unresolved medically; colon resection.

General Bowel Surgery

A. NURSING INTERVENTIONS: preoperative

  1. Laxatives and enemas until clear to evacuate intestines
  2. Laboratory work to include CBC, electrolytes, coagulation studies, and chest x-ray
  3. Prophylactic antibiotics to sterilize the colon given immediately preoperatively

B. NURSING INTERVENTIONS: postoperative

  1. Insert NG tube.
  2. Give IV fluids.
  3. Patient-controlled analgesia, epidural, and all pain management measures
  4. Perform aseptic wound care to prevent infection.
  5. Provide ambulation early to decrease risks of complications: increased peristalsis, decreased risk of thrombophlebitis, decreased risk of atelectasis.

Colostomy and Ileostomy

A. Types of Intestinal Ostomies (See Table I-6: Comparison of Colostomy and Ileostomy.)

B. NURSING INTERVENTIONS

  1. Preoperative care
     a. Provide emotional support (anticipatory grieving).

TABLE 1-6
COMPARISON OF COLOSTOMY AND ILEOSTOMY

	COLOSTOMY	ILEOSTOMY
Defined:	Portion of the colon brought through the abdominal wall, creating a temporary or permanent opening for exit of waste products	Portion of the ileum brought through the abdominal wall, creating a temporary or permanent opening for exit of waste products
Areas:	Involves large bowel	Involves small bowel
Indications:	Inflammatory or obstructive process of the lower intestinal tract; trauma to intestinal tract; cancer of the rectum or sigmoid where anastomosis is not possible	- Crohn's disease - Ulcerative colitis
Stool:	Semiformed to formed	Liquid
Control:	May be controlled by diet and/or irrigation depending on location in colon, may be able to control evacuation	No control, must wear appliance at all times Severe risk of dehydration with increased output

    b. Inform client of impending surgery (ileostomy/colostomy) and address concerns.

2. Postoperative care
    a. Provide general postoperative care.
    b. Provide psychological support.
    c. Insert NG tube.
    d. Initial stoma appears bloody and edematous. Stoma appears pink and above skin level once healed.
    e. Teach self-care to client.
       1) Type of equipment to use and how
       2) Skin care
       3) Diet: decrease fat- and odor-forming foods
       4) Irrigation: same time each day; make sure it fits into client's lifestyle; same as an enema

Hepatitis A, B, and C

A. Definition: an inflammation of the liver; manifestations prognosis, and treatment depend on the cause

B. See Table 1-7 for Comparison of Hepatitis A, B, and C. (Focus on client teaching: prevention of transmission.)

C. Hepatitis D (HDV): a defective virus that occurs only in clients with HBV infections; typical clients include IV drug users and their sexual partners; clients with coinfection of HBV and HDV have greater risk for liver failure and cirrhosis; clients with HBV should be tested for HDV

Cirrhosis

A. Definition: chronic, progressive liver disease where normal cells are replaced by scar tissue; causes include Laennec's cirrhosis (alcohol induced), postnecrotic cirrhosis (hepatitis, exposure to chemicals), biliary cirrhosis (chronic biliary obstruction), and cardiac cirrhosis (severe right-sided heart failure)

B. Functions of the Liver
1. Synthesis of clotting factors (fibrinogen, prothrombin, factors VII, IX, X)
2. Metabolism of hormones (aldosterone, antidiuretic hormone, estrogen, testosterone)
3. Synthesis of albumin (maintains normal colloid osmotic pressure)
4. Carbohydrate metabolism
5. Protein metabolism
6. Fat metabolism through bile production
7. Filtration removes bacteria and toxins, antigens, drugs
8. Storage: blood, fat, and water-soluble vitamins (A, D, E, K, B), as well as minerals (copper and iron)

C. Manifestations
1. Early stage (same as those for hepatitis)
    a. Enlarged liver with fatty infiltration
    b. Jaundice
    c. Gastrointestinal disturbances
    d. Abdominal discomfort

2. Late stage
   a. Liver becomes smaller and nodular
   b. Spleen enlarges: splenomegaly
   c. Ascites, distended abdominal veins; back-up of pressure in the portal system
   d. Bleeding tendencies; decreased vitamin K, prothrombin, anemia
   e. Esophageal varices, internal hemorrhoids; back-up of pressure in portal area
   f. Dyspnea from ascites and anemia
   g. Pruritus from dry skin
   h. Clay-colored stools: no bile in stool
   i. Tea-colored urine: bile in urine
3. End stage
   a. Hepatic encephalopathy stages
      1) Prodromal: slurred speech, vacant stare, restless; involves neuro deterioration
      2) Impending: asterixis (flapping tremors), apraxia, lethargy, confusion
      3) Stuporous: marked mental confusion, somnolence
      4) Coma: unarousable, fetor hepaticas, seizures, high mortality rate

D. NURSING INTERVENTIONS: goal is to treat the manifestations and maximizes liver functions

1. Encourage client to rest.
2. Avoid hepatotoxic medications (acetaminophen [Tylenol]) and alcohol.
3. Provide high-calorie, low-protein (20 to 40 g/day), low-fat, low-sodium diet. Maintain protein restriction during stages I & II of encephalopathy; no protein allowed during stages III & IV.
4. Fat-soluble vitamin supplements and folic acid may need to be given IV.
5. Restrict fluids.
6. Give albumin IV (temporary solution).
7. Weigh client daily.

TABLE I-7
COMPARISON OF HEPATITIS A, B, C

	HEPATITIS A (Infectious Hepatitis)	HEPATITIS B (Serum Hepatitis)	HEPATITIS C
Cause	Virus transmitted by fecal-oral contact; often seen contaminated water or shellfish	- Virus transmitted through infected blood or unprotected sex with infected persons, infants born to infected mother - Responsible for 80% of primary hepatocellular cancer cases	- Transmitted via blood transfusions (5 to 10%), IV drug abuse (40%), health care worker exposure (5%), promiscuous homosexual activity (10%), other sources not available
Manifestations	Fever, fatigue, malaise, nausea vomiting, anorexia, right upper quadrant pain, dark urine, acholic stools, jaundice, pruritus, hepatomegaly	- Some will develop manifestations similar to type A - Chronic carrier state 5 to 10%, may result in cirrhosis	Same as Type B, but 80% develop chronic infection; higher cirrhosis and cancer rate
Nursing Interventions	Enteric precautions, bedrest, low-fat diet, fluids, avoid acetaminophen and other liver-toxic medications	- Similar to A with special emphasis on blood precautions - Support for antiviral therapy side effects, which include fatigue, flu-like manifestations, neutropenia, depression; encourage membership in support groups	Same as Type B
Prevention	Good sanitation; if in contact with infected client, administer immune serum globulin within 2 to 7 days; hepatitis A vaccine is available	Mandatory screening of blood donors-use of disposable needles and syringes; administer hepatitis B immune globulin 2 to 7 days after exposure; hepatitis B vaccine: series of three injections over 6 months	No sharing of needles by drug users; care to avoid accidental needlesticks (health care workers); safe sexual practices

8. Measure abdominal girth.
9. Maintain skin integrity.
10. Monitor I&O.
11. Assess for bleeding, hemorrhoids.
12. Administer diuretics: spironolactone (*Aldactone*), furosemide (*Lasix*).
13. Administer neomycin: changes intestinal bacteria to decrease breakdown of protein, thereby reducing ammonia levels.
14. Administer lactulose (*Cephulac*): decreases ammonia levels.
15. Administer thiamine (vitamin B$_1$) daily.

Bleeding Esophageal Varices

A. Definition: esophageal varices are dilated veins found in the lower esophagus that occur secondary to portal hypertension; bleeding may result because of coughing, trauma, or vomiting; bleeding esophageal varices is a medical emergency

B. NURSING INTERVENTIONS

1. Maintain client airway before insertion of Sengstaken-Blakemore tube.
2. Care of client with Sengstaken-Blakemore tube
   a. Maintain traction and manometer pressure as ordered.
   b. Keep scissors by bedside, cut ports if respiratory obstruction occurs.
   c. Oral suctioning or will aspirate; cannot swallow saliva.
   d. Administer propranolol (Inderal) to decrease portal pressure.
   e. Deflate gastric balloon as ordered.
3. Position in semi-Fowler's.
4. Monitor vital signs.
5. Monitor I&O.
6. Administer vitamin K (Phytonadione).
7. Administer vasopressin (*Pitressin*): vasoconstrictor with IV nitroglycerine to prevent vasoconstriction of coronary arteries.
8. Receive endoscopic sclerotherapy.
   a. Sclerosing agent introduced via endoscope
   b. Thromboses and obliterates the distended veins

C. Surgical Interventions

1. Portosystemic shunts: splenorenal, portocaval
2. Transesophageal ligation
3. TIPS: transjugular intrahepatic portosystemic shunt (angiographic method of creating shunt) to relieve pressure

Gallbladder Disease

A. Definitions

1. Cholecystitis: inflammation of the gallbladder
2. Cholelithiasis: stones in the gallbladder

3. At-risk: fair, fat, forty, fertile, female

B. Manifestations

1. Right upper-quadrant or epigastric pain, shoulder pain
2. Nausea and vomiting
3. Fat intolerance
4. Murphy's sign: Have client take deep breath and palpate the right subcostal area. If the client has extreme pain and stops breathing on inspiration, this is a positive Murphy's sign and indicative of acute cholecystitis.
5. Jaundice: indicates obstruction

C. NURSING INTERVENTIONS

1. Relieve pain.
2. Maintain fluid and electrolytes balance.
3. Administer antiemetic PRN.
4. Maintain low-fat diet

D. Cholecystectomy: postoperative

1. Nursing care same as any abdominal surgery
2. Penrose drain in gallbladder area
3. T-tube to gravity after cholecystostomy and choledochostomy: to prevent total loss of bile drainage, tube may be elevated above level of abdomen
4. Resume regular diet as tolerated

E. Laparoscopic Cholecystectomy

1. Preferred procedure for uncomplicated cases
2. Common client report: pain in shoulder from gas in abdominal area needed to visualize organs

3. **NURSING INTERVENTION:** Postoperative instructions are important as client needs to assess self at home.

Pancreatitis

A. Definition: inflammation brought about by the digestion of this organ by the very enzymes it produces; clients at greatest risk are those suffering from alcohol abuse, and clients with other liver and gallbladder diseases

B. Manifestations

1. Extreme upper-abdominal pain radiating into back
2. Persistent vomiting
3. Abdominal distention
4. Weight loss
5. Steatorrhea: bulky, pale, foul-smelling stools
6. Elevated serum amylase and lipase
7. Pleural effusion

C. NURSING INTERVENTIONS

 1. Rest the organ.
   a. Administer anticholinergics, antacids, pancreatic extracts such as pancrelipase (*Viokase*).
   b. NPO with NG tube in place: no ice chips or hard candies, as these will stimulate the pancreas.
   c. IV fluids may require total parenteral nutrition in moderate or severe cases.
   d. Provide pain relief.
   e. Administer fat-soluble vitamins.
   f. Teach home care management/teaching.
      1) Avoid alcohol.
      2) Give IV fluids and TPN via central line.
      3) Teach client manifestations of complications to report (fever, nausea, vomiting, respiratory distress).

SECTION V
REVIEW OF MUSCULOSKELETAL DISORDERS

Rheumatoid Arthritis and Osteoarthritis

See Table I-8 for Comparisons.

Fractures

A. Definition: a complete or incomplete discontinuity of bone caused by a direct or indirect force
   1. Prevention through safety measures
   2. Identify populations at risk and intervene through teaching

TABLE I-8
COMPARISON OF RHEUMATOID ARTHRITIS AND OSTEOARTHRITIS

	RHEUMATOID ARTHRITIS (systemic)	OSTEOARTHRITIS (local and unilateral - wear and tear)
Onset:	20 to 50 years	Middle to older age
Sex:	Women 3:1	Women 20:1
Defined:	Chronic systemic disease of unknown cause, with recurrent inflammation involving the synovium or lining of the joints	Degeneration of the articular cartilage in the joints caused by prolonged wear and tear of joint surfaces
Joints involved:	Any finger joint, cervical, spine; systemic disease can involve heart, lung, etc.	Distal interphalangeal joints (Heberden's nodes); weight bearing joints: hips, knees, spine
Joints appearance:	Bilateral involvement; tenderness, swelling, warm, redness, subcutaneous nodules; every bone prominence; remission and exacerbation; increased symptoms in morning, decreasing with moderate activity	Normal on exam; grating (crepitus) during movement; pain and stiffness worsen after inactivity or after exercise
Other symptoms:	Serum laboratory results reflect positive rheumatoid factor, antinuclear antibody assay, C-reactive protein and elevated erythrocyte sedimentation rate	Pain, stiffness, swelling, deformed joints, cracking/ creaking with movement
Treatment:	Treatment aimed at symptomatic relief; exercise, physical therapy, weight management, NSAIDs, corticosteroids, disease-modifying antirheumatic medications such as methotrexate (Rheumatrex)	Pain management, corticosteroid therapy, ice and heat application; range-of-motion, isometric exercises; maintain ideal body weight; joint replacement surgery

B. Types of Fractures
1. Closed
2. Comminuted
3. Complete
4. Compression
5. Depressed
6. Greenstick
7. Compound/Open
8. Spiral
9. Pathological
10. Transverse

C. First Aid
1. Maintain airway
2. Prevent shock
3. Immobilize fracture
4. Assess circulation, movement, and sensation (CMS), also known as the five Ps.
   a. Pain
   b. Pallor
   c. Pulselessness
   d. Paresthesia
   e. Paralysis
5. Monitor for fat embolism up to 2 weeks following long bone fractures of femur and humerus.
   a. Manifestations of fat embolism; synonymous with a pulmonary embolus
      1) Restlessness
      2) Altered mental status
      3) Tachypnea
      4) Tachycardia
      5) Fever
      6) Petechiae

D. Traction
1. Definition: the use of a pulling force to treat muscles or skeletal disorders
2. Types (must be maintained continuously to be effective)
   a. Skin
      1) Buck's traction (5 to 10 lb maximum)
      2) Pelvic (up to 20 lb maximum)
   b. Skeletal
      1) Thomas splint with Pearson attachment
      2) Crutchfield tongs
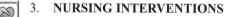 3. **NURSING INTERVENTIONS**
   a. General
      1) Maintain proper body alignment.
      2) Maintain weights hanging freely.
      3) Prevent complications of prolonged bedrest.
      4) Monitor for vascular occlusion; CMS checks.

   b. Skin
      1) Provide general care as above.
      2) Detect pressure points.

3) Provide daily rewrapping.
4) Maintain countertraction; usually bed on shock blocks.
   c. Skeletal
      1) Inspection
      2) Skin/pin care
   d. Muscles
      1) Strengthening exercises for uninvolved extremities
      2) Preparation for crutch walking

E. Casts
1. Applied to maintain immobilization while the fracture heals
 2. **NURSING INTERVENTIONS**
   a. Assess neurovascular integrity.
   b. Cast should be allowed to air dry.
   c. Apply ice to manage pain.
   d. Maintain skin integrity.
   e. Monitor compartment syndrome findings.
   f. Prevent complications of immobility.
   g. Compartment syndrome is a serious complication of fractures.
      1) Severe pain at rest with burning and tightness
      2) Impaired CMS
      3) Tissue swelling
      4) Paralysis is late finding with increased risk of amputation
      5) If untreated, results in paralysis in about 6 hr; may require amputation of extremity

F. Hip Fractures
1. Classification
   a. Fracture of the neck of femur (intracapsular)
   b. Fracture of trochanteric region of femur (extracapsular)
   c. Subtrochanteric fracture
2. Treatment
   a. Skin traction for immobilization (preoperative); decrease pain and muscle spasms
   b. Trochanter roll (prevents external rotation)
   c. Open reduction and internal fixation
   d. Total hip replacement
      1) The replacement of a severely damaged hip with an artificial joint
      2) Other indications for total hip replacement include arthritis, femoral neck fractures, failure of previous reconstructive surgery, and congenital hip disease
      3) Most prostheses consist of a metal femoral component topped with a spherical ball fitted into a plastic acetabular socket

4) **NURSING INTERVENTIONS**
   a) Preoperative care
      (1) Immobilization
      (2) Anticoagulation therapy
   b) Postoperative care
      (1) Maintain proper leg position.
         (a) Use abduction pillow.
         (b) Never flex operative hip more than 90°.
         (c) Maintain limited flexion during transfers and in sitting position.
         (d) Do not cross legs.
         (e) Hips should be higher than knees when sitting.
         (f) Use high-seated chair and raised toilet seat.
      (2) Exercise regularly.
      (3) Prevent infection.
      (4) Prevent deep-vein thrombosis formation.
         (a) Ankle and foot exercises
         (b) Elastic stockings and continuous passive motion
         (c) Anticoagulant
      (5) Observe for complications.
         (a) Dislocation of hip prosthesis
         (b) Excessive wound drainage
         (c) Thromboembolism
         (d) Infection
         (e) Heel pressure ulcer
         (f) Complications of immobility
         (g) Hemorrhage

G. Osteoporosis
1. Definition: demineralization of the bones; leading cause in crippling hip fractures in women
2. Risk factors
   a. Immobility
   b. Decreased calcium diet
   c. Menopause, men older than 65, amenorrhea at any age
   d. Thin and light-haired women
   e. Smoking
   f. Steroid use
3. Prevent by
   a. Weight-bearing exercises
   b. Adequate calcium intake: 1,200 mg premenopause; 1,500 mg postmenopause

4. **NURSING INTERVENTIONS**
   a. Increase calcium and vitamin D intake.
   b. Prevent falls.
   c. Engage in weight-bearing exercises.
   d. Assess bone density.
   e. Bisphosphonate therapy
      1) Alendronate (Fosamax)
      2) ibandronate (Boniva)

3) zoledronic acid (Reclast)
f. Hormone therapy
   1) Calcitonin (Calcimar)
   2) Raloxifene (Evista)

H. Pelvic Fractures

1. **NURSING INTERVENTIONS**
   a. Major assessments
      1) Bladder injuries: watch for hematuria
      2) Bowel injuries: watch for signs of peritonitis
      3) Bleeding
   b. Immobilization
      1) Bed rest
      2) Pelvic sling (may be removed intermittently)

Amputation

A. Definition: Surgical removal of extremity; most commonly related to advanced peripheral arterial disease; above or below the knee amputation is most common site

B. Preoperative Care
1. Psychological adjustment; "anticipatory grieving"
2. Preoperative teaching
3. Increase upper-body strength
4. Trapeze on bed

C. Postoperative Complications
1. Infection
2. Hematoma
3. Tissue necrosis
4. Thrombophlebitis
5. Flexion deformity

D. Nursing Interventions

1. Elevate surgical extremity.
2. Apply ice for first 24 hr.
3. Manage phantom pain.
4. Perform range-of-motion exercises.
5. Teach transfer techniques.
6. Instruct on pulmonary toilet measures.
7. Promote neurovascular integrity.

E. Rehabilitation
1. Exercise
   a. Stretch flexor muscles and upper extremities to prevent flexion deformity.
   b. Maintain range of motion.
   c. Avoid prolonged sitting in bed or chair; will enhance flexion deformities.
   d. Maintain proper alignment of extremity.
2. Stump conditioning
   a. Stump shrinking with wrapping
   b. Stump "toughening"
   c. Compression dressing

Gout

A. Definition: inflammatory type of arthritis caused by deposits of urate crystals in and around the joints; there is an hereditary error in purine metabolism that results in excessive uric acid production; risk factors are alcoholism, chemotherapy, heredity

B. Manifestations
1. Severe pain, usually in great toe
2. Joints are red, warm, painful, and swollen
3. Large accumulations of crystals in the joints (tophi) and connective tissue
4. Joint damage and deformity increase with each attack
5. Monarticular or polyarticular
6. Hyperuricemia - greater than 7 mg/dL
7. Sporadic and usually diet related

C. Treatment
1. NSAIDS
   a. Can cause bone marrow suppression and liver damage
   b. Indomethacin (*Indocin*)
   c. Probenecid (*Benemid*)
2. Allopurinol (*Zyloprim*) to prevent recurrence
3. Colchicine (*Colchicine*) during acute attack
   a. Reduces uric acid
   b. Can use during acute phase
4. Corticosteroid short-term therapy to manage pain and inflammation
   a. Provide bed rest during acute attacks.
   b. Keep covers away from affected joints.
   c. Apply heat or cold.
   d. Increase fluid intake 2,000 mL per or more each day to prevent stone formation.
   e. Limit intake of high purine foods (organ and red meats), wine.
   f. Limit alcohol intake.
   g. Develop weight loss strategies.

Total Knee Replacement

A. Definition: implantation of metal or acrylic prosthesis designed to provide functional, painless joint stability to clients experiencing severe pain and functional disabilities related to joint destruction

B. Postoperative Care
1. Monitor for swelling, manifestations of infection
   a. Apply ice to control edema and bleeding.
   b. Apply compression dressing.
   c. Assess for pain.
2. Assess neurovascular status.
3. Assess Hemovac, Jackson-Pratt drains for quality/quantity drainage.

4. Premedicate prior to using passive motion device.
5. Provide physical therapy for strength and range-of-motion exercises.
6. Review weight-bearing status per orders.
7. Review progressive ambulation with assistive devices.
8. Monitor client for complications.
   a. Infection
   b. Loosening/wear of prosthetic components

SECTION VI

REVIEW OF ENDOCRINE SYSTEM FUNCTIONS AND DISORDERS

Pituitary Gland

See Table I-9 Pituitary Gland: Hormones Produced and Functions.

Endocrine System Disorders

A. Disorders of Anterior Pituitary
1. Acromegaly
   a. Definition: hypersecretion of growth hormone that occurs in adulthood; commonly associated with benign pituitary tumors
   b. Manifestations
      1) Enlargement of skeletal extremities (e.g., nose, jaw, hands, feet)
      2) Protrusion of the jaw and orbital ridges
      3) Course features
      4) Visual problems, blindness
      5) Hyperglycemia, insulin resistance
      6) Hypercalcemia
   c. Treatment
      1) Irradiation of pituitary
      2) Transsphenoidal hypophysectomy: removal of pituitary gland
         a) Assess for signs of increased cranial pressure, adrenal insufficiency, hypothyroidism, and temporary diabetes insipidus.
         b) Elevate head of bed to 30°.
         c) Avoid coughing, sneezing, and blowing nose.
         d) Check for cerebrospinal fluid in nasal packing.
      3) Bromocriptine (*Parlodel*) with surgery or radiation
    d. **NURSING INTERVENTIONS**
      1) Provide emotional support.
      2) Provide symptomatic care.

TABLE I-9
PITUITARY GLAND: HORMONES PRODUCED AND FUNCTIONS

ENDOCRINE GLAND	HORMONE PRODUCED	FUNCTION
Pituitary gland		Controlled primarily by the hypothalamus; termed "master gland" as it directly affects the function of other endocrine glands
Anterior lobe	- Adrenocorticotropic hormone (ACTH)	- Concerned with growth and secretory activity of adrenal cortex, which produces steroids
	- Thyrotropic hormone (TSH)	- For growth and secretory activity of thyroid; controls release rate of thyroxine, which controls rate of most chemical reactions in the body; target is thyroid gland
	- Somatotropic hormones (STH or GH)	- Promote growth of body tissue
	- Gonadotropic hormones and estrogen secretion; follicle-stimulating hormone (FSH)	- Stimulate development of ovarian follicles, seminiferous tubules, and sperm maturation
	- Luteinizing hormone (LH)	- Works with FSH in final maturation of follicles; promotes ovulation and progesterone secretion
	- Prolactin	- Maintains corpus luteum and progesterone secretion
	- Melanocyte stimulating hormone (MSH)	- Produces the characteristic skin darkening

2. Gigantism
   a. Definition: hypersecretion of growth hormone that occurs in childhood
   b. Manifestations
      1) Proportional overgrowth in all body tissue
      2) Overgrowth of long bones: height in childhood may reach 8 or 9 ft
   c. Treatment (same as acromegaly)
   d. Nursing responsibilities (same as acromegaly)
3. Dwarfism
   a. Definition: hyposecretion of GH during childhood resulting in adult height less than 4 feet 10 inches.
   b. Manifestations
      1) Disproportionate head and extremities to torso
      2) Progressive bowed legs and lordosis
      3) Delayed adolescence

   c. Treatment
      1) Limb-lengthening surgery
      2) Human growth hormone injections
      3) Adaptive measures to meet activities of daily living
   d. Nursing responsibilities (same as acromegaly)

B. Disorder of Posterior Pituitary
   1. Diabetes insipidus
      a. Definition: Hyposecretion of antidiuretic hormone (ADH) due to several causes; insufficient production of vasopressin, head injury/tumors, idiopathic or genetic
      b. Manifestations
         1) Polyuria
         2) Polydipsia
         3) Hypernatremia
         4) Weight loss
         5) Dehydration/dry skin

c. Medication treatment
  1) Hydrochlorothiazide (*HCTZ*)
  2) Vasopressin (*desmopressin/DDAVP*)
  3) Lypressin (*Diapid*) nasal spray

 d. **NURSING INTERVENTIONS**
  1) Obtain daily weights.
  2) Monitor urine-specific gravity.
  3) Assess blood pressure and heart rate.
  4) Maintain fluid and electrolyte balance.
  5) Avoid foods with diuretic action.

2. Syndrome of inappropriate secretion of antidiuretic hormone
  a. Definition: inappropriate, continued release of antidiuretic hormone resulting in water intoxication; caused by neoplastic tumors, respiratory disorders, drugs
  b. Manifestations
    1) Mental confusion/irritability
    2) Lethargy/seizures
    3) Dilutional hyponatremia
    4) Weight gain
    5) Anorexia, nausea and vomiting
    6) Weakness
  c. Treatment
    1) Correct hyponatremia with fluid restriction and hypertonic solutions.
    2) Give demeclocycline (*Declomycin*) to inhibit vasopressin receptors.
    3) Treat underlying cause with surgery, chemotherapy and/or radiation.

Adrenal Gland

See Table I-10 for Hormones Produced and Functions.

A. Disorders of Adrenal Cortex

1. Addison's disease
  a. Definition: hyposecretion of adrenal cortex hormones, (insufficiency of cortisol, aldosterone and androgens); discontinuing steroid medications abruptly
  b. Manifestations
    1) Fatigue and muscle weakness
    2) Anorexia and weight loss
    3) Hyperpigmentation
    4) Hypotension and syncope
    5) Hypoglycemia, hyponatremia, hyperkalemia
    6) Craving salty foods
    7) Irritability and depression
    8) Joint and muscle pain
    9) Diminished libido
  c. Treatment
    1) Medications: hydrocortisone (Cortef) to replace cortisol
    2) Fluid and electrolyte balance
    3) High protein, high carbohydrate diet

 d. **NURSING INTERVENTIONS**
  1) Observe for addisonian crisis (sudden extreme weakness; severe abdominal, back, and leg pain; hyperpyrexia; coma; death) secondary to stress caused by infection, trauma, surgery, pregnancy or stress.
  2) Observe for side effects of hormone replacement; this will be the same symptoms as hypersecretion of this gland.
  3) Provide emotional support.
  4) Provide teaching (lifelong medications, prompt treatment of infection, illness, stress management).
  5) Monitor fluid and electrolyte balance regularly.

2. Cushing's syndrome
  a. Definition: hypersecretion of the glucocorticoids; overdose of steroid medications. May also be the result of adenoma of pituitary gland stimulating increased production of adrenocorticotropic hormone
  b. Manifestations
    1) Upper-body obesity, moon face, buffalo hump, and neck fat
    2) Poor skin integrity
    3) Purple striae
    4) Osteoporosis
    5) Hyperglycemia, hypernatremia, hypokalemia
    6) Hirsutism
    7) Amenorrhea
    8) Elevated triglycerides
    9) Hypertension
    10) Erectile dysfunction
    11) Immunosuppression
    12) Peptic ulcer
  c. Treatment
    1) Adrenalectomy: unilateral or bilateral (may be laproscopic approach)
    2) Chemotherapy: bromocriptine (*Parlodel*); mitotane (*Lysodren*), or aminoglutethimide (*Cytadren*)
    3) High-protein, low-carbohydrate, low-sodium diet with potassium supplement
    4) For pituitary adenoma, may need transsphenoidal adenomectomy
  d. **NURSING INTERVENTIONS**
    1) Protect from infection.
    2) Protect from accidents and falls due to osteoporosis.
    3) Provide client education concerning lifelong self-administration of hormone suppression therapy.

TABLE I-10
ADRENAL GLAND: HORMONES PRODUCED AND FUNCTIONS

HORMONE PRODUCED	FUNCTION
Cortex:	- Cannot live without the secretions from this gland; therefore if missing, hormones must be replaced

- Glucocorticoids
  - Cortisol
  - Cortisone
  - Corticosterone
	- Affect carbohydrate, fat, and protein metabolism; affect stress reactions and the inhibition of the inflammatory process

- Mineralocorticoids
  - Aldosterone
  - Corticosterone
  - Deoxycorticosterone
	- Regulate sodium and electrolyte balance

- Sex Hormones
  - Androgens
  - Estrogens
	- Influence the development of sexual characteristics

Medulla:
  - Catecholamines
    - Epinephrine
    - Norepinephrine
	- Stimulate "fight or flight" response to danger, sympathetic nervous system response

4) Steroid replacement
  a) Purpose
    (1) Anti-inflammatory and antiautoimmunity reaction
    (2) Enables one to tolerate high degree of stress
  b) Indications
    (1) Crisis (e.g., shock, bronchial obstruction)
    (2) Long-term therapy (e.g., postadrenalectomy, arthritis, leukemia)
  c) Side effects due to prolonged use (refer to Cushing's manifestations)
  d) Dosage schedule
    (1) Large dosages should be given at 0800 (⅔ morning, ⅓ night) to simulate the normal excretion by the body
    (2) Should be taken same time every day
    (3) Withdraw steroids by tapered dosages or may get symptoms of Addison's disease
    (4) Can be given with antacids to minimize gastrointestinal upset and ulceration
5) If postoperative transsphenoidal adenomectomy, client will have nasal packing; avoid coughing, straining, bending, and observe for cerebrospinal fluid leakage

3. Aldosteronism (Conn's syndrome)
  a. Definition: hypersecretion of aldosterone from adrenal cortex (usually due to a tumor)
  b. Manifestations
    1) Hypokalemia and hypernatremia
    2) Hypertension from hypernatremia
    3) Muscle weakness and cardiac problems related to hypokalemia
  c. Treatment
    1) Surgical removal of tumor/adrenal gland
    2) Potassium replacement
    3) Antihypertensive medications: spironolactone (*Aldactone*)
   d. **NURSING INTERVENTIONS**
    1) Provide quiet environment.
    2) Monitor blood pressure and cardiac activity.
    3) Monitor potassium level.

B. Disorders of Adrenal Medulla
  1. Pheochromocytoma
    a. Definition: Benign tumor of adrenal medulla that causes hypersecretion of epinephrine and norepinephrine
    b. Manifestations (sudden onset): seen in young women and men

1) Hypertensive crisis
2) Tachycardia
   a) Diaphoresis
   b) Apprehension
   c) Palpitations secondary to tachycardia
   d) Nausea, vomiting
   e) Orthostatic hypotension
   f) Headache
3) Pallor
4) Flight or fight
5) Hyperglycemia
6) Headache

c. Treatment
   1) Immediate surgical removal of tumor
   2) Alpha and beta-blocker medication to diminish effect of norepinephrine prior to surgery

d. **NURSING INTERVENTIONS**
   1) Provide high-calorie, nutritious diet (avoid caffeine).
   2) Promote rest.
   3) Preoperative: control hypertension (this is essential; high risk for hypertensive crisis).

Thyroid Gland

See Table I-11 for Hormones Produced and Functions.

A. Disorders of Thyroid Gland

1. Myxedema: highest incidence between ages 50 to 60; more common in women
   a. Definition: Hyposecretion of thyroxine (T_4) and triiodothyronine (T_3)
   b. Manifestations
      1) Fatigue and weakness
      2) Increased sensitivity to cold
      3) Constipation
      4) Dry skin, brittle hair and nails
      5) Unexplained weight gain

6) Deepened, hoarse voice
7) Joint pain and stiffness
8) Hyperlipidemia
9) Depression
10) Heavy menstrual cycle
11) Facial edema
12) Goiter
13) Weight gain
14) Puffy appearance (nonpitting)
15) Anemia
16) Increased cholesterol and lipids
17) Menstrual disorders

c. Treatment
   1) Synthetic thyroid-replacement hormone levothyroxine (Synthroid)
      a) Administer medication on empty stomach.
      b) Monitor for toxicity: palpitations, insomnia, increased appetite, and tremors.

d. **NURSING INTERVENTIONS**
   1) Directed toward manifestations of decreased metabolism
      a) Provide warm environment.
      b) Provide low-calorie, low-cholesterol, low-saturated-fat diet.
      c) Increase roughage.
      d) Moderate fluids.
      e) Avoid sedatives.
      f) Plan rest periods.
      g) Weigh client.
   2) Observe for overdosage manifestations of thyroid preparations (these will be the same as the manifestations of hyperthyroidism with the exception of exophthalmus).

2. Cretinism
   a. Definition: hyposecretion of thyroid hormones in the fetus or neonate

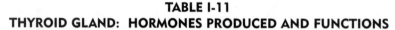

TABLE I-11
THYROID GLAND: HORMONES PRODUCED AND FUNCTIONS

HORMONES PRODUCED	FUNCTION
Thyroxine (T_4)	Acts as a catalyst; influences metabolic rate, growth, and development (Normal range 1.0 to 2.3 ng/dL)
Triiodothyronine (T_3)	Controls rate of body metabolism, growth, and nutrition (Normal range 80 to 200 ng/dL)
Thyrocalcitonin	Assists in control of calcium levels; decreases (Calcitonin normal level < 19 ng/dL)

b. Diagnosed shortly after birth through newborn screening; testing for thyroid hormones is mandated in all 50 states

c. Can lead to severe, irreversible mental retardation if not treated

d. Requires lifelong hormone replacement therapy

3. Hyperthyroidism (Graves' disease, diffuse toxic goiter)

a. Definition: Hypersecretion of thyroxine from immune system, attacking thyroid gland; more common in women older than 20 years of age

b. Manifestations
   1) Anxiety and irritability
   2) Insomnia and fatigue
   3) Tachycardia
   4) Tremors
   5) Diaphoresis
   6) Sensitivity to heat
   7) Weight loss; despite food intake
   8) Exophthalmos and photosensitivity
   9) Diarrhea
   10) Light or absent menstrual cycle

c. Treatment
   1) Beta-blocker medication to manage tachycardia, anxiety, and tremors
      a) Nadolol (Corgard), propranolol (Inderal), atenolol (Tenormin), metoprolol (Lopressor)
      b) Propylthiouracil (*Propyl-Thyracil*): blocks thyroid hormone production
         (1) Can cause agranulocytosis
         (2) Client must have frequent CBCs performed
      c) Iodides: decrease vascularity; inhibit release of thyroid hormones
         (1) Lugol's solution (use is decreasing because this medication is expensive and inactivates thyroid medications in the bowel)
         (2) Saturated solution of potassium iodide (*SSKI*); used prior to thyroidectomy
      d) Beta blockers: relief of tachycardia, new onset palpitations
   2) Antithyroid medication block production of thyroxine
      a) Methimazole (Tapazole)
   3) Radioactive iodine treatment shrinks thyroid gland prior to surgery
      a) Saturated solution of potassium iodide (SSKI)
   4) Thyroidectomy requires lifelong intake of levothyroxine (Synthroid) and calcium

 d. **NURSING INTERVENTIONS**
   1) Provide adequate rest.
   2) Provide cool, quiet environment.
   3) Provide high-caloric (4,000 to 5,000 cal/day), high-protein, carbohydrate, vitamin diet without stimulants, extra fluids.
   4) Weigh client daily.
   5) Provide emotional support; activities, and nothing repetitive.
   6) Provide eye protection: ophthalmic medicine; tape eyes at night; decrease sodium and water.
   7) Elevate head of bed.
   8) Be alert for complications.
      a) Corneal abrasion
      b) Heart disease
      c) Thyroid storm (usually occurs after thyroid surgery)

e. Thyroidectomy
   1) Definition: removal of the thyroid gland, either total or partial
   2) Preoperative goals
      a) Thyroid function in normal range: saturated solution of S*SKI*
      b) Signs of thyrotoxicosis are diminished
      c) Weight and nutritional status normal

 3) **NURSING INTERVENTIONS** (postoperative care)
      a) Place client in semi-Fowler's position.
      b) Check dressing, especially the back of the neck.
      c) Observe for respiratory distress: tracheostomy tray, oxygen, and suction apparatus at bedside.
      d) Be alert for signs of hemorrhage.
      e) Limit talking and note any hoarseness; may indicate injury to laryngeal nerve.
      f) Observe for signs of tetany: Chvostek's sign and Trousseau's sign (parathyroid glands may accidentally be removed).
      g) Have calcium gluconate IV at bedside.
      h) Observe for thyroid storm (life-threatening); increase release of thyroid hormone
         (1) Fever
         (2) Tachycardia
         (3) Delirium
         (4) Irritability
         (5) Important to assess temperature routinely
      i) Gradually increase range of motion to neck; support when sitting up.

TABLE I-12
PARATHYROID GLAND: HORMONES PRODUCED AND FUNCTIONS

HORMONES PRODUCED	FUNCTION
Parathyroid hormone (PTH)	Controls calcium and phosphate metabolism

Parathyroid Gland

See Table I-12 for Hormones Produced and Functions.

A. Disorders of Parathyroid Gland
1. Hypoparathyroidism
   a. Definition: Hyposecretion of calcitonin resulting in hypocalcemia and hyperphosphatemia
   b. Manifestations
      1) Paresthesia
      2) Muscle cramps and tetany
      3) Chvostek's sign; muscle spasms and twitching around mouth, throat, and cheeks
      4) Trousseau's syndrome; pressure from blood pressure cuff induces muscle spasms in distal extremity
      5) Alopecia
      6) Dry skin, brittle hair, and nails
      7) Painful menstruation
         a) Poor development of tooth enamel
         b) Lethargic
         c) Thin hair, brittle nails
         d) Mental retardation
         e) Circumoral paraesthesia with numbness and tingling of fingers
   c. Treatment
      1) Acute: IV calcium gluconate
      2) Chronic
         a) Oral calcium salts
         b) Vitamin D and aluminum hydroxide gel (*Amphojel*)
         c) High-calcium, low-phosphorous diet
    d. **NURSING INTERVENTIONS**
      1) Provide quiet room with no stimulus.
      2) Assess for increased signs of neuromuscular irritability.
2. Hyperparathyroidism (causes are tumor or renal disease)
   a. Definition: hypersecretion of calcitonin resulting in hypercalcemia and hypophosphoremia
   b. Manifestations (causes loss of calcium from the bones to the serum)
      1) Kidney stones and hyperuricemia
      2) Osteoporosis
      3) Hypercalcemia and hypophosphoremia
      4) Abdominal pain, nausea, and vomiting

5) Muscle weakness
6) Fatigue
7) Polyuria and polydipsia
8) Hypertension
   c. Treatment
      1) Subtotal surgical resection of parathyroid gland
      2) Hydration and diuretics - furosemide (*Lasix*) promotes excretion of excess calcium
      3) Plicamycin (*Mithracin*) or gallium nitrate (*Ganite*)
    d. **NURSING INTERVENTIONS**
      1) Force fluids.
      2) Provide a low-calcium, low vitamin D diet.
      3) Prevent constipation and fecal impaction.
      4) Strain all urine.
      5) Provide safety measures to prevent breaks.
      6) Calcitonin; binds phosphate; in renal failure

Pancreas

See Table I-13 for Hormones Produced and Functions.

A. Disorder of the Pancreas
1. Diabetes mellitus
   a. Definition: chronic disorder of carbohydrate metabolism characterized by an imbalance between insulin supply and demand; either a subnormal amount of insulin is produced or the body requires abnormally high amounts
      1) Insulin-dependent diabetes mellitus (type 1), usually juvenile onset
      2) Noninsulin dependent diabetes mellitus (type 2), usually adult onset
         a) Of the 21 million Americans with diabetes mellitus, approximately 90% have type 2
         b) Caused by the dual defects of insulin resistance and beta-cell secretory dysfunction
   b. Glycemic control
      1) Maintaining tight glycemic control substantially reduces the risk for the onset or progression of the chronic complications of diabetes mellitus

TABLE I-13
PANCREAS: HORMONES PRODUCED AND FUNCTIONS

HORMONES PRODUCED	FUNCTIONS
Insulin	Decreases blood glucose by: - Stimulating active transport of glucose into muscle and adipose tissue - Promoting the conversion of glucose to glycogen for storage - Promoting conversion of fatty acids into fat - Stimulating protein synthesis
Glucagon	Increases blood glucose by converting glycogen to glucose

2) Glucose control is monitored on a day-to-day basis by capillary blood glucose levels
  a) Normal preprandial (fasting) blood glucose is less than 100 mg/dL
  b) Normal postprandial blood glucose is less than 140 mg/dL
3) Glucose control is monitored on a long-term basis by the HbA1c (glysosylated hemoglobin)
  a) Normal (nondiabetic) HbA1c level is less than 6%
  b) American Diabetes Association goal is a HbA1c level of less than 7%
  c) American College of Endocrinology goal is a HbA1c level of less than 6.5%

c. Manifestations: "3 Polys"
1) Polyuria
2) Polydipsia
3) Polyphagia
4) Weight loss

 d. **NURSING INTERVENTIONS**
1) Balance diet, insulin, and exercise.
2) Administer insulin therapy.
  a) Insulin is the hormone necessary to "open the door" for glucose to enter the cell and be used for energy.
  b) When mixing insulins:
    (1) Draw up the Regular first, then NPH ("clear then cloudy").
    (2) Do not mix long-acting insulins (glargine, detemir) with any other insulin or solution. If giving at the same time as a rapid-acting insulin, the nurse must use a separate syringe and a different site.
  c) Insulin pump
    (1) External device that provides a basal dose of Regular insulin with a bolus dose before meals; does not read blood glucose

    (2) Needles are inserted into subcutaneous abdominal tissue (changed every 24 to 48 hr)
    (3) Complications
      (a) Insulin overdosage
      (b) Continued insulin injections during hypoglycemia
3) Sulfonylurea medications stimulate pancreas to produce insulin.
  a) Glipizide (*Glucotrol*)
  b) Chlorpropamide (*Diabinese)*
  c) Glyburide (*DiaBeta*)
  d) Metformin (*Glucophage*)
  e) Glimepiride (*Amaryl*)
4) Maintain diet therapy.
  a) Provide the body with adequate nutrients for cell growth and function.
  b) Maintain a balance between the amount of glucose in the body and the amount of insulin present to use that glucose.
  c) Monitor caloric requirements prescribed by provider in conjunction with the health care team.
5) Monitor for complications
  a) Hypoglycemia (occurs quickly; the most serious diabetic problem is no food for the brain)
    (1) Causes: decreased dietary intake, excess insulin, increased exercise
    (2) Manifestations
      (a) Tachycardia
      (b) Diaphoresis
      (c) Tremors
      (d) Weakness, fatigue
      (e) Irritability, anxiety
      (f) Confusion
    (3) **NURSING INTERVENTIONS**
      (a) Give hard candy (if conscious).
      (b) Give ½ cup fruit juice or milk.

TABLE I-14
INSULIN PREPARATIONS

INSULIN PREPARATION	ONSET OF ACTION	PEAK	DURATION OF ACTION	TYPE
Lispro/aspart/glulisine (NovoLog, Humalog, Apidra)	5 to 15 min	1 to 2 hr	4 to 5 hr	Rapid acting
Human regular (Humulin R, Novolin R)	30 to 60 min	2 to 4 hr	8 to 10 hr	Short acting
NPH (Humulin L, Lente Iletin II, Novolin, NPH)	1 to 2 hr	4 to 8 hr	10 to 20 hr	Intermediate acting
Glargine/detemir/insulin zinc suspension, extended (ultralente) (Lantus, Humulin U Ultralente, Novolin de Ultralente)	1 to 4 hr	Relatively flat	Up to 24 hr	Long acting

(c) Give 8 oz skim milk.

(d) Follow with snack or carbohydrates if next meal is more than 1 hr away.

(e) For severe hypoglycemia (blood glucose of less than 20 mg/dL), the client is likely to be unable to swallow. If unconscious, or seizing, administer 1 mg of glucagon IM or subcutaneous.

b) Diabetic ketoacidosis (DKA)

(1) Definition: Complication of diabetes mellitus due to deficient insulin production; exacerbated hyperglycemia causes production of ketones resulting from fat being used for energy; most common is type 1 diabetes mellitus

(2) Causes: illness, infection, lack of insulin, surgery, fever, and substance abuse

(a) Exacerbated polyuria, polydipsia, polyphagia

(b) Anorexia, nausea, and vomiting

(c) Metabolic acidosis

(d) Kussmaul's respirations

(e) Fruity, scented breath

(f) Level of consciousness changes

(g) Ketonuria

 (3) **NURSING INTERVENTIONS**

(a) Vascular support

(b) Fluid and electrolyte replacement

(c) Regular insulin IV therapy

c) Lipodystrophy: indurated areas of subcutaneous tissue secondary to injecting cold insulin or not rotating sites

d) Hyperglycemic hyperosmolar nonketotic coma

(1) Extremely high glucose levels cause dehydration

(2) No ketosis; elevated BUN

(3) Treatment: replace fluids; give insulin and electrolytes

6) Health teaching

a) Foot care: cleanse feet daily in warm soapy water; rinse and dry carefully; inspect, don't break blisters; trim nails to follow natural curve of toe; always wear breathable shoes such as leather; no crossing of the legs; no cream between toes; inspect visually daily

b) Injection techniques (IntraSite rotation)

c) Dietary management

d) No smoking

e) Stress management (stress increases blood glucose)

7) Long-term complications

a) Diabetic neuropathy: causes pain in legs, then no feeling; safety issues ensue; causes impotence in men

b) Renal: affects microcirculation of kidneys and can cause renal failure

c) Cardiovascular: clients with diabetes mellitus are four times more likely to have a myocardial infarction; unknown cause, but also increases occurrence of hypertension and decreased peripheral circulation

d) Eyes: number one cause of blindness and increases occurrence of cataracts

e) Infections: increased glucose in body fluids makes them an ideal medium for growth of micro-organisms, urinary tract infections, cellulitis

f) **NURSING INTERVENTIONS**
   (1) Assess for each complication early.
   (2) Teach client to maintain control of the illness and to consistently keep blood glucose within normal ranges.

TABLE I-15
BLOOD VALUES

NORMAL VALUES
RBC: female 4.2-5.4 mil/mm³, male 4.6-6.2 mil/mm³
Hgb: female 12-16 gm/dL, male 13-18 gm/dL
Hct: female 37%-48%, male 45%-52%
Note: 3x Hgb = Hct

SECTION VII

REVIEW OF BLOOD DISORDERS

Anemia

A. Definition: a deficiency of RBCs that is characterized by a decreased RBC count and a below-normal Hgb and Hct; this results in a decrease in oxygen to the cells directly related to the degree of anemia present

B. Causes
1. Acute or chronic blood loss (e.g., gastrointestinal ulcers)
2. Greater than normal destruction of RBCs (e.g., spleen diseases)
3. Abnormal bone marrow function (e.g., chemotherapy)

4. Decreased erythropoietin (e.g., renal failure)
5. Inadequate maturation of RBCs (e.g., cancer)

C. Manifestations
1. Fatigue
2. Weakness
3. Dizziness
4. Pallor: first seen in conjunctival area (Caucasian) and oral area (dark and black-skinned population)
5. Cardiac, if decreased oxygen to heart
6. Decreased activity tolerance
7. Decreased Hgb, Hct, RBC levels
8. Shortness of breath and dyspnea

D. NURSING INTERVENTIONS

1. Encourage activity as tolerated.
2. Protect skin from breakdown and decrease pressure.
3. Remove the cause or minimize as much as possible.
4. Provide oxygen therapy as needed.
5. Maximize rest and delivery of oxygen to tissues.
6. Administer blood products as necessary.

E. Blood Transfusions
1. Equipment
   a. Y-type tubing with filter
   b. NS
   c. Blood

2. **NURSING INTERVENTIONS**

   a. Check ID, name, blood type; information verified by two nurses.
   b. Take baseline vital signs, including temperature.
   c. For the first 15 min, stay with the client and infuse no more than 25 mL if possible, monitoring for reaction.
   d. Infuse within 4 hr.
   e. Monitor for transfusion reaction.
      1) Allergic (pruritus, respiratory distress, urticaria), flushing; if expect a minor reaction to something in the blood, may give diphenhydramine (*Benadryl*) if ordered, and continue to infuse
      2) Hemolytic: ABO incompatibility (flank pain, chest pain, fever, chills, tachycardia, tachypnea)
   f. Treat transfusion reaction.
      1) Stop blood immediately.
      2) Maintain IV access with NS.
      3) Take vital signs.
      4) Notify provider.
      5) Follow facility policy (e.g., send urine sample, CBC, send bag and tubing to laboratory for analysis).

F. Classifications

1. Hypoproliferation anemia; bone marrow is unable to produce adequate numbers of cells
    a. Anemia secondary to renal disease (lack of erythropoietin); treat by administering synthetic erythropoietin (*Procrit*, *Epogen*)
    b. Iron deficiency anemia
        1) Due to chronic blood loss (e.g., bleeding ulcer); treat the ulcer by methods discussed in gastrointestinal section; if due to a tumor in gastrointestinal tract, remove
        2) Due to nutritional deficiency; administer iron preparations
        3) Common in infants, young adult women, older adults
    c. Aplastic anemia (treat by eliminating the cause, administering steroid therapy, bone marrow transplantation, antibiotics, and splenectomy)
        1) Lack of precursor cells in the bone marrow with a decrease in all blood cell components (WBC: leukopenia; platelet: thrombocytopenia; RBC: anemia) due to medications, virus, toxins, irradiation
        2) Manifestations
            a) Hypoxia, fatigue, pallor (related to anemia)
            b) Increased susceptibility to infection (related to leukopenia)
            c) Hemorrhage, ecchymosis/leukopenia (related to thrombocytopenia)
         3) **NURSING INTERVENTIONS**
            a) Provide general nursing interventions as previously listed.
            b) Provide protective isolation.
            c) Provide psychological support.
            d) Monitor for manifestations of infection.
2. Megaloblastic anemia (deficiency of B_{12} and folic acid)
    a. Pernicious anemia: a vitamin B_{12} deficiency due to a lack of the intrinsic factor in the gastric juice or deficiency in diet
    b. Causes
        1) Atrophy of the gastric mucosa/hypochlorhydria
        2) Total gastrectomy
        3) Malabsorption (secondary to Crohn's disease, pancreatitis)
        4) Malnutrition
    c. Manifestations (low Hgb and Hct)
        1) Numbness, tingling of extremities
        2) Paresthesia/hypoxemia
        3) Gait disturbances
        4) Behavioral problems

 d. **NURSING INTERVENTIONS**
    1) Administer cobalamin (Vitamin B_{12}) 1,000 mcg IM daily for 2 weeks, then weekly until Hct level is therapeutic, and then monthly for lifetime.
    2) Cobalamin (Nascobal) is available intra-nasally. Self administer the medication weekly, then for lifetime.
    3) Promote rest and eat a balanced diet.
    4) Limit the consumption of alcohol.
3. Hemolytic anemia, due to excessive RBC destruction
    a. Causes
        1) Trauma
        2) Lead poisoning
        3) Tuberculosis
        4) Infections
        5) Transfusion reactions
        6) Toxic agents
     b. **NURSING INTERVENTIONS**
        1) Provide general nursing interventions as previously listed.
        2) Give steroids as needed.
        3) Treat underlying disease to remove the cause.
4. Congenital anemias
    a. Sickle cell anemia (See also page 175.): defective Hgb molecule that assumes a sickle shape when oxygen in venous blood is low; the sickle cells become lodged in the blood vessels, especially the brain and the kidneys as they have a constant need for oxygen
    b. Manifestations
        1) Severe pain
        2) Swelling
        3) Fever
        4) Jaundice
        5) Susceptibility to infection
        6) Hypoxic damage to organs
    c. Risk factors that will cause an attack by enhancing sickling in the cells
        1) Stress
        2) Dehydration
        3) Hypoxia
        4) High altitudes
     d. **NURSING INTERVENTIONS** (symptomatic)
        1) Hydrate.
            a) Autosomal recessive inheritance
            b) More common in African-American clients
        2) Provide oxygen therapy.
        3) Administer hydromorphone (Dilaudid) for pain management.
        4) Encourage rest.

5) Client teaching
a) Identify triggers
b) Immunizations
c) Haemophilus influenzae vaccination
d) Genetic counseling

Administering Iron Preparations

A. Oral
1. Dilute liquid preparations in juice or water and administer with a plastic straw to avoid staining teeth.
2. Orange juice facilitates absorption.
3. Avoid antacids, coffee, tea, dairy products, or whole grain breads concurrently and for 1 hr after administration as they decrease absorption.
4. Monitor for constipation and gastrointestinal upset.

B. Intramuscular
1. Use large bore needle (19 to 20 gauge, 3 inch needle).
2. Use one needle to draw up iron; change needle before administering (to prevent staining).
3. Use Z-track (to buttocks only, never arm).
4. Do not massage.

SECTION VIII

REVIEW OF CARDIOVASCULAR SYSTEM DISORDERS

Cardiovascular System in Failure

A. Deficits Present in at Least One Area
1. Adequately pumps blood to all parts of the body, thus good working cardiac muscles and conduction system
2. Good circulating blood volume to meet body's needs
3. Peripheral vascular resistance must be sufficient to maintain adequate blood pressure
4. Normal heart rate 60 to 100/min

Diagnostic Procedures

A. Laboratory Tests
1. Blood electrolytes (See Table I-1.)
2. Sedimentation rate (less than 20 mm/hour); increased with myocardial infarction
3. Blood coagulation tests
   a. PTT (16 to 40 seconds); most significant to monitor if client is on heparin therapy
   b. PT (11 to 14 seconds); most significant to monitor if client is on warfarin sodium (*Coumadin*) therapy
   c. Clotting time (10 min)
   d. INR
      1) Normal is 1
      2) Universal test not affected by variations in laboratory norms
      3) If client requires anticoagulation, the desired value is an increased value of approximately 2 to 3
4. BUN (7 to 20 mg/dL); reflects renal function; levels increase with myocardial infarction
5. Total serum cholesterol desirable; less than 200 mg/dL. Risk for cardiac or stroke event with levels greater than desirable levels
   a. Low-density lipids; desirable less than 140 mg/dL
   b. High-density lipids; desirable greater than 40 mg/dL for men, 50 mg/dL for women
   c. Triglycerides desirable less than 150 mg/dL
6. Blood cultures
7. Enzymes (indicates actual death of myocardial muscles; heart attack)
   a. Creatine phosphokinase MB Isoenzyme (CPK-MB) is an enzyme that increases within 5 hr after myocardial infarction, peaks at 24 hr
   b. Troponin is a protein considered to be the gold standard in diagnosing MI. A series of three tests completed over 12 hr and can remain elevated for 1 to 2 weeks following an event.

B. Central Venous Pressure (normal = 5 to 10 cm water)
1. Provides an indication of pressure in the right atrium
2. Trends are more important than values

C. Electrocardiogram (ECG)
1. Definition: a record showing the electrical activity of the heart
2. Interpretation
   a. P wave: atrial depolarization
   b. QRS complex: ventricular depolarization
   c. T wave: ventricular repolarization
   d. PR interval: 0.12 to 0.20 seconds
   e. QRS: 0.08 to 0.10 seconds
3. Atrial dysrhythmias (degree impacts on ventricular function and heartbeat)
   a. Atrial dysrhythmias (degree impacts on ventricular function and heartbeat)
      1) Atrial fibrillation
         a) Irregular, rapid rate
         b) Often asymptomatic with increased risk for stroke event
         c) Managed with cardioversion, beta-blocker medication, and warfarin (Coumadin)

2) Atrial tachycardia
   a) Heart rate exceeds 100/min
   b) Occurs with hypoglycemia, hypokalemia, digoxin toxicity, anxiety, and stimulants
   c) Treated by removing the cause
3) Atrial bradycardia
   a) Rate below 60/min
   b) Normal in athletes
   c) Significance related to how it affects cardiac output
   d) Treated by administering anticholinergic medication (Atropine)
4) AV heart block
   a) Definition: Cardiac electrical conduction transmission is blocked from sinoatrial node to the AV node causing bradycardia, syncope, and palpitations drops
   b) First degree
      (1) Delayed transmission of impulse through the AV node
      (2) Prolonged PR interval (greater than 0.20)
      (3) No treatment necessary
   c) Second degree
      (1) Some impulses pass through the AV node, some do not
      (2) May be a 2:1, 3:1, or 4:1 block
      (3) May process to more lethal heart block
      (4) Pacemaker may be necessary
   d) Third degree
      (1) No impulses pass through AV node
      (2) Atria and ventricles essentially beat independently of each other
      (3) Ventricular pacemaker takes over and the ventricles are a very slow and unreliable source to generate cardiac heart rate
      (4) Indication for a pacemaker
b. Ventricular dysrhythmias
   1) Premature ventricular contraction
      a) Ventricle contracts prematurely manifesting palpitations
      b) Side effects: slowing of the heart rate, decreased blood pressure
      c) Could lead to cardiac arrest or ventricular tachycardia, so must treat
      d) Treatment: antiarrhythmic medications
         (1) Procainamide hydrochloride (*Pronestyl*)
         (2) Lidocaine (*Xylocaine*)
   2) Ventricular tachycardia
      a) Pulse rate above 150

   b) Severely affects cardiac output
   c) Treatment: cardioversion
3) Ventricular fibrillation
   a) Most serious dysrhythmia
   b) Synonymous with cardiac arrest; treatment CPR and defibrillation

D. Arteriography/Angiography
1. Definition: injection of contrast medium into the vascular system to outline an area of the body; when it is done to the vessels around the heart, it is usually done with cardiac catheterization
2. Purpose: obtain information regarding coronary anatomy, structural abnormalities of the coronary artery
3. Assess circulation, movement, and sensation bilaterally. May require the use of Doppler on affected extremity.

E. Cardiac Catheterization
1. Definition: a diagnostic procedure; catheter is introduced into the right or left side of the heart through either the femoral or brachial artery
2. Purpose
   a. Measure oxygen concentration, saturation, tension, and pressure in various chambers of the heart.
   b. Detect shunts.
   c. Obtain blood samples.
   d. Determine cardiac output and pulmonary blood flow.
   e. Determine need for cardiac bypass surgery.
3. **NURSING INTERVENTIONS**
    a. Prior to catheterization:
      1) Know approach: right (venous) or left (arterial).
      2) Keep client NPO for 6 hr.
      3) Mark distal (baseline) pulses.
      4) Explain procedure to client and what to expect.
         a) May have metallic taste in mouth
         b) May feel flushed when dye is injected
      5) Assess client for history of allergy to dye, shellfish.
      6) Verify that client consent has been obtained.
   b. After catheterization:
      1) Monitor blood pressure and apical pulse every 15 min for 2 to 4 hr.
      2) Perform neurovascular assessment every 15 min, every 2 to 4 hr.
      3) Check puncture sites for bleeding.
      4) Apply sandbag to area to maintain hemostasis.
      5) Assess for chest pain.
      6) Keep extremity extended 4 to 6 hr.

7) Maintain bed rest; no hip flexion; no sitting up in bed.
8) Increase fluid intake to flush body of dye.

Disorders

A. Angina

1. Definition: Symptom of myocardial ischemia caused by arterial stenosis or blockage, uncontrolled blood pressure, or cardiomyopathy
 2. **NURSING INTERVENTIONS**
   a. Assess pain.
      1) Location: jaw and/or arm as well as chest
      2) Character
      3) Duration: goes away with rest and/or nitroglycerine (*Nitro-Bid*)
      4) Precipitating factors (once identified, eliminate or minimize to avoid attacks)
   b. Provide education to client to help adjust to living style to prevent episode of angina.
      1) Avoid excessive activity in cold weather.
      2) Avoid overeating.
      3) Stop smoking.
      4) Avoid constipation.
      5) Rest after meals.
      6) Exercise.
      7) Decrease stress.
   c. Teach client that anything that decreases cardiac output or increases workload of heart can cause chest pain.
   d. Teach client how to cope with an attack: use of nitroglycerin - peripheral vasodilation decreases myocardial oxygen demand; coronary artery vasodilation increases supply of oxygen to myocardium.
      1) When to take
         a) Daily to prevent angina (if indicated)
         b) As needed at onset of chest pain
         c) If client knows an activity can cause pain, should take nitroglycerin prophylactically before activity (e.g., sexual intercourse)
      2) How often
         a) Daily as prescribed
         b) For attack
            (1) ASAP at onset of attack
            (2) Every 5 min x 3 doses
            (3) If chest pain still not relieved, call 911
      3) Storage: dark, dry, replace every 6 months
      4) Side effects: headache; hypotension
      5) Types: tablets, ointment, patch, spray
         a) If given daily for prevention, client must be nitroglycerine free daily for 12 hr to prevent tolerance
         b) If patch user: "On" upon waking, "off" at bedtime

6) Never take nitroglycerin (*Nitrostat*) without sitting down and stopping activity.
7) Erectile dysfunction therapy contraindicated with the use of nitrates.

B. Myocardial Infarction

1. Definition: process by which myocardial tissue is destroyed due to reduced coronary blood flow and lack of oxygen; actual necrosis of heart muscle (myocardium) occurs
2. Causes
   a. Atherosclerotic heart disease
   b. Coronary artery embolism
3. Manifestations
   a. Chest pain
      1) Unrelieved with nitroglycerin or rest
      2) Crushing quality, radiates to jawline, left arm, neck, and/or back
      3) Diabetics and women report no pain
   b. Diaphoresis, nausea, vomiting, anxiety, fear
   c. Vital sign changes: tachycardia, hypotension, dyspnea, dysrhythmias
   d. Laboratory changes: elevated troponin and CK-MB enzymes, elevated LDH
   e. ECG changes: ST elevation, T-wave inversion
 4. **NURSING INTERVENTIONS:** aimed at resting myocardium
   a. Early
      1) Administer oxygen
      2) Medications
         a. Antidysrhythmics - lidocaine (*Xylocaine*), amiodarone HCL (*Cordarone*)
         b. Analgesics - morphine sulfate
         c. Anticoagulants - heparin IV
         d. Thrombolytics within 6 hr of cardiac event - tissue plasminogen activator (*TPA*), streptokinase (*Streptase*), alteplase recombinant (*Activase*)
         e. Vasodilators - nitroglycerine
         f. Beta blockers - metoprolol (*Lopressor*)
         g. Calcium channel blockers - verapamil HCL (*Calan*), nifedipine (*Procardia*)
      3) Frequently monitor the client's vital signs, O₂ saturation, ECG
      4) Provide emotional support.

b. Later
1) Administer stool softeners to prevent straining with bowel movement and/or Valsalva maneuver; decrease myocardial workload.
2) Provide soft, low-fat, low-cholesterol, low-sodium diet.
3) Use bedside commode: causes less energy expenditure than using a bedpan.
4) Promote self-care to tolerance; stop at the onset of pain.
5) Plan for cardiac rehabilitation.
   a) Initiate exercise program: stop if fatigue or chest pain occurs.
   b) Encourage stress management.
   c) Teach modifiable risk factors reduction.
      (1) Obesity
      (2) Stress
      (3) Diet
      (4) Hypertension
      (5) Smoking
      (6) Lack of exercise
   d) Recognize nonmodifiable risk factors.
      (1) Heredity
      (2) Race
      (3) Age
      (4) Sex
      (5) "Type A" personality
   e) Bleeding precautions with anticoagulant therapy.
   f) Initiate long-term medication therapy.
      (1) Antiarrhythmics: quinidine (*Quinora*), lidocaine (*Xylocaine*)
      (2) Anticoagulants: heparin, aspirin, warfarin (*Coumadin*), enoxaparin (*Lovenox*)
      (3) Antihypertensives: metoprolol (*Lopressor*), hydrochlorothiazide (*Hydrodiuril*), and calcium-channel blockers
      (4) Vasodilators - nitroglycerin (*Nitro-Bid*) and calcium-channel blockers

C. Heart Failure

1. Definition: inability of the heart to meet tissue requirements for oxygen (not pumping effectively); usually the body tries to compensate by increasing the rate (tachycardia), increasing the size of the muscle and increasing the length of the heart fibers; all these changes are aimed at increasing cardiac output
2. Left-ventricular failure: inadequate ejection of blood into the systemic circulation, usually associated with myocardial infarction, hypertension
   a. Manifestations (primarily respiratory symptoms)
      1) Dyspnea and paroxysmal nocturnal dyspnea
      2) Moist cough
      3) Crackles, wheezing
      4) Orthopnea
   b. Pulmonary edema results, causing excessive quantity of fluid in pulmonary interstitial spaces or alveoli evidenced by:
      1) Moist crackles, frothy sputum
      2) Severe anxiety
      3) Marked dyspnea and cyanosis
      4) Edema in pulmonary system
    c. **NURSING INTERVENTIONS**
      1) Administer morphine sulfate for pain: decreases respiratory rate and increases effective breathing; causes pooling of blood in the peripheral vessels, thus decreasing cardiac return and decreasing the work of the heart.
      2) Administer furosemide (*Lasix*) for diuretic.
      3) Deliver high-flow oxygen therapy.
      4) Monitor client for possible intubation.
      5) Maintain bed rest in semi-Fowler's position.
      6) Administer digitalis (*Digoxin*) to increase efficiency of the myocardium as a pump.
3. Right-ventricular failure: congestion due to blood not adequately pumped from systemic system to the lungs; also related to COPD/CAL;
   a. Manifestations (primarily systemic symptoms)
      1) Peripheral edema (dependent in nature)
      2) Distended neck veins
      3) Weight gain (greater than 2 lb in 1 day)
      4) Enlarged liver
      5) Elevated central venous pressure, wedge pressures
      6) Hypotension (from decreased cardiac output)
      7) Tachycardia
    b. **NURSING INTERVENTIONS**
      1) Provide psychological support for relief of anxiety and stress.

2) Deliver oxygen.
3) Decrease fluid intake to decrease preload.
4) Improve myocardial contraction with digitalis, dobutamine hydrochloride (*Dobutrex*).

c. Digitalis therapy
1) Purpose: decrease heart rate, improve ventricular filling, stroke volume, and coronary artery perfusion; improve strength of contraction
2) Manifestations of toxicity - check digitalis level in serum; 0.8 to 2.0 ng/mL is normal
3) **NURSING INTERVENTIONS**
   a) Monitor potassium levels; decreased levels enhance digitalis toxicity.
   b) Monitor apical heart rate: verify if greater than 60/min before each dose.

   c) Monitor client for digitalis toxicity.
      (1) Normal digitalis level in serum is 0.8 to 2.0 ng/mL
      (2) Manifestations of digoxin toxicity
         (a) Early - nausea, vomiting, anorexia, bradycardia, depression
         (b) Late - frequent PVCs, green-yellow halos in visual field, hyperkalemia, photophobia, diplopia
   d) Client teaching: assess pulse; report signs of toxicity; keep laboratory appointments; St. John's Wort and licorice increase the risk of toxicity; low-sodium/high-potassium diet

D. Valvular Disorders
1. Definition: results in narrowing of valve that prevents or impedes blood flow (stenosis) or impaired closure that allows backward leakage of blood (regurgitation); affects mitral, aortic, or tricuspid: stenosis or insufficiency; rheumatic fever history frequent causative factor (or infection such as endocarditis)
2. Manifestations
   a. Right-sided heart failure (mitral stenosis, mitral regurgitation, tricuspid stenosis)
   b. Left-sided heart failure (aortic stenosis, insufficiency)
   c. Murmurs

d. Decreased cardiac output
3. **NURSING INTERVENTIONS**
    a. Consume a diet low in sodium.
   b. Adhere to digoxin and diuretic therapy.
   c. Use prophylactic antibiotic therapy to prevent endocarditis.
4. Surgical management
   a. Heart valve replacement (can actually hear the click)
   b. Mitral commissurotomy (valvulotomy)
    1) **NURSING INTERVENTIONS**
      a) Provide routine postoperative care.
      b) See postoperative care for client after cardiac surgery.
   2) **NURSING INTERVENTIONS** (rehabilitation)
      a) Allow activities as tolerated.
      b) Implement cardiac diet: low-sodium, low-cholesterol.
      c) Administer medications (anticoagulant therapy) for lifetime.
      d) Instruct client in lifelong need for antibiotics prior to any invasive procedures and dental work.

E. Aortic Aneurysm
1. Definition: local distention of the artery wall, usually thoracic or abdominal (four times more common)
2. Watched until it gets above 5 cm, then rate of rupture increases, so surgery is required
3. Cause
   a. Infections (mycotic)
   b. Congenital
   c. Atherosclerosis or hypertension
4. Manifestations (frequently asymptomatic)
   a. Thoracic: pain, dyspnea, hoarseness, cough, dysphagia
   b. Abdominal: abdominal pain, persistent or intermittent low back or flank pain; may be asymptomatic; pulsating abdominal mass; shock
5. Treatment: usually surgery
   a. Preoperative: careful monitoring because of a possible rupture; prepare for abdominal surgery
   b. Postoperative: same as abdominal surgery, careful monitoring of peripheral circulation below level of aneurysms
   c. Postoperative complications
      1) Myocardial infarction
      2) Emboli
      3) Renal failure
      4) Spinal cord ischemia

F. Hypertension

1. Definition: persistent blood pressure above 140/ systolic and 90/diastolic; called "silent killer"
   a. Primary hypertension
      1) 90% have this kind
      2) Hereditary disease
      3) More common among African Americans
      4) Cause unknown
      5) Late manifestations: headaches, fatigue, dyspnea, edema, nocturia, blackouts
      6) Usually no signs or symptoms are displayed until end-organ involvement occurs
   b. Secondary hypertension
      1) Due to identifiable problem
      2) Pheochromocytoma
      3) Renal pathology
    c. **NURSING INTERVENTIONS**
      1) Counsel client on weight control methods.
      2) Teach client to stop smoking.
      3) Educate client to avoid stimulants (decrease alcohol and caffeine intake); moderate amount of alcohol is actually good: less than 1 oz of alcohol OR 24 oz of beer a day.
      4) Promote a program of regular physical exercise.
      5) Promote lifestyle with reduced stress.
      6) Maintain salt-restricted diet.
      7) Teach risk factors.
2. Antihypertensive medications
   a. Potassium-depleting diuretics
      1) Loop diuretic-furosemide (Lasix), bumetanide (Bumex)
      2) Thiazide-hydrochlorothiazide (HCTZ), chlorothiazide (Diuril)
    4) **NURSING INTERVENTIONS**
      a) Administer potassium supplements as prescribed.
      b) Teach dietary sources of potassium.
      c) Be aware of possible interaction of low potassium and digitalis (*Digoxin*) preparations.
   b. Potassium-sparing diuretics
      1) Spironolactone (*Aldactone*)
      2) Triamterene (*Dyrenium*)
      3) Watch for increased potassium level.
   c. Beta blockers
      1) Propranolol HCl (*Inderal*)
      2) Atenolol (*Tenormin*)
      3) Metoprolol (*Lopressor*)
    4) **NURSING INTERVENTIONS**
      a) Watch for major side effect of bradycardia.
      b) Monitor daily pulse.
      c) Monitor for manifestations of heart failure.

      d) Noncardioselective beta blockers may be contraindicated in asthmatics.
      e) Watch for reflex tachycardia due to decreased cardiac output and hypotension.
   d. Central-acting alpha blockers (sympatholytics)
      1) Clonidine HCL (*Catapres*)
         a) Constipation
         b) Sexual dysfunction
         c) Dry mouth
         d) Depression
      2) Guanfacine HCL (*Tenex*)
         a) Rebound hypertension
         b) Drowsiness
         c) Bradycardia
      3) Methyldopa (*Aldomet*)
         a) Aplastic anemia
         b) Thrombocytopenia
   e. Angiotensin-converting enzyme (ACE inhibitors)
      1) Captopril (*Capoten*)
      2) Enalapril (*Vasotec*)
      3) Lisinopril (*Zestril*)
      4) Major side effects
         a) Cough
         b) Headache
         c) Angioedema of face and limbs
   f. Calcium-channel blockers
      1) Nifedipine (Procardia)
         a) Headache/dizziness
         b) Bradycardia
         c) Peripheral edema
      2) Verapamil (Calan), diltiazem (Cardizem)
         a) Flushing
         b) Arrhythmias
         c) Constipation

G. Thrombophlebitis

1. Definition: clot in the vein with inflammation of the wall
2. Precipitating factors
   a. Stasis
   b. Hypercoagulability
   c. Damage to intima of blood vessels/trauma
   d. Pregnancy or estrogen (oral contraceptives)
   e. Malignancy or obesity
3. Manifestations
   a. Edema of affected limb
   b. Local swelling, bumpy, knotty
   c. Red, tender, local induration
 4. **NURSING INTERVENTIONS**
   a. Maintain bed rest.
   b. Elevate leg and apply moist warm compresses.
   c. Administer anticoagulant therapy.
   d. Initiate antiembolism stockings/support hose.

e. Administer pain medication.
f. Increase fluids.
g. Encourage deep breathing.
h. Assist client with range of motion.
i. Teach client
   1) Avoid eating an excessive amount of green leafy vegetables while on warfarin (*Coumadin*).
   2) Provide care to area of phlebitis.
   3) Watch for bleeding.

H. Varicose Veins
1. Precipitating factors
   a. Prolonged standing
   b. Pregnancy
   c. Obesity
   d. Heredity
2. Manifestations (accentuated by gravity)
   a. Enlarged, tortuous veins in lower extremities
   b. Pain
   c. Edema (after upright)
 3. **NURSING INTERVENTIONS** (teaching)
   a. Avoid prolonged sitting or standing.
   b. Wear supportive antiembolism stockings, especially during flights and pregnancy.
   c. Avoid crossing legs.
   d. Engage in daily exercise.
   e. Maintain ideal body weight.
   f. Elevate lower extremities to reduce edema.
   g. Provide postoperative care to promote circulation: thigh-high antiembolism stockings, ambulation, and elevation.
      1) Monitor circulation (elastic stockings to entire leg postoperative only).
      2) Elevate feet.
      3) Stand, lie down.
4. Ulcers
   a. Arterial: looks punched-out; no edema present
   b. Venous: around ankle usually, reddened and bluish, edema present many times

I. Arterial Disorders of the Peripheral Vascular System
1. Intermittent claudication
   a. Definition: Pain/cramping in lower extremities due to atherosclerosis of lower extremity arteries (popliteal); muscles do not receive adequate blood supply
   b. Manifestations
2. Classic manifestations
   a. Pain with walking
   b. Calf muscle atrophy
   c. Skin appears shiny with hair loss; thickened toenails
   d. Poor neurovascular integrity
   e. Necrotic ulcers
   f. Tingling and numbness of toes
   g. Cool extremities

h. Difficulty assessing pulses; grade pulses to assess changes
i. Surgical interventions
   1) Femoral popliteal bypass surgery
   2) Angioplasty
   3) Stenting
3. Client teaching
   a. Stop smoking.
   b. Consume a low-fat diet.
   c. Take pentoxifylline (*Trental*) and cilostazol (*Pletal*).
   d. Avoid crossing legs.
4. Arteriosclerosis obliterans: usually affects aorta or the arteries of the lower extremities
   a. Risk Factors
      1) Diabetes mellitus
      2) Hypertension
      3) Coronary artery disease
      4) Cerebrovascular disease
      5) Renal failure
      6) Smoking
   b. Surgical management
      1) Vascular grafts
      2) Patch grafts
      3) Endarterectomy
 c. **NURSING INTERVENTIONS**
      1) Frequently check extremities for pulses, color and temperature.
      2) Observe for paralysis of lower extremities after operation upon thoracic aorta.
      3) Ensure adequate circulating blood volume through arterial repair: I&O; central venous pressure.
      4) Teach client: avoid dependent positions, elevate extremities, use of support hose/antiembolism stockings.
      5) Administer heparin.
5. Buerger's disease (thromboangiitis obliterans)
   a. Definition: recurring inflammation of the arteries and veins of lower and upper extremities resulting in thrombus and occlusion (cause unknown)
   b. Characteristics
      1) Occurs in men ages 20 to 40 years
      2) Most common manifestations: pain in legs relieved by inactivity, numbness and tingling of toes and fingers in cold weather/intermittent claudication
      3) Cessation of smoking important; client teaching is same as arteriosclerosis
      4) Ulcerations and gangrene with amputation are common

6. Raynaud's syndrome
   a. Definition: vasospastic or obstructive condition of arteries that occurs with exposure to cold or stress and primarily affects the hands
   b. Characteristics
      1) Arteriolar vasoconstriction results in coldness, pallor, and pain
      2) Occasional ulceration of the fingertips
      3) Color changes from white to blue to red (can be bilateral or symmetrical)

   c. **NURSING INTERVENTIONS**
      1) Teach client to avoid cold (keep extremities warm); gloves.
      2) Educate client to stop smoking; limit caffeine.
      3) Administer nifedipine (*Procardia*); medication of choice.
      4) Arrange for sympathectomy.

Cardiac Surgery

A. Pacemaker
1. Definition: electronic device that provides repetitive electrical stimuli to the heart muscle to control heart rate
2. Types
   a. Permanent pacemakers
      1) Ventricular demand: fires at preset rate when client's heart rate drops below a predetermined/preprogrammed rate
      2) Ventricular fixed: fires constantly at preset/preprogrammed rate, regardless of the client's own heart rate
      3) Dual chamber: stimulates both the atria and the ventricles
      4) Atrial demand: fires as needed when the atria do not originate a rhythm
      5) Variable rate: senses oxygen demands and increases firing rate to meet the client's needs
   b. Temporary pacemakers
      1) Transcutaneous (skin); external, for use in emergency pacing situations
      2) Transvenous

3. **NURSING INTERVENTIONS**
   a. Teach client preoperatively.
   b. Postoperative care
      1) Monitor ECG and pulse rate.
      2) Check wound for hematoma, infection.
      3) Administer analgesics as necessary.
      4) Maintain electrically safe environment; client will need to avoid large generators, magnets, magnetic resonance imaging machines.
      5) Observe for hiccoughs; indicates pacemaker is malpositioned and is pacing the diaphragm.

      6) Maintain sterile technique at insertion site for wound care
   c. Monitor for complications after pacemaker insertion.
      1) Observe for local infection (will have to remove pacemaker).
      2) Monitor for hematoma.
      3) Monitor for dysrhythmia.
      4) Prevent accidental dislodging of the electrode; client must be careful using arm on the affected side until site is completely healed; no raising the arm high over the head.
      5) Observe for signs of pacemaker malfunction (failure to capture, sense, or pace).
   d. Teach client
      1) Carry ID information at all times.
      2) Batteries will need to be changed at intervals (3 to 15 years for lithium batteries).
      3) Instruct on how to transmit data via telephone from pacemaker to provider.
      4) Wear loose-fitting clothes.
      5) Avoid contact sports.
      6) Lower limit: All permanent pacemakers are set at a definitive lowest rate whereby the pacemaker will fire and stimulate the heart if the pulse rate drops below this predetermined/preprogrammed rate. The nurse must know this rate to assess and teach the client. If the pulse ever drops below this rate, it must be reported.

B. Percutaneous Transthoracic Cardiac Angioplasty
1. Definition: variety of procedures used to treat clients with plaque in the arteries of the heart; most commonly, a balloon is passed into the diseased vessel and is then inflated, compressing the plaque and dilating the narrowed coronary artery so that blood can flow more easily
   a. Done through a left cardiac catheterization
   b. A stent is often placed into the vessel to hold it open

   c. **NURSING INTERVENTIONS**
      1) Follow procedure that is the same as postangioplasty care.
      2) Monitor for complications: vasospasm, dysrhythmia, or rupture of coronary vessel leading to a myocardial infarction.

C. Coronary Artery Bypass Graft
1. Done to replace damaged coronary arteries and re-establish perfusion in areas of myocardium
2. Most procedures in use require open chest/heart approach with bypass machine, however, latest techniques may not use bypass; resulting in shorter recovery for some clients

a. Preoperative care; general care
b. Psychological support: may need to be done on an emergency basis
c. Postoperative care
   1) Chest tubes
   2) General postoperative care including pain management and care of wound
   3) Will have endotracheal tube for a day postoperative; prepare client about and provide sterile technique when caring for tube and suctioning
   4) Assess all systems since they all can be affected by decreased cardiac output; (e.g., vital signs, urine output, circulation in legs, chest pain).
   5) Assess for complications: myocardial infarction, pleural effusion, dysrhythmia.

Shock

A. **Definition:** lack of oxygen and nutrients at the cellular level (due to impaired tissue perfusion) for cellular metabolism, regardless of the etiology

B. **Types**
1. Cardiogenic: failure of the heart to pump adequately
2. Hypovolemic: decreased blood volume
3. Distributive (vasogenic)
   a. Neurogenic: increased size of vascular bed due to loss of vascular tone
   b. Anaphylactic: hypersensitivity reaction
   c. Septic: systemic reaction vasodilation due to infection

C. **General Manifestations** (related to decreased tissue perfusion)
1. Tachycardia
2. Tachypnea
3. Oliguria
4. Cold, moist skin
5. Color ashen: pallor
6. Hypotension
7. Metabolic acidosis
8. Decreased level of consciousness
9. Septic shock: initially warm, flushed skin, fever

D. **NURSING INTERVENTIONS**

1. Position client in a modified Trendelenburg.
2. Secure a large bore IV line (16 or 18 g).
3. Administer oxygen.
   a. Record vital signs every 5 min.
   b. Promote rest; decrease movement.
   c. Monitor urine output.
4. Treat underlying cause.

E. **Emergency Medications**
1. Atropine: increases heart rate
2. Dopamine (*Intropin*): vasoconstrictor; increases blood pressure and tissue and renal perfusion
3. Epinephrine HCl (*Adrenalin*): increases body reaction to stress
4. Isoproterenol (*Isuprel*): increases heart rate and cardiac output
5. Dobutamine (*Dobutrex*): inotropic; increases force of myocardial contraction in cardiogenic shock
6. Norepinephrine levarterenol (*Levophed*): vasoconstrictor; increases tissue perfusion
7. Sodium bicarbonate: decreases acidosis

Cardiopulmonary Resuscitation (CPR)

A. **Indications**
1. Absence of palpable carotid pulse
2. Absence of breath sounds

B. **Purpose**
1. Establish effective circulation and respiration
2. Prevent irreversible cerebral anoxic damage

C. **Procedure**
1. Determine unresponsiveness, make sure scene is safe.
2. Activate Emergency Response System and get an Automated External Defibrillator (AED).
3. Open airway (head tilt/chin lift), check breathing.
4. Give two breaths.
5. Check pulse (carotid artery pulse).
6. Follow American Heart Association 2006 recommendations:
   a. Ratio of 30 compressions to 2 ventilations for one or two rescuers
   b. Compression rate of 100/min for all age groups

D. **Complications**
1. Fractured ribs
2. Punctured lungs
3. Lacerated liver
4. Abdominal distension

E. **Stop CPR When:**
1. Provider pronounces client dead
2. Exhausted
3. Help arrives
4. Heartbeat returns

F. **Automated External Defibrillator (AED)**
1. Computerized defibrillator analyzes cardiac rhythm once pads are placed on client's chest
2. Mechanical voice tells rescuer if/when to deliver shock to client

3. Do not have to be a professional rescuer, but must be trained in use of machine
4. Do not use AED on children ages 1 to 12 months.

G. Obstructed Airway
1. Conscious
   a. Establish that victim is choking.
   b. Perform Heimlich maneuver until successful or client becomes unconscious.
2. Unconscious
   a. If a conscious choking victim becomes unresponsive, look for foreign object in pharynx and remove it if you see it. Do not blind finger sweep.
   b. Begin CPR. Every time you open the airway to give breaths, open the victim's mouth wide and look for the object. Remove it only if you see it.
   c. If you do not see the object, continue CPR.
   d. If you encounter a victim who is choking that you do not know has an airway obstruction, activate the emergency medical service system and start CPR.

SECTION IX

REVIEW OF GENITOURINARY SYSTEM DISORDERS

Assessment of the Client

A. Functions of the Kidney
1. Regulates acid-base balance
2. Excretes metabolic wastes (creatinine, urea)
3. Regulates blood pressure: renin (stimulated by decreased blood pressure or blood volume) stimulates production of angiotensin I, which is converted to angiotensin II in the lungs; angiotensin II is a strong vasoconstrictor and also stimulates aldosterone secretion; vasoconstriction and sodium reabsorption result in increased blood volume and increased blood pressure
4. Secretes erythropoietin
5. Converts vitamin D to its active form for absorption of calcium
6. Excretes water-soluble medications and medication metabolites

B. History
1. Has there been renal disease in the past?
2. Is there a family history of renal disease?
3. Age: developmental issues; incontinence and prostatic problems
4. Gender: incontinence increased in women; benign prostate hypertrophy: older men

C. Manifestations
1. Pain (usually in acute conditions): flank radiating to upper thigh, testis, or labium
2. Changes in voiding: hematuria, proteinuria, dysuria, frequency, urgency, burning, nocturia, incontinence, polyuria, oliguria, anuria
3. Thirst, fatigue, edema (generalized)

Diagnostic Tests
KEY INFORMATION
A. Urinalysis
1. Specific gravity: range tested 1.010 to 1.025
2. Color: yellow/amber
3. Negative glucose, protein, RBCs, and WBCs
4. pH: 5 to 8
5. First voided morning sample preferred; 15 mL
6. Send to laboratory immediately or refrigerate.
7. If clean catch, get urine for culture prior to starting antibiotics.
   a. Cleanse labia, glans penis
   b. Obtain midstream sample

B. Renal Function Tests (several tests over a period of time are necessary)
1. BUN: 7 to 20 mg/dL
2. Creatinine: 0.5 to 1.0 mg/dL
3. 24-hour creatinine clearance: 75 to 120 mL/min
   a. Have client void and discard specimen.
   b. Draw at the start serum creatinine.
   c. Collect urine for the next 24 hr (refrigerate).
   d. Have client void at the completion of the 24 hr.
4. Uric acid (serum): 3.5 to 7.8 mg/dL
5. Prostate-specific antigen: greater than 10 increases risk of prostate cancer

C. Radiologic Test
1. Kidneys, ureters, bladder (x-ray): shows size, shape and position of kidneys, ureters, and bladder; no preparation necessary (except to ensure that client is not pregnant)
2. IV pyelography (IVP): visualizes urinary tract

   a. **NURSING INTERVENTIONS**
      1) Ensure that informed consent has been obtained.
      2) Assess client's creatinine level.
      3) Discontinue food for 8 hr before test, fluids permitted.
      4) Administer laxatives (as prescribed) to clear bowel.
      5) Give enema or suppository on morning of test (as necessary).
      6) Check for allergies to iodine or shellfish.

7) Provide client information: may experience flushing, warmth, nausea, metallic or salty taste, sensation of urinary incontinence.

8) Have emergency equipment available during procedure.

9) Encourage fluids after procedure to flush out dye.

3. Renal angiography: visualization of renal arterial supply; contrast material injected through a catheter

 a. **NURSING INTERVENTIONS:** same as IVP plus

1) Femoral or brachial artery approach.
2) Locate and mark peripheral pulses.
3) Have client void before procedure.
4) Teach client: procedure takes ½ to 2 hr; client will feel heat along vessel.

 b. **NURSING INTERVENTIONS** (after procedure)

1) Maintain bed rest for 6 to 8 hr.
2) Monitor vital signs until stable.
3) Observe for swelling and hematoma.
4) Palpate peripheral pulses/vascular checks.
5) Monitor urinary output.

D. Cystoscopy

1. Diagnostic uses: inspect bladder and urethra; insert catheters into ureters; see configuration and position of urethral orifices

2. Treatment uses: remove calculi from urethra, bladder and ureter; treat lesions of bladder, urethra, prostate

 3. **NURSING INTERVENTIONS** (general preoperative care)

a. Maintain NPO if general anesthesia; liquids if local anesthesia.
b. Administer preoperative cathartics/enemas.
c. Teach client deep breathing exercises to relieve bladder spasms.
d. Monitor for postural hypotension.
e. Inform client that pink-tinged or tea-colored urine is common following the procedure; bright, red urine or clots should be reported to provider.
f. Inform client that postprocedural pain may be present.
   1) Leg cramps due to lithotomy position
   2) Back pain and/or abdominal pain
   3) Warm sitz baths comforting
g. Push fluids/analgesics.
h. Monitor I&O; make sure no obstruction.

E. Renal Biopsy

 1. **NURSING INTERVENTIONS** (prebiopsy)

a. Obtain bleeding, clotting, and prothrombin times.

b. Obtain results of prebiopsy x-rays of kidney, IVP.
c. Inform pregnant client that ultrasound may be used.
d. Keep client NPO for 6 to 8 hr.
e. Position client prone with pillow under abdomen, shoulders on bed.

 2. **NURSING INTERVENTIONS** (postbiopsy)

a. Keep client supine, on bed rest for 24 hr.
b. Monitor vital signs every 5 to 15 min for 4 hr, then decrease if stable.
c. Maintain pressure to puncture site 20 min.
d. Observe for pain, nausea, vomiting, blood pressure changes.
e. Encourage fluid intake.
f. Assess Hct and Hgb 8 hr after procedure.
g. Monitor urine output.
h. Educate client to avoid strenuous activity, sports, and heavy lifting for at least 2 weeks.

F. Catheterization

1. Purpose: to empty contents of bladder, obtain a sterile specimen, determine residual urine, allow irrigation of bladder, bypass an obstruction; procedure is sterile

2. **NURSING INTERVENTIONS**

 a. Maintain closed system.
b. Measure output each shift.
c. Keep drainage bag below bladder.
d. Have client increase fluid intake.
e. Ensure that there are no dependent loops.
f. Discontinue as soon as possible due to increased risk for urinary tract infection.

Specific Disorders and Nursing Interventions

A. Cystitis

1. Definition: inflammation of the urinary bladder
2. Etiology: ascending infection after entry via the urinary meatus; acute infections usually *Escherichia coli*
   a. More common in females
   b. Benign prostate hypertrophy in men
3. Manifestations
   a. Frequency and urgency
   b. Dysuria
   c. Suprapubic tenderness; pain in region of bladder or flank pain
   d. Hematuria
   e. Fever/malaise/chills
   f. Cloudy, foul-smelling urine

 4. **NURSING INTERVENTIONS**

a. Obtain urine for culture and sensitivity (before initiating antibiotic therapy).

b. Give antimicrobial medications - sulfonamides are the medications of choice unless allergic; (e.g., cotrimoxazole, sulfamethoxazole-trimethoprim [*Bactrim*] and nitrofurantoin microcrystal [*Macrodantin*])

c. Maintain acidic urine pH.

d. Force fluids (greater than 3,000 mL per day).

e. Give urinary analgesics: phenazopyridine (*Pyridium*).

f. Apply heat to perineum for comfort.

g. Teach client
   1) Practice good perineal care.
   2) Wear cotton underwear.
   3) Avoid bubble baths (can be irritating to urethra).
   4) Maintain a high fluid intake.
   5) Encourage client to void after sexual intercourse.
   6) Encourage client to drink cranberry juice, which may be helpful for some clients.

B. Glomerulonephritis

1. Definition: type of acute renal failure that results from inflammatory disease involving the renal glomeruli of both kidneys; thought to be an antigen-antibody reaction that damages the glomeruli of the kidney (usually in children); good prognosis if treated

2. Etiology: group A beta-hemolytic streptococcal infection; usually client reports a history of sore throat, pharyngitis, or tonsillitis 2 to 3 weeks prior to renal manifestations

3. Manifestations
   a. Hematuria (cola or tea-colored urine), proteinuria, chills, weakness, pallor, nausea, vomiting
   b. Edema (especially facial and periorbital; ascites)
   c. Oliguria or anuria
   d. Hypertension
   e. Headache
   f. Increased BUN; elevated BUN is azotemia
   g. Flank pain/abdominal pain
   h. Anemia

 4. **NURSING INTERVENTIONS**
   a. Protect kidney. Recognize and treat infection.
   b. Maintain bed rest.
   c. Administer penicillin for streptococcal infection (substitute other antibiotics for clients with penicillin allergy).
   d. Administer corticosteroids for inflammatory disease.
   e. Treat other manifestations symptomatically (e.g., antihypertensives for increased blood pressure).

f. Reduce dietary protein and sodium; increase calories.

g. Restrict fluids.

C. Nephrosis

1. Definition: clinical disorder associated with protein-wasting; secondary to diffuse glomerular damage

2. Etiology: likely to have an autoimmune etiology; the glomerular membrane becomes more permeable to protein

3. Manifestations
   a. Insidious onset of pitting edema (generalized edema is anasarca)
   b. Proteinuria
   c. Anemia
   d. Hypoalbuminemia
   e. Anorexia and malaise
   f. Nausea
   g. Oliguria
   h. Ascites

 4. **NURSING INTERVENTIONS**
   a. Preserve renal function.
   b. Maintain bed rest (during severe edema only).
   c. Maintain low-sodium, low-potassium, moderate-protein, high-calorie diet.
   d. Protect client from infection.
   e. Monitor I&O.
   f. Weigh client daily.
   g. Measure abdominal girth.

5. Medication therapy
   a. Loop diuretics: furosemide (*Lasix*)
   b. Steroids: prednisone (*Deltasone*)
   c. Immunosuppressive agents: cyclophosphamide (*Cytoxan*)

D. Urolithiasis (Urinary calculi)

1. Definition: stones in the urinary system

2. Etiology
   a. Obstruction and urinary stasis
   b. Uric acid stones (excessive purine intake)
   c. Dehydration
   d. Immobilization
   e. More common in men ages 20 to 40
   f. Tend to recur
   g. Most stones are calcium phosphate or oxalate, also struvite, cystine

3. Manifestations (based on location, size of stone)
   a. Pain: severe renal colic (ureter); dull, aching (kidney); radiates to the groin
   b. Nausea, vomiting, diarrhea, or constipation
   c. Hematuria
   d. Manifestations of urinary tract infection

 4. **NURSING INTERVENTIONS**
   a. Goals: to eradicate the stone, determine stone type and prevent nephron destruction.

b. Force fluids: at least 3,000 mL per day (IV or by mouth).
c. Strain all urine.
d. Provide pain control.
e. Maintain proper urine pH (depends on stone type).
f. Avoid foods high in oxalates if calcium oxalate stone (spinach, black tea, rhubarb, chocolate).
g. Administer allopurinol (*Zyloprim*) for uric acid stones.
h. Lithotripsy (crush stone through sound waves)
   1) Conscious sedation used for procedure
   2) May have bruised flank postprocedure
   3) Prophylactic antibiotic postprocedure
   4) Increase fluids to at least 3,000 mL per day
   5) Strain all urine postproduction

E. Acute Renal Failure (ARF)
1. Definition: abrupt reversible cessation of renal function; may be result of trauma, allergic reactions, kidney stones, shock
2. Etiology: obstructed blood flow to renal tissue; three types of conditions occur due to which part of the kidney is involved
  a. Prerenal: disrupted blood flow enroute to kidneys.; hypovolemic shock, dehydration, heart failure, burn injury, and anaphylaxis
  b. Renal: renal tissue damage; trauma, hypokalemia, acute glomerulonephritis, hemolytic uremic syndrome (infection caused by *Escherichia coli*; common in children), substance abuse
  c. Postrenal: renal filtration of urine compromised; kidney stones, prostate hypertrophy, tumors, and strictures
3. Manifestations: three phases
  a. Oliguric phase (8 to 15 days): sudden onset, less than 400 mL in 24 hr, edema, elevated BUN, creatinine and potassium; decreased specific gravity; acidosis; heart failure; dysrhythmias
  b. Diuretic phase: urine output slowly rises followed by diuresis of up to 4,000 to 5,000 mL per day, indicating recovery of damaged nephrons; hypotension and fluid and electrolyte imbalances are a concern
  c. Recovery phase: may take up to a year until urine function returns to normal (baseline); older adults at increased risk for residual impairment

4. **NURSING INTERVENTIONS**
  a. Treat, eliminate, or prevent cause.
  b. Correct metabolic acidosis, hyperkalemia, Hyperphosphatemia, hypocalcemia.
    1) Kayexalate (an ion exchange resin given orally or by enema).
    2) IV glucose and insulin or calcium carbonate (causes potassium to enter cells).
    3) Calcium IV or sodium bicarbonate to stabilize cell membrane.
  c. Implement diet.
    1) Oliguric phase: low-protein, high-carbohydrate, restrict potassium intake.
    2) Diuresis phase: low-protein, high-calorie, restrict fluids as indicated.
  d. Administer phosphate binders to lower phosphorus while replacing calcium (Phos-Lo, Calcium acetate).
  e. Remain on bed rest in oliguric phase.
  f. Weigh client daily.
  g. Monitor I&O; replacement is usually based on previous output.
  h. Implement and maintain dialysis (as ordered) until renal function returns.
  i. Assess for pericarditis; friction rub.

F. Chronic Renal Failure
1. Definition: a slower or progressive failure of the kidneys to function that results in death unless hemodialysis or transplant is performed; irreversible
2. Etiology
  a. Diabetes mellitus (first leading cause)
  b. Uncontrolled hypertension (second leading cause)
  c. Chronic glomerulonephritis
  d. Pyelonephritis
  e. Congenital kidney disease
  f. Renal vascular disease
3. Stages of renal failure
  a. Diminished renal reserve (creatinine 1.6 to 2.0)
  b. Renal insufficiency (creatinine 2.1 to 5.0)
  c. Renal failure (creatinine > 8.0)
  d. Uremia: end stage (creatinine > 12.0)
4. Manifestations (progressively worsen)
  a. Fatigue
  b. Headache
  c. Nausea, vomiting, diarrhea
  d. Hypertension
  e. Irritability
  f. Convulsions/coma
  g. Anemia
  h. Edema
  i. Hypocalcemia/hyperkalemia
  j. Pruritus, uremic frost
  k. Pallid, gray-yellow complexion
  l. Metabolic acidosis; elevated BUN and creatinine; decreased glomerular filtration rate

5. **NURSING INTERVENTIONS**

   a. Goal: help the kidneys maintain homeostasis.
   b. Maintain bed rest.
   c. Implement renal diet: low-protein, low-potassium, high-carbohydrate, vitamin and calcium supplements, low-sodium, low-phosphate.
   d. Treat hypertension.
   e. Maintain strict I&O; fluid replacement: 500 to 600 mL more than 24-hr urine output.
   f. Monitor electrolytes, especially potassium.
   g. Administer phosphate binders.
   h. Contraindicated to administer antacids with magnesium or enemas with phosphorous
   i. Maintain dialysis.
   j. Administer diuretics in early stages.
   k. Provide skin care (collects kidney wastes).
   l. Provide emotional support to client and family.
   m. Assess for and prevent bleeding tendencies.
   n. Evaluate need for kayexalate orally to keep potassium levels down.
   o. Care for anemia: administer epoetin alfa/erythropoietin (*Epogen, Procrit*) to stimulate RBC formation; transfuse as necessary.

G. Dialysis
1. Goals
   a. Remove end products of metabolism (urea and creatinine) from the blood.
   b. Maintain a safe concentration of the serum electrolytes.
   c. Correct of acidosis and restore blood buffer system.
   d. Remove excess fluid from the blood.
2. Hemodialysis
   a. Definition: process of cleansing the blood of accumulated waste products; used for end-stage renal failure and those clients who are acutely ill and require short-term treatment; uses diffusion, osmosis, and filtration

   b. **NURSING INTERVENTIONS**
      1) Weigh client before and after procedure.
      2) Monitor client continuously during procedure; blood pressure may "bottom out".
      3) Provide care to access site to prevent clotting and infection.
      4) Assess bruit and thrill to determine patency of shunt.
      5) Provide adequate nutrition.
      6) Monitor for hypotension.
      7) Maintain fluid restrictions.
      8) Withhold regular morning medications prior to dialysis.
      9) Observe for psychological and physiological complications.

3. Peritoneal dialysis
   a. Definition: substitute for kidney function during failure that uses the peritoneum as a dialyzing membrane; usually short term; peritoneal catheter inserted by provider
   b. **NURSING INTERVENTIONS**
      1) Have client void (if applicable) prior to procedure.
      2) Weigh client daily.
      3) Monitor vital signs, baseline electrolytes.
      4) Maintain asepsis.
      5) Keep accurate record of fluid balance.
      6) Procedure
         a) Warm dialysate (1 to 2 L of 1.5, 2.5, or 4.25% glucose solution)
         b) Allow to flow in by gravity
         c) 5 to 10 min inflow time; close clamp immediately
         d) 30 min of equilibration (dwell time)
         e) 10 to 30 min of drainage (clear yellow)
      7) Continue treatment for 2 full days.
      8) Monitor for complications: peritonitis, bleeding, respiratory difficulty, abdominal pain; bowel, or bladder perforation.
4. Continuous Ambulatory Peritoneal Dialysis (CAPD)
   a. Definition: dialyzing method involving almost continuous peritoneal contact with a dialysis solution for clients with end-stage renal disease
   b. Procedure (slightly different from acute peritoneal dialysis)
      1) Permanent indwelling catheter inserted into peritoneum
      2) Fluid infused by gravity (1.5 to 3 L)
      3) Dwell time: 4 to 10 hr
      4) Dialysate drains by gravity: 20 to 40 min
      5) Four to five exchanges daily, 7 days a week (some clients may elect to do at night with automatic cycling machines; 10 to 14 hr, three times per week)
   c. Complications
      1) Peritonitis (rebound tenderness, fever, cloudy outflow)
      2) Bladder perforation (yellow outflow)
      3) Hypotension
      4) Bowel perforation (brown outflow)
   d. Advantages
      1) More independence
      2) Free dietary intake; better nutrition
      3) Satisfactory control of uremia
      4) Least expensive dialysis
      5) Decreased likelihood of transplant rejection
      6) More closely approximates normal renal function

H. Urinary Tract Surgery

1. Kidney Transplantation
   a. Indicated for individual with irreversible end-stage renal disease
   b. Requires well-matched donor: screened for ABO blood group, tissue-specific antigens, human leukocyte antigen suitability, and histocompatibility
      1) Living donors: most desirable are donors who match client closely
      2) Cadaver donors
   c. Preoperative management
      1) Regain normal metabolic state
      2) Tissue typing
      3) Immunosuppressive therapy
      4) Hemodialysis within 24 hr
      5) Teaching and emotional support
    d. **NURSING INTERVENTIONS** (postoperative management)
      1) Maintain homeostasis until kidney is functioning.
      2) Administer immunosuppressive medications: azathioprine (*Imuran*), cyclosporine (*Sandimmune*), steroids.
      3) Monitor for rejection: oliguria, edema, fever, tenderness over graft site, fluid and electrolyte imbalance, hypertension, elevated BUN, creatinine, elevated WBC.
      4) Monitor for infection.
      5) Maintain protective isolation.
      6) Provide emotional support; monitor for depression.

2. Urinary diversion: remove bladder and transplant ureters into a pouch under the abdominal skin; can be either continent or incontinent; care is of a stoma plus general interventions
    a. **NURSING INTERVENTIONS**
      1) Monitor vital signs (hemorrhage and shock are frequent complications).
      2) Provide pain control.
      3) Be alert for manifestations of paralytic ileus (very common).
      4) Provide adequate fluid replacement.
      5) Weigh client daily.
      6) Maintain function and patency of drainage tubes.
         a) Indwelling urinary catheter (dependent position, tape tubing to thigh)
         b) Nephrostomy tube
            (1) Never clamp
            (2) Irrigate only with order of 10 mL NS
            (3) Assess for leakage of urine
         c) Ureteral catheters
            (1) Each one drains ½ of the urinary system, so expect only ½ of the urinary output from each one
            (2) Bloody drainage expected after surgery, but should clear
            (3) Never irrigate
            (4) Surgical implant; make sure secure
            (5) Aseptic technique required

I. Benign Prostatic Hyperplasia (BPH)

1. Definition: enlargement of the prostate
2. Etiology: unknown, usually accompanies aging process in the male
3. Manifestations
   a. Difficulty starting stream/dribbling
   b. Decrease in force of urinary stream
   c. Urinary tract infection
   d. Nocturia
   e. Hematuria
4. Diagnosis
   a. Digital rectal exam
   b. Prostate-specific antigen for diagnosis
   c. Cystoscopy
5. Treatments
   a. Urinary antibiotics
   b. Alpha-blocker medications to promote urinary flow: terazosin (*Hytrin*), tamsulosin (*Flomax*), alfuzosin (*Uroxatral*), doxazosin (*Cardura*)
   c. Enzyme inhibitors to shrink prostate gland: dutasteride (*Avodart*), finasteride (*Proscar*)
   d. Transurethral resection of prostate surgery (TURP)
    1) **NURSING INTERVENTIONS** (Preoperative)
      a) Insert indwelling urinary catheter.
      b) Give antibiotics as prescribed.
    2) **NURSING INTERVENTIONS** (Postoperative)
      a) Observe for shock and hemorrhage.
      b) Teach client to avoid heavy lifting, prolonged sitting, constipation or straining with defecation; may cause a rebleed.
      c) Monitor continuous bladder irrigation (expect bloody drainage; monitor I&O carefully to ensure proper functioning.
      d) Encourage fluid intake (at least 3,000 mL per day).
      e) Assess for TURP syndrome: cluster of manifestations secondary to neurologic, cardiovascular, and electrolyte imbalance resulting from absorption of irrigating fluids through prostate tissue during surgery (hyponatremia, confusion,

bradycardia, hypo/hypertension, N/V, visual changes).

    f) Medicate for pain control: may need medication to decrease bladder spasms as well as narcotics.

    g) Maintain catheter taped tightly to leg (for hemostasis at surgical site by catheter balloon).

    h) Address sexual concerns.

      (1) May have temporary loss of sexual function or urinary control

      (2) Kegel exercises

      (3) If erectile dysfunction occurs, it may require medication for sexual relations

J. Prostate Cancer

1. Definition: slow growing cancer of the prostate gland

2. Risk factors
   a. Men after age 50
   b. African American
   c. Family history
   d. Elevated testosterone levels
   e. High-fat diet

3. Manifestations
   a. Asymptomatic in early stages
   b. Hematuria
   c. Prostate-specific antigen greater than 10
   d. Rectal exam: hard, pea-sized nodule

4. Treatment
   a. Radical prostatectomy
   b. External radiation therapy
   c. Internal radioactive seeds
   d. Hormone therapy

 5. **NURSING INTERVENTIONS**
   a. Preoperative
      1) Insert indwelling urinary catheter.
      2) Administer antibiotics as prescribed.
   b. Postoperative
      1) Observe for shock and hemorrhage.
      2) Teach client to avoid heavy lifting, prolonged sitting, constipation or straining with defecation; may cause a rebleed.
      3) Monitor continuous bladder irrigation; expect bloody drainage; monitor I&O carefully to ensure proper functioning.
      4) Encourage fluid intake (at least 3,000 mL per day).
      5) Assess for TURP syndrome (altered mental status, bradycardia, tachycardia and confusion) due to absorption of bladder irrigant through tissue planes of the wound.
      6) Medicate for pain control: may need medication to decrease bladder spasms as well as narcotics.
      7) Maintain catheter taped tightly to leg (for hemostasis at surgical site by catheter balloon).
      8) Address sexual concerns.
         a) Retrograde ejaculation
         b) Urinary incontinence
         c) Erectile dysfunction

TABLE I-16
SURGICAL APPROACHES FOR PROSTATECTOMY

APPROACH	ADVANTAGE	DISADVANTAGE	NURSING INTERVENTION
Transurethral (removal of prostatic tissue by instrument introduced through urethra)	Safer for client at risk; shorter period of hospitalization and convalescence	Not indicated for greatly enlarged prostate	Observe for hemorrhage, stricture, and incontinence
Open Surgical Removal			
- Suprapubic	- Technically simple	- Requires surgical approach through the bladder	- Strict aseptic care
- Perineal	- Offer direct anatomic approach	- Impotency and urinary incontinency; use drainage pads to absorb	- Avoid rectal tubes, thermometers, and enemas after perineal surgery
- Retropubic	- Most versatile procedure; affords direct visualization	- Cannot treat associated pathology in bladder	- Watch for evidence of hemorrhage

K. Incontinence
  1. Types
     a. Urge: Client cannot hold urine when stimulus to void occurs
     b. Functional: cannot physically get to the bathroom; doesn't know to go to the bathroom
     c. Stress: pressure such as coughing, straining, bearing down, laughing causes urine to escape; very common in middle-age women
  2. **NURSING INTERVENTIONS** (general)
      a. Use adult incontinency devices.
     b. Decrease fluid intake after 1800.
     c. Maintain toilet regimen: toilet routinely; use schedule.
     d. Perform Credé method as needed.
     e. Monitor for signs for cystitis.
     f. Teach client Kegel exercises for stress incontinence.
     g. Assure physical environment enhances ability to get to bathroom.
  3. Urine Retention
     a. Cause: actual obstruction of the urethra from acute or chronic causes; (e.g., edema, tumor, inflammation or inability of bladder to work; postanesthesia, stroke)
      b. **NURSING INTERVENTIONS**
        1) Stimulate relaxation of urethral sphincter
           a) Provide privacy.
           b) Place hands in warm water.
           c) Encourage guided imagery.
        2) Administer medications: bethanechol chloride (*Urecholine*).
        3) Position client; near normal, upright.
        4) Ensure adequate fluid intake.
  4. Medications
     a. Urge incontinence
        1) Anticholinergics: tolterodine (*Detrol*), Oxybutynin (*Ditropan*), Propantheline (*Pro-Banthine*)
     b. Stress incontinence
        1) Tricyclic antidepressant: imipramine (*Tofranil*)

SECTION X

REVIEW OF NEUROSENSORY DISORDERS

Neurological Assessment

A. History of Present Illness

B. Mental Status
  1. Level of consciousness (alert, lethargic, obtunded, stupor, coma)
  2. Orientation (person, place, time)
  3. Affect
  4. Mood
  5. Speech (language, vocabulary, word-finding ability)
  6. Cognition (judgment and abstraction ability)

C. Cranial Nerves (I thru XII)
  1. CN I: Olfactory - sensory smell
  2. CN II: Optic - sensory vision
  3. CN III: Oculomotor - motor eye
  4. CN IV: Trochlear - motor eye
  5. CN V: Trigeminal - sensory face, motor chewing
  6. CN VI: Abducens - motor eye
  7. CN VII: Facial - motor facial movements, sensory taste
  8. CN VIII: Acoustic - sensory hearing, balance
  9. CN IX: Glossopharyngeal - sensory posterior taste
  10. CN X: Vagus - sensory throat, motor swallow, and speak
  11. CN XI: Spinal accessory - motor shoulders
  12. CN XII: Hypoglossal - motor tongue

D. Motor System
  1. Muscles
     a. Size
     b. Symmetry
     c. Tone
     d. Strength
  2. Coordination
  3. Movement
     a. Voluntary control/involuntary movements
     b. Tremors
     c. Twitches
     d. Balance and gait
  4. Posturing
     a. Decorticate: an abnormal posturing indicated by rigidity, flexion of the arms, clenched fists, and extended legs; arms are bent inward toward the body with wrists and fingers bent and held on the chest; indicative of damage to the corticospinal tract (pathway between the brain and spinal cord)
     b. Decerebrate: abnormal body posture indicated by rigid extension of the arms and legs, downward pointing of toes, and backward arching of head; indicative of deterioration of structures of the nervous system, particularly of the upper brain stem

E. Reflexes
  1. Assessment Findings
     a. 0 to absent
     b. 1+ to diminished

    c.   2+ to normal
    d.   3+ to brisk
    e.   4+ to hyperactive

F. Motor Function
1. Assessment
   a. Babinski reflex
   b. Steady gait
   c. Muscle tone and strength
   d. Upper and lower extremity

G. Client's Response to Stimulus: Glasgow Coma Scale (normal 8 to 15; 7 or less indicates coma)
1. Best eye-opening response
   a. Spontaneously   = 4
   b. To speech   = 3
   c. To pain   = 2
   d. No response   = 1
2. Best motor response
   a. Obeys verbal command   = 6
   b. Localizes pain   = 5
   c. Flexion: withdrawal to pain   = 4
   d. Flexion: abnormal (decorticate)   = 3
   e. Extension: abnormal (decerebrate)   = 2
   f. No response to pain on any limb   = 1
3. Best verbal response
   a. Oriented x 3   = 5
   b. Conversation (confused)   = 4
   c. Speech: inappropriate   = 3
   d. Sounds: incomprehensible   = 2
   e. No response   = 1

H. Pupil Check
1. Pupils are compared for size equality, movement, and response to light
2. Normal finding: pupils equal and reactive to light

I. Vital Signs
1. Blood pressure or pulse changes may be indicative of increased intracranial pressure

Diagnostic Procedures

A. Lumbar Puncture
1. Procedure done to measure pressures within the cerebrospinal fluid and to collect a sample of fluid for testing; cerebrospinal fluid is used to diagnose neurological disorders, infections, and brain or spinal cord damage
 2. **NURSING INTERVENTIONS**
   a. Confirm that informed consent has been obtained.
   b. Have client empty bladder and bowel.
   c. Position client on side with knees pulled toward chest and chin tucked downward.
   d. Spinal needle inserted between third and fourth lumbar vertebrae.
   e. Spinal fluid pressure is measured and fluid is collected once needle is properly positioned.

    f.   Postprocedure
      1) Remove needle, cleanse back, apply bandage, and position client flat for 20 to 60 min.
      2) Encourage fluid intake if cerebrospinal fluid has been removed.
      3) Check puncture site for redness, swelling, and clear drainage.
      4) Assess movement of extremities.

B. Computed Tomography (CT scan)
1. Head CT: a computerized tomography image (with or without dye) is used to evaluate acute cranial-facial trauma, subarachnoid or intracranial hemorrhage, and headaches; also used to diagnose stroke and determine abnormal development of head and neck
 2. **NURSING INTERVENTIONS** (preprocedure)
   a. Verify that informed consent has been obtained.
   b. Check for allergies to iodine, contrast dyes, or shellfish.
   c. Instruct the client to lie still and flat.
   d. Have client remove metal objects, including hair clips and jewelry.
 3. **NURSING INTERVENTIONS** (postprocedure)
   a. Increase fluids due to diuresis from dye.
   b. Assess dye injection site and monitor distal pulses.

C. Cerebral Arteriogram
1. Injection of dye into the carotid arteries, via the femoral artery, to allow visualization of the cerebral arteries and to assess for brain lesions
 2. **NURSING INTERVENTIONS** (preprocedure)
   a. Verify informed consent has been obtained.
   b. Check for allergies to iodine, contrast dyes, or shellfish.
   c. Keep client NPO 4 to 6 hr before procedure.
   d. Mark distal peripheral pulses.
   e. Warn client that they may feel warmth in face during the procedure.
 3. **NURSING INTERVENTIONS** (postprocedure)
   a. Monitor for altered level of consciousness, sensory or motor deficits.
   b. Check for hematoma at postinsertion site; keep leg straight for 2 hr with sand bag to insertion site; maintain bedrest for 12 hr.
   c. Ice cap to decrease swelling.
   d. Check peripheral pulses, color, and temperature of extremities.

D. Myelogram
1. Injection of contrast medium or air into subarachnoid space to detect abnormalities of vertebrae and/or spinal cord
 2. **NURSING INTERVENTIONS** (preprocedure)
   a. Verify informed consent has been obtained.

b. Check for allergies to iodine, contrast dyes, or shellfish.

c. Maintain NPO 4 hr before procedure.

 3. **NURSING INTERVENTIONS** (postprocedure)

a. Keep client horizontal for 12 to 24 hr after procedure if oil-based dye is used; head of bed raised 15 to 30° if water-based dye is used.

b. Monitor vital signs.

c. Monitor output.

d. Encourage fluid intake.

e. Monitor for fever, stiff neck, and back pain.

E. Electroencephalogram (EEG)

1. A test to detect problems in the electrical activity of the brain; 16 to 25 electrodes are placed on the scalp over multiple areas of the brain to detect and record patterns of electrical activity and check for abnormalities (seizure disorders, confusion, evaluate head injuries, tumors, infections, degenerative diseases, and metabolic disturbances) or to confirm brain death

 2. **NURSING INTERVENTIONS** (preprocedure)

a. Verify informed consent has been obtained.

b. Verify with primary provider which medications should be administered to the client before EEG.

c. Avoid caffeine 8 hr before the test.

d. Instruct client to wash hair the night before the test; do not use any oils, sprays, or conditioners on hair before test.

e. Verify if test is to be done awake, asleep, or sleep-deprived.

F. Electromyography (EMG)

1. A test to assess the health of the muscles and the nerves controlling the muscles; a needle electrode is inserted through the skin into the muscle where electrical activity is detected

 2. **NURSING INTERVENTIONS** (preprocedure)

a. Verify informed consent has been obtained.

b. Explain there will be some discomfort due to insertion of needle into skeletal muscles.

G. Magnetic Resonance Imaging (MRI)

1. A noninvasive procedure that uses magnets and radio waves to construct clear, detailed pictures of the brain and nerve tissues without obstruction by overlying bone

 2. **NURSING INTERVENTIONS** (preprocedure)

a. Verify informed consent has been obtained.

b. Assess for claustrophobia.

c. Have client remove all removable metal objects (body piercings, jewelry) from self.

d. Have client remove metal valuables (credit cards, wrist watch) from pockets and self.

e. No special test, diet, or medications are required.

Increased Intracranial Pressure

A. Definition: increase in normal brain pressure due to an increase in the cerebrospinal fluid pressure; increased pressure within the brain matter caused by lesions or swelling within the brain matter itself; increased intracranial pressure causes compression of the brain structures and restricts blood flow through blood vessels that supply the brain

B. Causes

1. Head injury
2. Cerebrovascular accident
3. Brain tumor
4. Hydrocephalus
5. Ruptured aneurysm and subarachnoid hemorrhage
6. Cerebral edema
7. Subdural or epidural hematoma
8. Meningitis, encephalitis

C. Manifestations: may vary depending on cause and location; will affect the level of consciousness

1. Lethargic, drowsy, stupor; motor and sensory changes
2. Headache, irritability, restlessness
3. Nausea and vomiting, often projectile
4. Pupil changes: dilated, unequal, nonreactive
5. Diplopia
6. Changes in vital signs
   a. Widening pulse pressure; bradycardia with increased systolic blood pressure is Cushing's syndrome
   b. Irregular or decreasing respirations (Cheyne-Stokes respirations)
   c. Elevated temperature

D. NURSING INTERVENTIONS

1. Monitor vital signs and neurological function.

 2. Keep head of bed elevated 30 to 45°.

3. Keep head in neutral position to enhance drainage.

4. Avoid coughing, sneezing, and suctioning.

5. Maintain good respiratory exchange (hyperventilation causes CO_2 to decrease leading to vasoconstriction. This causes a decrease in the ICP; this may be used as an intervention); administer oxygen to increase supply to brain.

6. Administer oxygen to increase supply to brain.

7. Monitor fluid I&O; restrict fluids to prevent increased cerebral edema.

8. Administer medications as prescribed.
   a. Avoid opiates and sedatives (contraindicated).
   b. Barbiturates: (e.g., pentobarbital [*Nembutal*]) may be prescribed for uncontrolled increased intracranial pressure to place client into a barbiturate coma; client will require ventilatory support and close monitoring of cardiac status

c. Give acetaminophen (*Tylenol*) for fever.
d. Administer osmotic diuretics: (e.g., mannitol [*Osmitrol*]) and steroids (e.g., dexamethasone [*Decadron*]) to decrease cerebral swelling
e. Obtain order for antihypertensive medications or anticonvulsant medications if necessary.
9. Use hypothermia as ordered to decrease metabolism.
10. Decrease environmental stimuli.
11. Monitor intracranial pressure; intracranial pressure monitoring (ventriculostomy) requires intensive care.

Hyperthermia

A. Definition: body temperature above 105° F; may be caused by infection, cerebral edema, or excessive environmental heat
1. Clients may also experience nausea/vomiting, shivering
2. Increases risk of hypoxia due to increase in cerebral metabolism

B. Hypothermia Blanket
1. Protect skin
2. Manual temperature every 2 hr

C. NURSING INTERVENTIONS

1. Monitor vital signs.
2. Assess neuro status with each set of vital signs.
3. Monitor client for tachycardia, dysrhythmias.
4. Monitor for manifestations of dehydration.
   a. Monitor I&O.
   b. Monitor daily weight.
5. Prevent shivering.
   a. Decreases risk of increased intracranial pressure and oxygen consumption
   b. Chlorpromazine hydrochloride (*Thorazine*)
   c. Meperidine hydrochloride (*Demerol*)
6. Initiate seizure precautions.

Seizure Disorders

A. Definition: abnormal, sudden, excessive discharge of electrical activity within the brain due to genetics, trauma, tumors, toxicity, or infections

B. Classifications
1. Generalized (four types)
   a. Tonic-clonic (formerly grand-mal)
   b. Absence (formerly petit-mal seizures)
   c. Myoclonic
   d. Atonic or akinetic ("drop-attacks")
2. Partial seizures (two types)
   a. Complex (loss of consciousness)
   b. Simple (no loss of consciousness)

C. NURSING INTERVENTIONS

1. During seizure
   a. Maintain patent airway (turn to side after tonic phase).
   b. Protect from injury.
   c. Do not restrain.
   d. Do not put anything in client's mouth.
   e. Turn client's head to side to prevent aspiration.
2. Document
   a. Length of seizure
   b. Prodromal signs (irritability, mood change, insomnia) preceding aura (a sensory warning that the seizure is about to occur)
   c. Length of loss of consciousness (if any); incontinence
   d. Precipitating factors (if any)
   e. Respiratory difficulty
   f. Postictal phase (period of lethargy and limpness following seizure)
3. Teach client
   a. Take medications consistently; do not stop abruptly; keep laboratory appointments.
   b. Get adequate rest and exercise.
   c. Avoid alcohol.
4. Administer anticonvulsants
   a. Phenytoin (*Dilantin*) side effects: gum hypertrophy (client must visit the dentist routinely), ataxia, diplopia, hirsutism; monitor medication levels
   b. Carbamazepine (*Tegretol*) side effects: nystagmus, ataxia, blood dyscrasias; monitor CBC, liver function tests, medication levels
   c. Valproic acid (*Depakene*) and divalproex sodium (*Depakote*) side effects: nausea, bleeding problems, liver damage; monitor liver function tests, medication levels
   d. Phenobarbital (*Luminal*) side effects: drowsiness; monitor liver function test, medication levels
5. Monitor anticonvulsant levels: all anticonvulsants have variable absorption and excretion rates from one client to another; doses are tapered to maintain a therapeutic level
6. Institute seizure precautions for clients prone to multiple seizures and/or in poor control:
   a. Bed rest with padded side rails
   b. Oxygen and suction available at bedside

D. Status Epilepticus:
1. Definition: an emergency condition designated by prolonged or clustered seizures that develop into nonstop continuous seizures for 30 min or more; usually caused by sudden withdrawal of anticonvulsant medications; can lead to brain damage or death

2. **NURSING INTERVENTIONS**
   a. Initiate standard seizure precautions.
   b. Administer benzodiazepine and anticonvulsant therapy.
      1) Lorazepam (*Ativan*) is the medication of choice; dose: 4 mg IV every 2 min up to maximum dose of 8 mg
      2) Diazepam (*Valium*) may also be used in status epilepticus; dose: 5 to 10 mg IVP every 10 min up to maximum dose of 30 mg
      3) Phenytoin (*Dilantin*) 500 to 1,000 mg IV slowly
         a) Give no more than 50 mg/min.
         b) Do not mix with glucose; must be administered in NS only.
         c) Monitor for bradycardia and heart block.

Cerebrovascular Accident (CVA)

A. Definition: sudden loss of brain function resulting from a disruption of blood supply to the involved part of the brain; commonly referred to as a "stroke"; causes temporary or permanent neurological deficits

B. Risk Factors
1. Hypertension
2. Smoking
3. Obesity
4. Hypercholesterolemia
5. Diabetes mellitus
6. Peripheral vascular disease
7. A-V malformation
8. Aneurysm
9. Hemorrhage (cerebral)
10. Cocaine

C. Manifestations: severity of deficit determined by location and extent of tissue ischemia; symptoms manifest in cross reference pattern
1. Loss of motor balance, coordination
2. Slurred speech, aphasia
3. Hemiparesis, hemiplegia
4. Visual disturbance
5. Dysphagia
6. Cranial nerve disturbance

D. NURSING INTERVENTIONS (initially same as management of client who is unconscious)

1. Maintain adequate airway.
2. Monitor neurological function and vital signs routinely.
3. Maintain fluid and electrolyte balance.
4. Monitor for aspiration due to risk of dysphagia; feed slowly, from the front; place food on unaffected side.

5. Provide psychological support due to emotional lability; understand and help family to cope.
6. Establish means of communication due to aphasia (expressive, receptive, global): encourage client to talk; don't assume needs; don't speak in a loud voice; speak to client clearly and slowly.
7. Participate in acute and rehabilitation phases.
   a. Range of motion: prone to flexion contractures; keep extremities in position of extension or neutrality
   b. Hemiparesis, hemiplegia: will cause safety issues in the client; consult occupational or physical therapy
   c. Hemianopsia: place articles where one can see; encourages client to turn their head to actually be able to see items.
   d. Help client to achieve bowel and bladder control using regimen.
   e. Consult occupational or physical therapy to assist client with self-care deficits.

Transient Ischemic Attacks (TIA)

A. Definition: temporary episode of neurological dysfunction lasting only a few minutes or seconds due to decreased blood flow to the brain; may be a warning sign of an impending stroke, especially in first 4 weeks after TIA

B. Causes
1. Atherosclerosis
2. Microemboli from atherosclerotic plaque
3. Cerebral artery spasm

C. Manifestations
1. Sudden change in visual function
2. Sudden loss of sensory function
3. Sudden loss of motor function

D. Diagnostic Testing
1. Carotid Doppler studies
2. CT scan and/or MRI
3. Arteriography

E. Treatment
1. Antiplatelet medications
   a. Clopidogrel (*Plavix*)
   b. Dipyridamole (*Aggrenox*)
   c. Ticlopidine (*Ticlid*)
2. Anticoagulant medications
   a. Warfarin (*Coumadin*)
3. Angioplasty
   a. Carotid endarterectomy

F. Prevention
1. Stop smoking.
2. Consume a diet that is low in cholesterol and sodium.

3. Maintain ideal body weight.
4. Exercise.
5. Control hypertension and diabetes mellitus.
6. Limit alcohol intake.

Spinal Cord Injury

A. Definition: partial or complete disruption of nerve tracts and neurons resulting in paralysis, sensory loss, altered activity, and autonomic nervous system dysfunction

B. Risk Factors
1. Men ages 16 to 30
2. High-risk activities
   a. Driving while intoxicated
   b. Not wearing a seat belt
   c. No protective sports gear
   d. No firearm safety

C. Types
1. Contusion
2. Laceration
3. Compression of the cord

D. Level of Injury (determines manifestations)
1. Cervical: causes quadriplegia
   a. Respiratory problems (may be ventilator dependent)
   b. Paralysis of all four extremities
   c. Loss of bladder and bowel control
   d. Injury above C3 is usually fatal unless witnessed
2. Thoracic injury: causes paraplegia
   a. Loss of bladder and bowel control
   b. Paralysis of lower extremities and major control of body trunk
   c. Potential complication of autonomic dysreflexia - injury above T6
3. Lumbar
   a. Paralysis of lower extremities (remain flaccid)
   b. Loss of bladder and bowel control

E. NURSING INTERVENTIONS
 1. Immobilize client as ordered.
   a. Spinal board
   b. Halo traction
   c. Gardner-Wells traction tongs or Crutchfield tongs
2. Provide care resulting from spinal shock/neurogenic shock (flaccid paralysis below level of injury followed by spastic reflexes).
3. Maintain respiratory function.
4. Monitor for autonomic hyperreflexia or dysreflexia.
   a. Life-threatening syndrome
   b. Sudden, severe hypertension secondary to noxious stimuli below cord damage

1) Bowel or bladder distension
2) Pressure ulcers or points
3) Pain or spasms (labor pain)
   c. Remove stimuli to correct
   d. Manifestations
      1) Hypertension (250 to 300/100)
      2) Headache, flushing, nausea
      3) Blurred vision and restlessness
      4) Bradycardia
5. Initiate bladder management program.
6. Initiate bowel regimen.
7. Administer dexamethasone (*Decadron*) to reduce edema.
8. Consult with occupational or physical therapy regarding rehabilitation issues; self care deficits.

Head Injury

A. Definition: any trauma that leads to injury of the scalp, skull, or brain, ranging from a minor bump on the head to a devastating injury; classified as either closed or penetrating
1. Closed-head injury: head sustains a blunt force by striking against an object
   a. Concussion
   b. Contusion
   c. Fracture
      1) Basilar Skull Fracture
         a) Manifestations
            (1) Bleeding from nose, ears
            (2) Otorrhea, rhinorrhea: cerebrospinal fluid from the ears or nose; must differentiate between cerebrospinal fluid and mucus by assessing glucose content of drainage
         b) Raccoon eyes (periorbital edema and ecchymosis)
         c) Battle's sign (postauricular ecchymosis)
   d. Hematomas
      1) Epidural hematoma
         a) Bleeding into space between skull and dura
         b) Commonly involves the middle meningeal artery
         c) Typical presentation: client sustains injury and has a period of loss of consciousness; this is followed by a lucid interval, then a rapid deterioration in level of consciousness
         d) Emergency management: burr holes to relieve increasing intracranial pressure
      2) Subdural hematoma
         a) Bleeding below dura

b) Usually venous
c) May be acute, subacute, or chronic
d) Management: craniotomy
2. A penetrating head injury: an object breaks through the skull and enters the brain

3. **NURSING INTERVENTIONS**
   a. Assess frequently for signs of increased intracranial pressure.
   b. Implement same interventions for client experiencing increased intracranial pressure.

Laminectomy

A. Definition: a surgical procedure to remove a portion of a vertebra for treatment of severe pain and disability resulting from compression of spinal nerves by a ruptured disk or bony compression; an option to relieve persistent pain or to treat progressive neurological problems due to nerve compression

B. NURSING INTERVENTIONS

1. Observe for circulatory impairment.
2. Observe for loss of sensation in lower extremities.
3. Observe dressing for spinal fluid leakage and bleeding.
4. Log roll client.
5. Address sexual concerns.
6. Institute measures to decrease infection at the site.

Multiple Sclerosis

A. Definition: chronic, progressive disease of the CNS, characterized by small patches of demyelination in the brain and spinal cord (exact cause unknown, but thought to have an autoimmune basis)

B. Manifestations
1. Occurs in young adults 20 to 40 years of age
2. Nystagmus, blurred vision, diplopia
3. Slurred hesitant speech
4. Spastic weakness of extremities/paresthesia
5. Emotionally labile/depression
6. Fatigue
7. Difficulty with balance
8. Intention tremors
9. Spastic bladder
10. MRI shows sclerotic patches through the brain and spinal cord

C. Management
1. No cure or specific treatment; characterized by long periods of remissions and exacerbation
2. During exacerbation: give corticosteroids
3. Stress management techniques may be helpful to prevent exacerbations
4. Immunosuppressants - (e.g., azathioprine [*Imuran*]) or beta-interferon [*Betaseron*)])

5. Muscle spasticity and tremors: baclofen (*Lioresal*), gabapentin (*Neurontin*), clonazepam (*Klonopin*)
6. Urinary problems and constipation: oxybutynin (*Ditropan*), tolterodine (*Detrol*), propantheline (*Pro-Banthine*), psyllium (*Metamucil*)
7. Depression: amitriptyline (*Elavil*), imipramine (*Tofranil*), sertraline (*Zoloft*)
8. Sexual difficulties: sildenafil (*Viagra*)
9. Fatigue: amantadine (*Symmetrel*), modafranil (*Provigil*), fluoxetine (*Prozac*)

D. NURSING INTERVENTIONS

1. Encourage active and normal life as long as possible.
2. Teach client self-catheterization techniques.
3. Promote daily exercise.
4. Prevent injury.
5. Educate client to avoid stressors that exacerbate condition, (e.g., infections).
6. Teach client self-injection technique - for beta interferon (*Betaseron*).

Parkinson's Disease

A. Definition: chronic, progressive neurologic disorder affecting the brain centers responsible for control and regulation of movement; extrapyramidal tract; loss of pigmented cells of substantia nigra and depletion of dopamine

B. Manifestations
1. Bradykinesia
2. Rigidity
3. Resting tremor
4. Expressionless, fixed gaze; "mask-like"
5. Drooling
6. Constipation
7. Depression
8. Retropulsion, propulsion
9. Slurred speech
10. Oily skin and seborrheic dermatitis

C. Stages
1. Unilateral flexion of upper extremity
2. Shuffling gait
3. Progressive difficulty ambulating
4. Progressive weakness
5. Progressive, permanent disability

D. Management
1. Medication Therapy
   a. Antiparkinsonian agent: levodopa (*Dopar*); side effects: hypotension, gastrointestinal upset; administer on an empty stomach ½ to 1 hr before meals

b. Antiparkinsonian agent: carbidopa (*Lodosyn*); side effects: hypokinesia, hyperkinesia, psychiatric manifestations

c. Dopamine agonist: bromocriptine mesylate (*Parlodel*)

d. Anticholinergic: benztropine (*Cogentin*); trihexyphenidyl (*Artane*); side effects: dry mouth, mydriasis, constipation, confusion

e. Antiviral, antiparkinsonian: amantadine HCl (*Symmetrel*); side effects: tremor, rigidity, bradykinesia

2. Surgical procedures include: stereotaxic thalamotomy to decrease tremors, deep brain stimulation, and gamma knife procedures

E. NURSING INTERVENTIONS

1. Fall prevention
2. Clothing that fosters independence (no snaps, buttons, or zippers)
3. High-fiber diet
4. Care with physical, occupational, and speech therapy
5. Use of rocking chair

Amyotrophic Lateral Sclerosis (ALS)

A. Definition: rapidly progressive, invariably fatal neurological disease that attacks the nerve cells (neurons) that control the voluntary muscles. Also known as Lou Gehrig's disease

B. Progression

1. Most commonly affects clients 40 to 60 years of age; men more commonly affected than women
2. Presents with muscle weakness in extremities, slurred speech, and progresses to inability to swallow, chew, communicate, breathe, and perceive sensory or tactile stimulation
3. Greatest risk of respiratory failure or pneumonia within 3 to 5 years of onset
4. Eventually the client loses the ability to breathe without ventilatory support; death due to respiratory failure or pneumonia typically occurs within 3 to 5 years from the onset of symptoms
5. ALS does not affect the client's sensory or cognitive abilities; the client is still able to see, smell, taste, hear, and recognize touch

C. Manifestations

1. Twitching, cramping, and stiffness of muscles
2. Muscle weakness affecting an arm or leg
3. Slurred and nasal speech
4. Difficulty chewing and swallowing (dysphagia)
5. Overactive gag reflex
6. Difficulty forming words (dysarthria)

7. Fatigue
8. Difficulty with manual dexterity

D. Management

1. Etiology unknown; no known cure, treatment is symptomatic

 2. **NURSING INTERVENTIONS**

a. Schedule speech therapy to assist with communication and swallowing needs.

b. Have occupational therapy assist with adaptive devices to foster independence.

c. Have physical therapy maintain muscle strength and tone.

d. Support respiratory needs with mechanical respirator devices.

e. Administer medication to provide relief from excessive salivation, pain, muscle cramps, constipation, and depression.

f. Provide supportive services to client and family.

Myasthenia Gravis

A. Definition: disorder affecting the neuromuscular transmission of the voluntary muscle of the body; loss of acetylcholine receptors on the postsynaptic membrane of the neuromuscular junction (exact cause unknown, but thought to have an autoimmune basis)

B. Manifestations

1. Extreme muscular weakness: increased with fatigue and relieved by rest
2. Early manifestations: diplopia, ptosis, dysphagia

C. Management

1. Medication management

a. Anticholinesterase medications that increase the amount of acetylcholine in the neuromuscular function

1) Pyridostigmine (*Mestinon*); Neostigmine (*Prostigmin*)
2) Atropine is antidote

b. Steroids: (e.g., prednisone [*Deltasone*])

2. Thymectomy (excision of the thymus)

3. Crisis

a. Cholinergic; usually from overmedication; causes severe tremors

b. Myasthenic; from infection or spontaneous; drooling and severe ptosis; can actually cause respiratory arrest

c. Differentiate between the two with the Tensilon test: edrophonium (*Tensilon*) injected with a response expected in 30 seconds; if no response, it is cholinergic crisis

D. NURSING INTERVENTIONS

1. Maintain patent airway.
2. Plan activities early in day to avoid fatigue.
3. Teach client: action of medications, manifestations of crisis.
4. Give medications on time.

Guillain-Barré Syndrome

A. Definition: an acquired acute inflammatory disease of peripheral nerves resulting in demyelination characterized by ascending, reversible paralysis

B. Manifestations
1. Disease usually proceeded by an infection: respiratory or gastrointestinal
2. Initial manifestations: tingling of the legs that may progress to upper extremities, trunk and facial muscles; "ascending paralysis" is classic disease presentation
3. Progresses to paralysis, possible respiratory failure
4. Recovery after several months to one year; descending recovery: last lost, first recovered

C. Management
1. Immunotherapy: plasma exchange or IV immune globulin/IVIG

D. NURSING INTERVENTIONS

1. Support airway; monitor respiratory status, oximetry.
2. Monitor blood pressure and heart rate.
3. Provide nutrition, especially if problems with chewing and swallowing.
4. Manage bowel and bladder problems.
5. Collaborate with physical therapy to maintain muscle strength and flexibility.
6. Prevent complications of immobility: pneumonia; DVT; UTI.

Sensory Assessment

A. Assessment of Visual Acuity
1. Visual acuity: assessment of client's ability to see objects at certain distances
2. Common findings
   a. Myopia (nearsightedness): distant objects appear blurred
   b. Hyperopia (farsightedness): close objects appear blurred
   c. Presbyopia (farsightedness associated with aging): a progressive condition in which the lens of the eye loses its ability to focus with age
   d. Macular degeneration (loss of visual acuity associated with aging): a progressive disorder that involves the retina causing decreased vision, and potentially the loss of central vision

B. Treatment of Visual Acuity Problems
1. Abnormal refractory findings typically treated with corrective lens
2. Lasik surgery: a surgical procedure that permanently changes the shape of the cornea and (in most cases) restores 20/20 vision

C. Auditory Assessment
1. Audiology exam (audiogram) tests the client's ability to hear sounds at varying intensity and decibels
2. Common findings
   a. Presbycusis (hearing deficit associated with aging): a progressive disorder in which the client loses the ability to hear sounds at high frequencies; may lead to deafness

D. Treatment of Hearing Deficits
1. Typically involves the use of hearing aides to amplify desirable environmental sounds

Ménière's Disease

A. Definition: disorder of the inner ear that causes change in sensory perception due to increase fluid

B. Manifestations
1. Vertigo
2. Tinnitus
3. Hearing loss
4. Pressure in the ear

C. Management
1. Medication therapy
   a. Meclizine (Antivert) to manage vertigo
   b. Hydrochlorothiazide (HCTZ) to reduce inner ear fluid volume
   c. Dexamethasone (prednisone) to reduce inflammation
2. Modify diet.
   a. Select low sodium foods.
   b. Eat six small meals daily.
   c. Avoid caffeine.
3. Manage anxiety and stress.

D. NURSING INTERVENTIONS

1. Prevent falls.
2. Maintain a quiet environment.
3. Assist client with identifying triggers; bright lights, loud music, caffeine, stress, and nicotine.
4. Provide supportive services to client and family.

Detached Retina

A. Definition: occurs when the sensory retina separates from the pigment epithelium of the retina; vitreous humor fluid flows between the layers when a tear occurs in the retina; can be related to age and trauma

B. Manifestations
1. Sudden visual disturbances
   a. Flashes of light
   b. Blurred vision
   c. Floaters
   d. Curtain or shadow over visual field

C. Management
1. Immediate bed rest
2. Avoid coughing, sneezing, straining
3. Surgical intervention: scleral buckling, photocoagulation, cryosurgery

D. NURSING INTERVENTIONS: (postoperative)

1. Maintain bed rest with both eyes bandaged for 24 hr.
2. Avoid jarring or bumping head.
3. Teach client self administration of eye drops on schedule.

Cataract

A. Definition: Slow, progressive clouding of the lens

B. Manifestations
1. Diplopia and blurred vision
2. Photophobia
3. Frequent change in eyeglasses prescription
4. Halos around lights and colors appear pale

C. Management: surgical removal of the lens under local anesthesia, with intraocular lens implant

D. NURSING INTERVENTIONS

1. Preoperative (dilate the eye)
   a. Mydriatics
   b. Cycloplegics
2. Postoperative
   a. Keep client's operative eye covered.
   b. Elevate head of bed 30 to 45°, do not turn client onto operative side.
   c. Teach client: avoid bending at waist, lifting, sneezing, coughing; keep fingers away from eyes.
   d. Prevent vomiting/straining.
   e. Report severe pain immediately; may indicate a major complication postoperative: glaucoma.

Glaucoma

A. Definition: increased intraocular pressure; if uncorrected, may lead to atrophy of the optic nerve and eventual blindness

B. Manifestations
1. Acute (closed angle)
   a. Results from an obstruction to the outflow of aqueous humor
   b. Severe pain in and around eye
   c. Lights have a rainbow of colors around them
   d. Cloudy and blurred vision
   e. Pupils dilate
   f. Nausea and vomiting
   g. Within hours may develop gastrointestinal, sinus, neuro, and dental manifestations
2. Chronic (open angle)
   a. Insidious onset
   b. Tired feeling in eye
   c. Slowly decreasing peripheral vision
   d. Halos around lights
   e. Progressive loss of visual field

C. Management
1. Administer medications
   a. Medication action
      1) Pupil contracts, iris is drawn away from cornea
      2) Aqueous humor may drain through lymph spaces (meshwork) into Schlemm's canal
   b. Types (avoid all anticholinergic medications)
      1) Pilocarpine hydrochloride (*Pilocar*); lasts 6 to 8 hr; medication of choice for glaucoma
      2) Acetazolamide (*Diamox*); decreases production of aqueous humor; side effect: gastric distress
      3) Mannitol (*Osmitrol*), IV (systemic); reduces intraocular pressure by increasing blood osmolality; indications: useful in treatment of acute attacks of pressure and preoperatively
      4) Isosorbide (*Isordil*), oral; cautions: safer than IV medication for cardiac clients; may cause diuresis, which is troublesome in men with prostatitis
2. Surgical care
   a. Procedures
      1) Iridencleisis
      2) Thermosclerectomy
      3) Trabeculectomy
   b. Local anesthetic usually used

3. **NURSING INTERVENTIONS**
   a. Promote safety when ambulating.
   b. Administer stool softeners.

c. Teach client
   1) Glaucoma is controllable, not curable
   2) Avoid emotional upsets, constrictive clothing, extreme exertion and lifting, colds.
   3) Encourage moderate exercise, regular bowel habits, daily use of medicines, medical checkups and Medic-Alert bracelet; monitor fluid intake.

SECTION XI

REVIEW OF ONCOLOGY NURSING

Neoplastic Diseases

A. Characteristics
1. Etiology
   a. Healthy cells transformed into malignant cells upon exposure to certain etiological agents: viruses, chemical and physical agents
   b. Failure of immune response
2. Pathophysiology
   a. Rapid cell division
   b. Malignant cells metastasize
     1) Extending directly into adjacent tissue
     2) Permeating along lymphatic vessels
     3) Traveling through lymph system to nodes
     4) Entering body circulation
     5) Diffusing into body cavity
3. Classification of tumors
   a. Classified according to type of tissue from which they evolve
     1) Carcinomas begin in epithelial tissue (e.g., skin, gastrointestinal tract lining, lung, breast, uterus)
     2) Sarcomas begin in nonepithelial tissue (e.g., bone, muscle, fat, lymph system)
   b. Type of cell in which they arise; cell type affects appearance, rate of growth, and degree of malignancy (e.g., epithelial basal cells are basal cell carcinoma; bone cells are osteogenic carcinoma; gland epithelium are adenocarcinoma)
4. Staging
   a. Describes extent of tumor
   b. Describes extent to which malignancy has increased in size
   c. Indicates involvement of regional nodes
   d. Indicates metastatic development

B. Manifestations Suggesting Malignant Disease
(ACS 7 Warning Signs) – Client teaching mnemonic: "CAUTION"
1. C: Change in bowel or bladder habits
2. A: A sore that does not heal
3. U: Unusual bleeding or discharge
4. T: Thickening or lumps in breast or elsewhere
5. I: Indigestion or difficulty swallowing
6. O: Obvious change in wart or mole
7. N: Nagging cough or hoarseness

C. Cancer Therapy
1. Objective: to cure the client and to ensure that minimal functional and structural impairment results from the disease; if cure is not possible:
   a. Prevent further metastasis.
   b. Relieve manifestations.
   c. Maintain high quality of life as long as possible.
2. Surgery
   a. Radical
   b. Prophylactic
   c. Palliative
3. Chemotherapy
   a. Medications interfere with cell division; combination of medications usually given
   b. Classification of medications
     1) Alkylating agents: uracil mustard (*Nitrogen mustard*), cyclophosphamide (*Cytoxan*)
     2) Antimetabolite: fluorouracil (*5-FU*), methotrexate (*MTX*) (*Folex*)
     3) Antibiotics: doxorubicin hydrochloride (*Adriamycin*), bleomycin (*Blenoxane*), dactinomycin (*Actinomycin D*)
     4) Plant alkaloids: vincristine (*Oncovin*), vinblastine (*Velban*)
     5) Hormones: estrogen, progesterone, tamoxifen citrate (*Tamofen*)
     6) Miscellaneous: procarbazine (*Matulane*)
     7) Biological modifiers (*Procrit, Neupogen*)
     8) Immunomodulators (MP3)
     9) Liposome suspensions: used to decrease toxicity of medication delivery (amphotericin b liposome)
   c. Common side effects and interventions to counteract and cope with them
     1) Bone marrow depression: some is expected or medication is not working
       a) Leukopenia (WBC less than 1,000 mm^3): measures to enhance immune system: balanced diet, rest, handwashing, filgrastim (Neupogen) medication, protective isolation during hospitalization; routine laboratory work

TABLE I-17
NURSING INTERVENTIONS FOR CLIENT ON CHEMOTHERAPY

DRUGS	USES	SIDE EFFECTS	NURSING INTERVENTIONS
fluorouracil (5-FU)	Cancers of GI tract, breast, lung, uterus, ovary	Anorexia, nausea, bone marrow depression	Monitor CBC and platelets
mercaptopurine (6-MP)	Acute leukemia	Bone marrow depression	Monitor CBC and platelets
methotrexate (Folex) (Amethopterin, MTX)	Acute leukemia	Bone marrow depression	Methotrexate is excreted through the kidneys, so if renal function is impaired, the drug should not be given; folinic acid (Leucovorin) used to "rescue" non-cancerous cells after MTX treatment
chlorambucil (Leukeran)leukemia	Chronic lymphocytic	Bone marrow depression	Monitor CBC and platelets
cyclophosphamide (Cytoxan)	Acute lymphocytic leukemia	Bone marrow depression	Monitor CBC and platelets
mitomycin (Mutamycin)	Pancreas, stomach, breast cancer	Nausea, vomiting, bone marrow depression, severe skin reaction	Vitamin B$_6$ may reverse skin reaction
melphalan (Alkeran) stomatitis	Cancers of the breast, ovary, testicles; multiple melanoma	Unpredictable bone marrow depression, nausea, vomiting,	Monitor CBC and platelets; mouth care
vincristine sulfate and (Oncovin)	Cancers of the breast lung; acute leukemia	Alopecia, bone marrow depression	Monitor CBC and platelets; liquid diet for nausea

b) Anemia (Hgb less than 10): measures to enhance RBCs: oxygen therapy, iron-rich foods, blood transfusions, erythropoietin (Epogen), epoetin alfa (Procrit); routine laboratory work

c) Thrombocytopenia (platelets less than 50,000): measures to enhance platelet count: platelet transfusion, oprelvekin (Neumega), bleeding precautions, and avoiding use of aspirin and alcohol

2) Alopecia: hair loss 2 weeks after start of treatment. Apply ice to scalp during chemotherapy to slow hair loss. Use gentle shampoo, hats, scarves, and sunscreen. The American Cancer Society provides wigs and supportive services.

3) Gastrointestinal distress: Administer antiemetic prior to therapy. Eat small, favorite meals with high-calorie supplements. Select foods high in potassium. Drink cool beverages (e.g., flat ginger ale). Avoid unpleasant odors. Take loperamide (Imodium A-D) to manage diarrhea. Consume soft, bland, high-protein foods at room temperature for stomatitis, and use straw for fluids. Rinse mouth with a topical anesthetic, and use topical steroids and zinc supplements.

4) Elevated uric acid, crystal and urate stone formation: allopurinol (Zyloprim) therapy; increase fluid intake

5) Specific medications have specific toxic effects; most important are:
a) Doxorubicin hydrochloride (Adriamycin): irreversible cardiomyopathy
b) Cisplatin, cis-platinum (Platinol): renal toxicity
c) Vincristine sulfate (Oncovin): peripheral neuropathy

d. Emotional concerns: support client and family; support groups; help to live with this chronic disease
4. Radiation
    a. Purposes
        1) Curative (Hodgkin's disease)
        2) Palliative
    b. Types
        1) External: gamma rays
         a) **NURSING INTERVENTIONS**
            (1) Teach client about the procedure.
            (2) Give antiemetic before treatment if nausea is a problem: ondansetron (*Zofran*).
            (3) Give pain medication before treatment if needed.
            (4) Provide psychological support.
            (5) Provide skin care: dermatitis 3 to 6 weeks after start of treatment; teach client to wash with water; avoid lotions, powders, sunlight.
            (6) Treat "wet" reaction: cleanse with warm water; keep open; may use antibiotic cream.
        2) Internal: cesium needles
         a) **NURSING INTERVENTIONS**
            (1) Observe time, distance, and shielding, because the client is radioactive.
            (2) Follow institutional guidelines to protect yourself.
            (3) Limit visitors; private room; face area of body to be irradiated toward the outside of the building.
            (4) Very prone to inflammation in the site of radiation, (e.g., intrauterine may lead to proctitis and cystitis; oral insertion may lead to stomatitis).
                (a) Observe for signs of complications.
                (b) Treat specifically by resting the area; indwelling urinary catheter.
                (c) Alter diet as needed; increase fluids, low residue, soft.
                (d) Administer medications to decrease inflammation as necessary; steroids, urinary antiseptics, and aesthetics.
            (5) If radiation source falls out, do NOT touch it with bare hands.
                (a) Use lead forceps and put in lead container.

(b) Follow institution guidelines for radiation containment.

REVIEW OF IMMUNOLOGIC DISORDERS

Acquired Immune Deficiency Syndrome (AIDS)

A. Definition: infectious disease characterized by severe deficits in cellular immune function; manifested clinically by opportunistic infection and/or unusual neoplasms

1. Etiology: human immunodeficiency virus (HIV)
2. Risk factors
    a. Unprotected intercourse with an infected or high-risk partner
    b. IV drug abusers sharing needles
    c. Blood transfusions (hemophiliacs, surgical clients; blood supply testing for HIV began in 1985)
    d. Infants of infected mothers

KEY INFORMATION

 The disease has a long incubation period, sometimes up to 10 years until late in the infection

3. Manifestations
    a. Flu-like symptoms
    b. Swollen lymph glands
    c. Weight loss
    d. Chronic diarrhea and fever
    e. Night sweats
    f. CD4 lymphocyte count less than 200 (800 to 1,200 normal)
    g. Bacterial infections
        1) Pneumonia
        2) Tuberculosis
        3) Salmonellosis - severe diarrhea, abdominal pain and fever
    h. Viral infections
        1) Cytomegalovirus - can cause blindness
        2) Herpes simplex virus - genital and systemic
        3) Human papillomavirus (HPV)
    i. Fungal infections
        1) Candidiasis - tongue, esophagus, vagina
        2) Cryptococcal meningitis
    j. Parasitic infections
        1) *Pneumocystis carinii* pneumonia (PCP)
        2) Toxoplasmosis

k. Cancer
   1) Kaposi's sarcoma
   2) Non Hodgkin's lymphoma
l. Other
   1) AIDS dementia complex
   2) Wasting syndrome
    3) **NURSING INTERVENTIONS**
      a) Provide respiratory support.
         (1) Pulmonary toilet
         (2) Oxygen therapy
      b) Maintain fluid and electrolyte balance.
      c) Prevent spread of infection through use of universal precautions.
      d) Provide emotional support.
      e) Provide skin care.
      f) Provide high-nutrition, low-residue meals.
      g) Teach clients about abstinence, safer sex practices, monogamy, handwashing, use of condoms.
   4) Medication therapy: World Health Organization; highly active antiretroviral therapy guidelines (HAART) (NOTE: always follow the most current research findings, which are constantly being updated)
      a) Efavirenz (*Sustiva*), azidothymidine (*AZT*), and lamivudine (*Epivir*)
         (1) Common adverse effects: neutropenia, gastrointestinal distress, anemia, insomnia
         (2) Zidovudine (*AZT*) recommended for protecting the unborn fetus of HIV-positive pregnant women
            (a) Do not breastfeed
      b) Interferon (*Roferon*)
      c) Pneumocystis pneumonia prophylaxis: Pentamidine (*Pentam 300*)
      d) Antifungals: metronidazole (*Flagyl*) and amphotericin B (*Fungizone*)
      e) Antituberculosis medications as needed
      f) Acyclovir (*Zovirax*) herpes treatment
      g) Protease inhibitors: saquinavir (*Fortovase*), ritonavir (*Norvir*)
      h) Antivirals: zalcitabine, ddC, dideoxycytidine (*Hivid*), lamivudine (*Epivir*)

Systemic Lupus Erythematosus (SLE)

A. Definition: chronic inflammatory disease that involves the vascular and connective tissue of multiple organs; cause is unknown, may be autoimmune

B. Manifestations
1. Insidious onset
2. Characterized by remissions and exacerbations
3. Erythematous "butterfly rash" on both cheeks and across the bridge of the nose; rash worsens on exposure to sunlight (most common manifestation)
4. Polyarthralgia
5. Normochromic, normocytic anemia
6. Fever, malaise, weight loss
7. Positive for antinuclear antibodies
8. Raynaud's phenomenon

C. NURSING INTERVENTIONS
 1. Supportive (depends on organs involved)
2. Teaching
   a. Sleep uninterrupted and take daytime naps.
   b. Wear sunscreen and protective clothing.
   c. Exercise 30 min a day.
   d. Avoid smoking.
   e. Identify triggers (stress, oral contraceptives, sunlight, foods, and pregnancy).
   f. Select barrier contraceptive method; no IUD.

KEY INFORMATION
 Lupus nephritis occurs early in the disease
1. Manifestations
   a. Symptomatic relief
   b. Medications
      (1) NSAIDS
      (2) Antimalarial hydroxychloroquine (Plaquenil); Monitor vision and muscle weakness.
      (3) Corticosteroids
      (4) Dialysis
2. Treatment
   a. Symptomatic
   b. Salicylates, steroids
   c. Dialysis
3. Prognosis variable

SECTION XIII

REVIEW OF BURNS

Assessment

A. Extent of Body Surface
1. Adults: Rule of nines

a. Head and neck	9%
b. Anterior trunk	18%
c. Posterior trunk	18%
d. Arms (9%)	18%
e. Legs (18%)	36%
f. Perineum	1%

2. Babies and young children
   a. Head and neck   21%
   b. Arms and hands   10%
   c. Chest and stomach   13%
   d. Back   13%
   e. Buttocks   5%
   f. Legs and feet   13.5%
   g. Groin   1%

B. Depth of Burn
1. Superficial (formerly called first degree)
2. Partial thickness (formerly called second degree)
3. Full thickness (formerly called third degree)

C. Type of Burn
1. Thermal
2. Chemical
3. Electrical
4. Radiation

D. Pre-existing Physical and Psychological Status of Client
1. Age
2. Preburn weight
3. Medical history

E. Concomitant Injuries

Treatment

A. Prehospital Care
1. Stop thermal process.
   a. Stop drop and roll
   b. Cool water for 10 min
2. Establish airway.
3. Cover large areas with clean cloth to decrease pain.
4. Chemical burns: irrigate copiously.
5. Electrical burns: interrupt power source.
6. Transport to emergency facility.

B. Emergency Department
1. Establish and maintain client airway.
2. Assessment
   a. Time of injury
   b. How injury occurred
   c. Cause of burn
3. Administer 100% oxygen if burn occurred in enclosed area.
4. Maintain fluid balance.
5. Insert indwelling urinary catheter.
6. Insert NG tube as prescribed.
7. Administer tetanus toxoid.
8. Assist with escharotomy or fasciotomy if needed.

C. Hospital Care
1. Maintain patent airway.
2. Maintain aseptic area.
3. Provide fluid replacement therapy.
   a. Goal is to maintain vital organ perfusion
   b. Shock phase: 24 to 48 hr
      1) Fluid shifts from plasma to interstitial space
      2) Hct rises
      3) Metabolic acidosis
      4) Serum potassium rises
      5) Fluid loss is plasma
      6) Protein loss
      7) Monitor vital signs
      8) Monitor urine output (goal of 50 mL/hr)
      9) Fluid resuscitation:
         a) Parkland formula (most common) 4 mL/kg/% burn (4 mL per kg times % burn)
         b) Give half of total fluids in first 8 hr
         c) Give second half over remaining 16 hr
   c. Postshock phase (diuretic phase)
      1) Ensure capillary permeability stabilizes and fluid shifts from interstitial spaces to plasma.
      2) Observe for pulmonary edema.
      3) Check vital signs, central venous pressure.
      4) Monitor output.
      5) Check laboratory values (electrolyte shifts such as low potassium; high sodium).

D. NURSING INTERVENTIONS

1. Control client pain.
   a. Medication (morphine sulfate/PCA pump/ NSAIDS)
   b. IV administration due to poor absorption of tissues
2. Meet nutritional needs.
   a. NPO until bowel sounds heard (usually has NG tube)
   b. Caloric needs high: 6,000 to 8,000 calories per day; may use enteral or total parenteral nutrition
   c. Diet should be high in protein, carbohydrates, fats, and vitamins
   d. Prevent stress ulcers: antacids, H2-receptor antagonists
3. Prevent complications.
   a. Infection
      1) Asepsis: reverse isolation
      2) Wound care (debridement, hydrotherapy)
      3) Antimicrobial therapy
   b. Contractures and deformities
      1) Range of motion initiated first postburn day

2) Positioning: position of function (pressure garments and splints)
c. Respiratory difficulty
1) Airway
2) Cough, turn, deep breathe
3) Assess for inhalation injury
4) Give oxygen
d. Emotional support
1) Essential for long-term adjustment
2) Alteration in body image

Methods of Treating Burns

A. Open Air or Exposure Method
1. Allows for drainage of burn exudate
2. Eschar forms protective covering (may constrict circulation requiring escharotomy)
3. Use of topical therapy
4. Skin easily inspected
5. Range of motion easier
6. Asepsis essential
7. Disadvantages
   a. Painful
   b. Heat loss
   c. Difficult to manage burns of hands and feet

B. Closed Method
1. Gauze dressing wrapped distal to proximal
2. Decreased fluid and heat loss
3. Limited mobility may result in contractures
4. Wound assessment limited

C. Topical Antimicrobial
1. Silver sulfadiazine (*Silvadene*)
   a. Broad-spectrum coverage including yeast
   b. Can be washed with water
2. Mafenide acetate (*Sulfamylon*)
   a. Broad-spectrum coverage
   b. Penetrates tissue wall
   c. Never use a dressing
   d. Breakdown of medication provides heavy acid load, may cause metabolic acidosis
   e. Painful
3. Bacitracin

D. Biologic Dressings
1. Homograft or allograft (human tissue donors)
2. Xenograft or heterograft (animal sources)
3. Amniotic membrane
4. Biosynthetic (Biobrane) or synthetic (transparent film)

E. Skin Care After Discharge
1. Control and prevent recurring swelling.
   a. Wear pressure garment 23.5 hr per day.
   b. Engage in regular exercise per physical therapy.
   c. Elevate affected areas.
2. Keep skin moisturized.
3. Combat itching.
   a. Take cool baths.
   b. Wear cotton fabric.
   c. Avoid tight clothing.
4. Avoid sun exposure.
5. Expect skin color to change.
   a. Scars fade from deep red to almost a natural skin tone.
6. Take in extra calories and protein.
7. Prevent contractures with use of splints.

NOTES

MENTAL HEALTH
NURSING

UNIT CONTENT

SYMBOLS

 Key Points

 Nursing Interventions

 Points to Remember

SECTION I

OVERVIEW

A. Mental Health Nursing: core, heart, basis, art of nursing

1. Interpersonal process
   a. Communication
   b. Caring
2. Goal
   a. Dealing with emotional responses to stress and crisis
   b. Satisfying basic needs
   c. Learning more effective ways of behaving
   d. Developing a healthy lifestyle
   e. Achieving a realistic and positive self-concept
3. Responsibilities
   a. Therapeutic relationship
   b. Therapeutic environment
4. Nursing process
   a. Assessment
   b. Diagnosis
   c. Planning
   d. Implementation
   e. Evaluation
5. Roles
   a. Counselor
   b. Teacher
   c. Advocate
   d. Leader, coordinator, manager

B. Theoretical Models of Treatment

1. Medical-biologic model
   a. Oriented to diagnosing mental disturbances as medical diseases with specific classifiable manifestations
      1) Causes
         a) Biochemical
         b) Psychological conditions
         c) Psychophysiological conditions
         d) Structural problems
      2) Diagnosis
         a) History
         b) Physical
         c) Diagnostic and Statistical Manual of Mental Disorders
      3) Focus
         a) Accurate diagnosis
         b) Selection of treatment modalities
         c) Nurse's role as supportive, not therapeutic
   b. Treatment
      1) Physical or somatic
      2) Interpersonal
2. Psychoanalytical model (Sigmund Freud)
   a. Oriented to uncovering childhood trauma and repressed feelings that cause conflicts in later life

KEY INFORMATION

1) Psychopathology
   a) Alterations in psychosocial behavior
   b) Stress-related behaviors
2) Structure of the mind
   a) Id: contains instinctual primitive drives
   b) Ego: mediates demands of primitive id and self-critical superego
   c) Superego: values and mores that guide behavior
   d) Conscious: ability to recall or remember events without difficulty
   e) Unconscious: memories and thoughts that do not enter awareness
3) Freud's psychosexual stages
   a) Oral: 0 to 1 years
   b) Anal: 1 to 3 years
   c) Phallic: (oedipal) 3 to 6 years
   d) Latency: 6 to 12 years
   e) Genital: 12 years to young adult

   b. Treatment modalities: oriented to clarifying the meaning of unconscious and conscious events, feelings and behavior to gain insight
      1) Transference (unconscious projection of feelings onto others)
      2) Countertransference
      3) Free association
      4) Dream analysis
      5) Catharsis (talking it out)

 c. **NURSING INTERVENTIONS**
   1) Establish guidelines for understanding human behavior.
   2) Determine adaptive/maladaptive personality traits.
   3) Individualize teaching based on psychosexual development.

3. Psychosocial developmental model: (Erik Erikson) oriented to psychosocial tasks that are accomplished throughout the life cycle; an individual who experiences failure in any stage is likely to have greater difficulty achieving success in future stages of development
   a. Uses an interdisciplinary approach to treatment; wellness is on a continuum
   b. Developmental stages (See Table II-1.)

 c. **NURSING INTERVENTIONS**
   1) Identify client's present stage of psychosocial development.
   2) Assist client to complete that stage (See Table II-2.).
   3) Set goals toward advancing through next stage(s).

TABLE II-1
ERIKSON'S STAGES OF DEVELOPMENT

STAGE	TASK	BEHAVIOR
Infancy (Birth to 1 year)	Trust vs Mistrust	Hopefulness, trusting vs Withdrawn, alienated
Toddler (12 months to 3 years)	Autonomy vs Shame, doubt	Self-control vs Compliance and compulsiveness, uncertainty
Preschooler (3 to 5 years)	Initiative vs Guilt	Realistic goals: explores, tests reality vs Strict limits on self-worry
School age (5 to 12 years)	Industry vs Inferiority	Explores, persistent, competes vs Incompetent, low self-esteem
Adolescent (12 to 20 years)	Identity vs Role diffusion	Sense of self vs Confusion, indecision
Young adult (20 to 40 years)	Intimacy vs Isolation	Commitment in love/work/play vs Superficial, impersonal
Middle adult (40 to 60 years)	Generativity vs Stagnation	Productivity, caring about others vs Self-centered and indulgent
Older adult (Older than 65)	Integrity vs Despair	Sense of accomplishment vs Hopelessness, depression

TABLE II-2
ERIKSON'S STAGES DEFINED

STAGE	DEFINITION
INFANCY (Birth to 1 year) Trust vs. Mistrust	Infants learn to trust one consistent caregiver (not necessarily the mother)
TODDLER (12 months to 3 years) Autonomy vs. Shame & Doubt	Learning independence and self-control; how to affect the environment with direct manipulation
PRESCHOOLER (3 to 5 years) Initiative vs. Guilt	Personal exploration and setting goals that influence the environment, evaluating own behavior
SCHOOL AGE (5 to 12 years) Industry vs. Inferiority	Developing sense of self and competency, learning to create and manipulate
ADOLESCENT (12 to 20 years) Identity vs. role diffusion	Integrating life experiences for a sense of self (trying new roles to see "what fits", peer pressure creates tumultuous rebellions, examines own sexual identity
YOUNG ADULT (20 to 40 years) Intimacy vs. isolation	Developing intimate or committed relationships, commit to work/profession, seek balance in life
MIDDLE ADULT (40 to 60 years) Generativity vs. Stagnation	Establishing and guiding next generation "giving back" to society with creativity, being productive and concerned
OLDER ADULT (Older than 65) Integrity vs. despair	Life review (necessary); accepting one's life as fulfilling; worthwhile, successful; providing a legacy

4. Basic human needs model (Maslow): a hierarchy of needs; a belief that needs are fulfilled in a progressive order
    a. Levels
        1) Physiologic
            a) Oxygen
            b) Food
            c) Sleep
            d) Sexual expression
        2) Safety
            a) Avoiding harm
            b) Feeling secure
        3) Love and belonging
            a) Group identity
            b) Being cared about
            c) Caring for others
            d) Play
        4) Self-esteem
            a) Self-confidence
            b) Self-acceptance
        5) Self-actualization
            a) Self-knowledge
            b) Satisfying, interpersonal relationships
            c) Environmental mastery
            d) Stress management

**TABLE II-3
MASLOW'S PYRAMID**

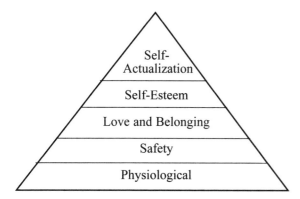

    b. Treatment
        1) Interdisciplinary: shared roles
        2) Developmental: interpersonal view of the self
        3) Goal: fill needs in progressive manner
     c. **NURSING INTERVENTIONS**
        1) Use needs and psychosocial development for assessment.
        2) Prioritize care based on needs according to hierarchy.
        3) Help client fulfill needs to relieve stress.
        4) Help client advance through stages to become more able to fulfill own needs.
        5) Help client develop new behaviors to reduce stress and prevent recurrences of mental illness and dysfunction.

5. Behaviorist model (behavior modification): "Maladaptive behavior is learned."
    a. Changes behavior by using learning theory: replaces nonadaptive behavior with more adaptive behavior
    b. Treatment
        1) Reconditioning: unlearning learned or maladaptive behavior
        2) Reinforcement: increases the probability of positive behavior recurring
            a) Positive reinforcement: per contract, use rewards to increase or reinforce desired behavior (e.g., adding something such as food, attention, phone privileges)
            b) Negative reinforcement: per contract, extinguish undesirable behavior by removing aversive consequences (e.g., removal of imposed restrictions)
        3) Positive punishment: decrease behavior by adding aversive consequences (e.g., quiet time)
        4) Negative punishment: decrease behavior by withdrawing a reward (e.g., privilege, such as an outing or calls)
    c. Main uses
        1) Children
        2) Clients who are severely regressed
        3) Personality disorders
        4) Anxiety disorders such as phobias
        5) Eating disorders
        6) Clients who are mentally disabled
    d. **NURSING INTERVENTIONS**
        1) Assess behavior.
        2) Implement specific behavioral interventions, either negative or positive reinforcement (contracts, role-play, progressive relaxation).
        3) Place emphasis on positive reinforcement as a primary nursing intervention.
        4) Evaluate progress and change behavioral interventions according to client's needs.

6. Community mental health model (psychosocial rehabilitation): individual interacting with environment
    a. Uses interdisciplinary team approach; nurse works as case manager and supervises the team
    b. Emphasis on providing treatment services in the least restrictive setting
    c. Treatment modalities
        1) Primary prevention: maintenance and promotion of health by teaching (e.g., risk factors, medication management, health promotion and wellness)

2) Secondary prevention: early diagnosis and treatment (e.g., crisis intervention, partial hospitalization, acute care hospitalization)
3) Tertiary prevention: rehabilitation, follow-up to avoid permanent disability (e.g., psychiatric day care)

 d. **NURSING INTERVENTIONS**
1) Provide holistic care.
2) Practice therapeutic use of self in the nurse/client relationship.
3) Use primary, secondary, and tertiary prevention.
4) Identify client needs, strengths, and community resources.

C. Treatment Modes

1. Crisis intervention
   a. Definitions
      1) Crisis: overwhelming feelings of helplessness when coping mechanisms are inadequate in response to an event; crisis lasts 4 to 8 weeks
      2) Crisis intervention: brief treatment used to assist client to effectively adapt to stressor; role of nurse is to provide safety, support, and to focus on client's strengths
   b. Type of crisis
      1) Situational: unanticipated, (e.g., death, divorce, termination from job)
      2) Transitional: maturational, anticipated (e.g., birth, marriage)
      3) Cultural/social (e.g., war)
   c. Responses to crisis
      1) Physiological (nervous system)
      2) Psychological (panic, fear, helplessness)
      3) Behavioral (extremes, talkative to withdrawn)
   d. Principles of crisis management
      1) Requires prompt intervention in calm, controlled atmosphere
      2) Focus on client strengthens positive coping skills
      3) Time limited (4 to 8 weeks)
    e. **NURSING INTERVENTIONS**
      1) Provide therapeutic interventions to keep client focused on immediate problem.
      2) Set specific goals for resolution.
      3) Help client develop more adaptive coping behaviors, sense of mastery.
      4) Use simple, concrete sentences with step-by-step direction to promote effective communication.
2. Group therapy
   a. Definition: collection of 7 to 10 individuals interacting together with a shared purpose
   b. Dynamics and concepts
      1) Content: work done to problem solve and

fulfill the group functions and goals
2) Process: what is happening in the group; interactions, seating, participation
3) Cohesiveness: feeling of belonging, helpfulness, problem solving, sharing
4) Norms: standards of behavior adhered to by group

 c. **NURSING INTERVENTIONS**
1) Assume leadership role.
2) Promote problem solving.
3) Direct group toward common goals and tasks.
4) Set limits and prevent scapegoating within group.
5) Clarify issues and promote consistency.
6) Support members.

d. Types of groups
1) Supportive, therapeutic
2) Task groups
3) Teaching groups
4) Psychotherapy
5) Peer support
6) Self-help groups
   a) 12-step (Alcoholics Anonymous [AA], Al-anon, Alateen, Overeaters Anonymous)
   b) Recovery, Inc.
   c) Ostomy Clubs

3. Family therapy
   a. Definition: psychotherapy in which the focus is on the family as the unit of treatment, not just one individual
   b. Concepts
      1) Systems approach: member with the manifestations, illness
      2) Scapegoating: the object of blame or displaced aggression, usually one member of the family
      3) Family involvement necessary for treatment

 c. **NURSING INTERVENTIONS**
1) Help family re-establish communication between members.
2) Help family redefine roles and rules.
3) Clarify ambiguous communication patterns between family members.
4) Support individual family members.
5) Teach family problem-solving techniques.
6) Help the family accept differences among the members.

4. Milieu therapy
   a. Definition: management of the client's environment to promote a positive living experience and facilitate recovery (holistic approach)

b. Concepts
  1) Client government: groups and meetings between client and staff to promote shared responsibility and cooperation
  2) Environment in the facility as close to the "real world" as possible and has potential for therapeutic value

 c. **NURSING INTERVENTIONS**
  1) Provide guidance in developing new ways of helping the client relate and learn to cope more effectively.
  2) Help client maintain strengths.
  3) Manage the client's day-to-day activities.
  4) Provide a positive, therapeutic environment through environmental manipulation.
  5) Assist in developing effective relationship and coping skills.

5. Adjunctive therapies
  a. Definition: therapies used to aid assessment, increase social skills, encourage expression of feelings, and provide opportunities to raise self-esteem, relieve tension, and be creative
  b. Types
    1) Dance: movement
    2) Recreational: picnic, volleyball
    3) Occupational: painting, hand work
    4) Art: clay, painting, drawing
    5) Alternative therapies: pet therapy, reminiscence therapy, music therapy

6. Interdisciplinary team approach
  a. Definition: A team with members of different disciplines involved in a formal arrangement to provide client services while maximizing educational interchange

b. Members of the team
  1) Nurse
  2) Primary care provider
  3) Social worker
  4) Psychologist
  5) Case manager
  6) Occupational therapist
  7) Recreational therapist
  8) Job coaches
  9) Mental health technicians

 c. **NURSING INTERVENTIONS:** The nurse should work collaboratively with the interdisciplinary team to promote and maintain health.

D. Mental Health/Mental Illness Continuum (See Table II-4.)
  1. Mental health
    a. Positive attitude toward self
    b. Growth, development, self-actualization, autonomy
    c. Ability to cope with stress
    d. Reality perception and environmental mastery
  2. Mental illness
    a. Inability to cope/manage stress
    b. Development of maladaptive behavior
    c. Disruption in ability to relate successfully with others
    d. Inability to meet basic needs in a socially acceptable way
  3. Defense mechanisms
    a. Definition: unconscious operations used to defend against anxiety or stress and relieve emotional conflict
    b. In contrast, coping mechanisms are conscious efforts to deal with daily frustrations and conflicts

TABLE II-4
MENTAL HEALTH/ILLNESS CONTINUUM

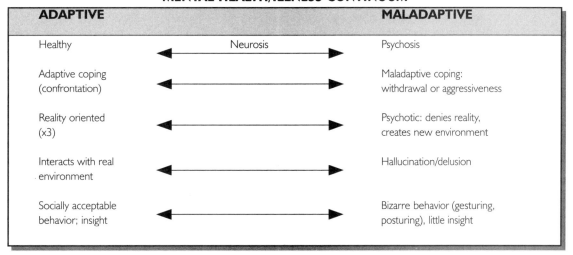

ADAPTIVE		MALADAPTIVE
Healthy	Neurosis	Psychosis
Adaptive coping (confrontation)		Maladaptive coping: withdrawal or aggressiveness
Reality oriented (x3)		Psychotic: denies reality, creates new environment
Interacts with real environment		Hallucination/delusion
Socially acceptable behavior; insight		Bizarre behavior (gesturing, posturing), little insight

c. Unconscious defense mechanisms (See Table II-17 of definitions at end of mental health content.)

1) Denial: avoidance of disagreeable reality by ignoring or refusing to recognize it

2) Rationalization: offering a socially acceptable or logical explanation for otherwise unacceptable impulses, feelings, and behaviors (e.g., "I don't pay taxes because the government wastes money.")

3) Displacement: transferring painful feelings to a neutral object (e.g., being angry at brother, so dog is kicked as a result)

4) Projection: attributing own thoughts or impulses to another person (e.g., "You made me take a wrong turn.")

5) Compensation: putting forth extra effort to achieve in areas of real or imagined deficiency (e.g., an unpopular student excels as a scholar)

6) Reaction formation: displaying overt behavior or attitudes in precisely the opposite direction of unacceptable conscious or unconscious impulses (e.g., feeling compassion for a person you dislike)

7) Identification: unconsciously adopting the characteristics of another, generally someone who possesses attributes that are admired or envied

8) Sublimation: directing energy from unacceptable drives into socially acceptable behavior (e.g., aggressive person becomes a star football player)

9) Regression: going back to an early level of emotional development (e.g., becoming dependent on someone else for all decisions)

10) Undoing: a compulsive response negating or reversing a previous unacceptable act (e.g., washing hands [of guilt] after touching germs)

11) Introjection: incorporating the traits of others (e.g., a client who is depressed causes the nurse to become depressed)

12) Isolation: splitting-off response in which person blocks feeling associated with unpleasant experience (e.g., planning out funeral details of a loved one)

13) Splitting: viewing people as all good or all bad, failure to integrate positive and negative qualities

14) Repression: unconscious, involuntary forgetting of unacceptable or painful thoughts, impulses, feelings, or actions (e.g., forgetting what was on a difficult exam)

d. Conscious defense mechanism: Suppression: deliberate forgetting of unacceptable or painful thoughts, impulses, acts

E. Nurse/Client Relationship: an interpersonal, collaborative helping process and organized sequence of events leading toward a mutually identified goal

1. Characteristics
   a. Professional vs. social
   b. Purposeful
   c. Nonjudgmental
   d. Designated setting and time
   e. Organized sequence of events
   f. Goal directed to facilitate client's growth vs. reciprocal
      1) Collaborative: contract that outlines and clarifies role expectations
      2) Confidential

2. Phases of the nurse/client relationship
   a. Preinteraction phase
      1) Gather data from secondary source.
      2) Avoid prejudgment.
      3) Assess nurse's feelings.
      4) Assess client's feelings.
   b. Orientation phase: assessment
      1) Introduction: purpose, roles, responsibilities
      2) Establishing trust
         a) Honesty
         b) Remaining nonjudgmental
         c) Empathy
         d) Offering self
      3) Assessing client
         a) Orientation
         b) Activities of daily living (degree of ability to perform)
         c) Physical status
         d) Memory (recent and remote)
         e) Emotional state
         f) Intellectual capacity
         g) Family history
         h) Spiritual history
         i) Alcohol and drug history (over-the-counter and prescription)
         j) Identifying problem
      4) Formulating contract
         a) Time of meeting
         b) Confidentiality
         c) Focus: goals that are behaviorally stated
   c. Working phase: planning and intervention
      1) Establish specific collaborative goals.
      2) Explore thoughts, feelings, and actions.
      3) Establish nursing diagnosis.
      4) Problem solve.

d. Termination phase: termination begins on admission or first contact; the nurse prepares the client for this eventuality during the first meeting.
1) Evaluate behavioral goals.
2) Transfer to other support systems.
3) Assess for separation reactions such as regression, acting out, anger, withdrawal.
4) Help express and work through feelings.
5) Be alert to nurse's response to separation.
6) Do not promise to continue the relationship or schedule future appointments.

KEY INFORMATION

 3) Communication tools
a) Listening: nonverbal, using eye contact
b) Offering self: "I'll stay with you."
c) Focusing: on "here and now" and on the client
d) Broad openings: "How are things going today?"
e) Clarifying: "What does that mean to you?"
f) Reflecting: directing back ideas, feelings, and content, "You feel tense when you fight."
g) Empathy: stating a feeling implied by the client
h) Summarizing: "Today we have discussed…"
i) Silence: sitting, conveying nonverbal interest
j) Sharing perceptions: "You seem angry."
k) Restating: repeating the main thought "You are sad."
l) Validating: "Are you saying…"
m) Giving information (e.g., answering a direct question, teaching)
4) Communication blocks
a) Falsely reassuring: "Don't worry."
b) Agreeing and disagreeing: "I think you did the right thing."
c) Advising: "You should . . ."
d) Judging: "That was good."
e) Belittling: "Everyone feels like that."
f) Defending: "All the doctors here are great."
g) Approving: good or bad
h) Focusing on nurse: "I feel that way, too."
i) Changing the subject
j) Ignoring a client
k) Changing client's words or assuming feelings

 5) **NURSING INTERVENTIONS:**
a) Avoid communication blocks.
b) Use open-ended questions and responses vs. closed.
c) Avoid "why" questions that the client is unable to answer.
d) Limit questions to one idea at a time.
e) Communicate client's nonverbal communication: "I notice you are shaking your legs."
f) Avoid invading the client's space.
g) Use touch carefully - can be interpreted as caring or as a threat.

SECTION II

ANXIETY

A. Definition: anxiety and apprehension are tension in response to a perceived physical or psychological threat (internal or external) resulting in feelings of helplessness and uncertainty

B. Responses
1. Psychological
   a. Fear
   b. Impending doom
   c. Helplessness
   d. Insecurity
   e. Low self-confidence
   f. Anger
   g. Guilt
2. Defense mechanisms
   a. Displacement
   b. Regression
   c. Repression
   d. Sublimation
3. Physiological: nervous system
   a. Dry mouth
   b. Elevated vital signs
   c. Diarrhea
   d. Increased urination
   e. Palpitations
   f. Diaphoresis
   g. Hyperventilation
   h. Fatigue
   i. Insomnia
   j. Sexual dysfunction
   k. Irritability
   l. Fidgeting, pacing
4. Behaviors
   a. Fight-or-flight response
   b. Talkative, giggly, angry, withdrawn

C. Levels of Anxiety (See Table II-5.)

KEY INFORMATION

 The initial nursing priority is to reduce the client's anxiety to a tolerable level, since learning cannot occur until the client's anxiety is manageable.

D. Maladaptive Responses to Anxiety

1. Anxiety disorders: characterized by fear that is out of proportion to external events with attacks lasting minutes to hours
   a. Panic disorders
      1) Definition: sudden onset of intense apprehension, fear, or terror (panic attacks)
      2) Physical manifestations
         a) Dyspnea
         b) Palpitations
         c) Chest pain
         d) Faintness, dizziness
         e) Fear of dying or going crazy (out of control)
         f) Choking
         g) Depersonalization or derealization
         h) Hyperventilation
       3) **NURSING INTERVENTIONS**
         a) Stay with client and remain calm.
         b) Provide reassurance and support.
         c) Remove anxiety-producing stimuli.
         d) Have client take deep breaths.
         e) Distract client from anxiety-producing stimuli.
         f) Provide a paper bag for hyperventilation.
   b. Generalized anxiety disorder
      1) Definition: excessive worry about numerous things out of proportion to the impact of the events
      2) Worries including finances, health, job responsibilities, interpersonal concerns
      3) Manifestations:
         a) Restlessness
         b) Irritability
         c) Poor concentration
         d) Sleep disturbance

TABLE II-5
LEVELS OF ANXIETY

LEVEL	PHYSIOLOGIC RESPONSE	COGNITIVE STATE	BEHAVIORAL CHANGES	NURSING INTERVENTIONS
Mild (+)	Slight discomfort, restlessness; tension relief; fidgeting, tapping	Perceptual field can be heightened; learning can occur.	* - Restlessness (inability to work toward goal) * - Examine alternatives	* - Listen to client. * - Promote insight, problem solving.
Moderate (++)	Increased pulse, respirations, shakiness, voice tremors, difficulty concentrating, pacing	Perceptual field narrows; client is selective in attention.	* - Focus on immediate events. * - Benefits from guidance of others.	* - Remain calm, and rational in discussion. * - Encourage relaxation exercises.
Severe (+++)	Elevated BP, tachycardia, somatic reports, hyperventilation, confusion	Perceptual field greatly reduced; attention scattered; cannot attend to events even when pointed out	- Feelings of increasing threat; purposeless activity * - Feeling of impending doom	* - Listen to client. * - Encourage expression of feelings. * - Establish concrete activity. Reduce stimuli by channeling energy into simple tasks.
Panic (++++)	- Immobility or severe hyper-activity; cool, clammy skin; pallor; dilated pupils; severe shakiness; chest pain * - Prolonged anxiety can lead to exhaustion.	- Perceptual field closed. * - Hallucinations or delusions may occur. * - Effective decision making is impossible.	- Mute or psychomotor agitation * - May strike out physically or withdraw - Loss of control	* - Isolate from stimuli. * - Stay with client. * - Remain very calm. * - Decrease demands. * - Protect client safety. * - Do not touch client.
* Important				

4) **NURSING INTERVENTIONS**
   a) Allow opportunity to discuss preceding events.
   b) Help client to identify the source of anxiety.
   c) Help client to identify his or her strengths.
   d) Assist the client in the development of positive coping skills.
   e) Teach cognitive therapy principles.

c. Phobic disorders
   1) Definition: persistent or irrational fear of a specific object, activity, or situation that leads to avoidance (e.g., fear of flying)
   2) Types
      a) Agoraphobia: fear of being in places or situations from which there is no escape
      b) Specific: irrational fear of object or situation
      c) Social (social anxiety disorder): irrational fear that social situations expose client to possible ridicule or embarrassment
   3) Defense Mechanisms
      a) Repression
      b) Displacement
      c) Avoidance

   4) **NURSING INTERVENTIONS**
      a) Teach client relaxation techniques.
      b) Avoid major decision making.
      c) Use behavior modification techniques.
      d) Avoid competitive situations.
      e) Provide gradual desensitization experiences.
      f) Assist client in verbalizing thoughts and feelings of anxiety.

d. Obsessive-compulsive disorder
   1) Definition: recurring obsessions or compulsions
      a) Obsessions: recurring thoughts of violence, contamination, doubt, and worry that cannot be voluntarily removed from consciousness
      b) Compulsions: recurring, irresistible impulse to perform acts (e.g., touching, rearranging, checking, opening and closing, washing)
      c) Obsessions and compulsions may occur together or separately
      d) Client's attempt to reduce anxiety
   2) Characteristics
      a) Irrational coping to handle guilt
      b) Feelings of inferiority and low self-esteem
      c) Compulsion to repeat act

   d) Repeating act to prevent severe anxiety
   e) Defense mechanisms
      (1) Displacement
      (2) Undoing
      (3) Isolation
      (4) Reaction formation

3) **NURSING INTERVENTIONS:** aimed at reducing client anxiety
   a) Distract: substitute.
   b) Do not interrupt compulsive act.
   c) Schedule time to complete ritual; gradually decrease the time and number of times ritual is performed.
   d) Provide safety.
   e) Maintain structure, schedules, activities.
   f) Demonstrate acceptance of individual.
   g) Encourage expression of feelings.
   h) Antianxiety medications may be used to relieve manifestations.

e. Posttraumatic stress disorder (PTSD)
   1) Definition: repeated re-experiencing of a highly traumatic event
   2) Traumatic events could including military combat, prisoner-of-war experiences, natural disasters, crime-related events, rape, or hostage events
   3) Manifestations
      a) Persistent re-experiencing of events (flashbacks)
      b) Persistent avoidance of the stimuli associated with trauma
      c) Feelings of detachment or emptiness
      d) Irritability
      e) Difficulty sleeping, nightmares
      f) Difficulty concentrating
      g) Hypervigilance and startle response

4) **NURSING INTERVENTIONS**
   a) Help client to identify community support systems.
   b) Teach client stress reduction techniques.
   c) Encourage client to attend a support group of other persons with PTSD and/or persons who have experienced the same or similar trauma to increase the client's social support.

2. Somatoform disorders: physical manifestations and reports without organic impairment (no real pathology) (e.g., soldiers paralyzed during war with no real injury)
   a. Conversion disorders (hysteria)
      1) Definition: alteration in physical function that is an expression of an unconscious psychological need

TABLE II-6
ANTIANXIETY AGENTS AND ADVERSE REACTIONS

CHEMICAL CLASS	GENERIC NAME	TRADE NAME	MEDICATION ALERTS
Benzodiazepine compounds	- chlordiazepoxide	- *Librium*	- Benzodiazepines: Warn clients about sedating effects; avoid activities requiring mental alertness; monitor for signs of drug dependence Withdrawal up to 2 weeks; client is at risk for seizure
	- diazepam	- *Valium*	
	- oxazepam	- *Serax*	
	- clorazepate	- *Tranxene*	
	- lorazepam	- *Ativan*	
	- alprazolam	- *Xanax*	
	- clonazepam	- *Klonopin*	
	- clomipramine	- *Anafranil*	- Anafranil, commonly used for OCD; should be cautiously used in clients with cardiovascular disease; is potentially fatal in overdose
Mephenesin-like compounds	meprobamate	*Miltown, Equanil*	
Sedating antihistamines	hydroxyzine	*Vistaril, Atarax*	Antihistamines tend to cause drying and sedation.
Beta-blockers	propranolol	*Inderal*	
(SSRI) Selective serotonin reuptake inhibitors	paroxetine	*Paxil*	Shown to be effective with social anxiety disorder; allow 2 to 3 weeks to note effects.
Anxiolytics	buspirone	*BuSpar*	BuSpar-nonsedating; allow 2-3 weeks to note effects; do not use concurrently with alcohol or history of hepatic disease.

ADVERSE REACTIONS	NURSING INTERVENTIONS
Dry mouth	Provide candies, fluids.
Blurred vision	Will disappear within a week
Urinary retention	Monitor I&O; monitor for distention, run water
Drowsiness or sedation	Instruct client not to operate machines; do not give with other CNS depressants.
Ataxia	Use side rails if needed; stay with client if out of bed.
Tremors	Observe severity.
Hypotension	Take blood pressure often.
Tolerance	Observe for proper usage and effect; withdraw gradually.

MEDICATION INTERACTIONS

- CNS depressants: action potentiated, avoid alcohol and concurrent use of MAOIs
- Tolerance does develop; discontinue slowly to minimize symptoms and rebound symptoms of insomnia or anxiety.
- Older adults are more vulnerable to adverse reactions; safety risk.
- Possible paradoxical reactions can occur in children and older adults.
- Stopping suddenly could cause seizures or death.

2) Characteristics of manifestations
   a) Sensory: blindness, deafness, loss of sensation in extremities
   b) Motor: mutism, paralysis of extremities, ataxia, dizziness
   c) Visceral: headaches, difficulty breathing
   d) Convulsive disorder with atypical seizure response
   e) Little concern about manifestations: *la belle indifference*
   f) Defense mechanism: repression of conflict and conversion of anxiety into manifestations
   g) Primary gain: suppressing conflict
   h) Secondary gain: sympathy or avoidance of unpleasant activity gained

 3) **NURSING INTERVENTIONS**
   a) Redirect client away from manifestations.
   b) Encourage client to express feelings.
   c) Use stress-reduction techniques.
   d) Teach client relaxation techniques.
   e) Understand that the symptoms are real to the client.
   f) Engage client in schedule of daily activities to decrease time spent focusing on symptoms and counter secondary gain.

b. Hypochondriasis
  1) Definition: exaggerated preoccupation with physical health, not based on real organic disorders; no pathology
  2) Characteristics
   a) Multiple manifestations
   b) Worried/anxious about manifestations
   c) Seeks medical care frequently from multiple health care providers

 3) **NURSING INTERVENTIONS**
   a) Help client express feelings.
   b) Set limits on rumination.
   c) Do not "feed into" the manifestations.

3. Psychophysiological/psychosomatic disorders
a. Definition: stress-related medical disorders with true pathology; psychosocial factors predispose client to episodes of illness and influence the progression of manifestations; can be fatal if not treated adequately; these disorders are characterized by increasing anxiety in addition to the physical manifestations; clients are often first treated in medical facilities
b. Defense mechanisms
  1) Repression
  2) Introjection

c. Types
  1) Migraine
  2) Ulcerative colitis
  3) Peptic ulcer
  4) Eczema
  5) Cancer
  6) Rheumatoid arthritis
 d. **NURSING INTERVENTIONS**
  1) Care for physical signs of client.
  2) Educate client about body/mind relationship.
  3) Teach client relaxation techniques (e.g., biofeedback imagery, progressive relaxation).
  4) Assist client to express thoughts and feelings.
  5) Encourage self-health promotion and regulation activities (e.g., relaxation, exercise).
  6) Promote positive lifestyle changes.

4. Dissociative disorders (hysterical neuroses)
a. Definition: splitting off an idea or emotion from one's consciousness; "psychological flight" from anxiety (common with abused children)
b. Types
  1) Dissociative identity disorder
  2) Dissociative fugue
  3) Dissociative amnesia
  4) Depersonalization disorder
 c. **NURSING INTERVENTIONS**
  1) Assess client to rule out organic pathology.
  2) Help client recognize when dissociation occurs.
  3) Help client express feelings.
  4) Initiate individual, group, and family psychotherapy.

5. Somatic treatment for maladaptive responses to anxiety, insomnia, and stress-related conditions
6. Antianxiety agents: anxiolytic, minor tranquilizers (See Table II-6.)
7. Expressive therapy for maladaptive responses to anxiety
a. Client with poor concentration: group work, simple tasks
b. Client with hyperactivity: decrease external stimuli, one-to-one interaction, walks, noncompetitive activities

KEY INFORMATION
 Antianxiety medications are not a cure for anxiety, but a temporary means to reduce anxiety; antianxiety medications can be highly lethal in overdose; monitor clients who are suicidal closely; older adults clients are easily sedated and at risk for falls with benzodiazepines.

SECTION III

SCHIZOPHRENIA

A. Definition: group of psychotic disorders characterized by regression, thought disturbances (including delusions and hallucinations), bizarre dress and behavior, poverty of speech, abnormal motor behavior, and withdrawal

B. Overview

1. Bleuler's four A's
   a. Autism: preoccupation with self and inner experience
   b. Affect: feeling tone is flat, blunted, or inappropriate
   c. Ambivalence: conflicting strong feelings that may confuse, frighten, or immobilize
   d. Loose association: disrupted or disorganized thinking
2. Appearance: disheveled
3. Other major manifestations
   a. Delusions: fixed false beliefs; can be paranoid, grandiose, or somatic delusions
   b. Hallucinations: sensory perceptions without any environmental stimuli (e.g., hearing voices, seeing spiders, smelling foul)
   c. Illusions: misidentification of actual environmental stimuli; client may see an electrical cord as a snake
   d. Ideas of reference: personalizing environmental stimuli (e.g., client believes static on telephone is wiretapping)
   e. Neologisms: nonsense words
   f. Circumstantiality: can't come to point, includes nonessential details
   g. Blocking: interruption of speech due to distracting thoughts, words, ideas, subjects
   h. Regressive behavior: behavior appropriate at earlier stage of development
   i. Echolalia: repetition of words or phrases heard from another person
   j. Echopraxia: imitation of movement or gestures of another person
   k. Pressured speech: words rush out quickly
   l. Poor interpersonal relationships
   m. Declining ability to work, socialize, care for self
4. Characteristics and defense mechanisms
   a. Depersonalization: feeling alienated from self, no ego boundaries
   b. Projection
   c. Regression
   d. Denial
   e. Fantasy world

C. Schizophrenic Disorders

1. Types
   a. Disorganized: incoherent, severe thought disturbance, shallow, inappropriate, often silly behavior and mannerisms
   b. Catatonic (psychomotor)
      1) Stupor: lessening of response
      2) Excitement: increase in activity
      3) Waxy flexibility: bizarre posturing
      4) Negativism: doing the opposite of what is being asked
      5) Mutism: continuous refusal to speak
      6) Severe withdrawal
   c. Paranoid (can be dangerous)
      1) Hallucination: grandiose or persecutory
      2) Delusions: persecution and grandeur
      3) Emotions: angry, suspicious, argumentative, mistrust, excessive religiosity of a punitive nature
   d. Undifferentiated
      1) Mixed characteristics
      2) Meets criteria of more than one type
 2. **NURSING INTERVENTIONS**
   a. Provide physical care.
   b. Promote client safety.
   c. Increase client trust with a one-on-one nurse/client relationship.
   d. Orient client to reality.
   e. Provide structure to the client's day.
   f. Involve client's family.
   g. Keep interactions simple and concrete; often nonverbal and short.
   h. Help work through regressive behavior.
   i. Decrease bizarre behavior, anxiety, agitation, aggression.
   j. Deal with hallucinations.
      1) Distract client.
      2) Do not confront; do not deny.
      3) Point out that others do not share the same perception, but acknowledge that the hallucination is real to the client.
      4) Seek to establish feelings.
      5) Avoid leaving client alone (Client will hallucinate more.).
      6) Engage client in activities (e.g., current events discussion groups).
   k. Provide least restrictive environment and avoid restraining.
   l. Provide care in a firm matter-of-fact manner that allows client participation.
   m. Provide consistency, positive reinforcement, and unconditional acceptance of client.

D. Paranoid Personality Disorder

1. Definition: insidious development of a permanent and unshakable delusional system accompanied by preservation of clear and orderly thinking

2. Characteristics
   a. Projection: unacceptable feelings attributed to others
   b. Delusions of grandeur and/or persecution
   c. Ideas of reference (e.g., personalizing environmental stimuli)
   d. Resistance to treatment
   e. Loneliness and distrust (failed Erikson's Stages)
   f. Refusal to eat
   g. Suspiciousness and fear
   h. Emotional expressions that are appropriate to content of delusional system
   i. Argumentative and hostile
3. **NURSING INTERVENTIONS**
    a. Persecutory delusions
      1) Do not argue or confront.
      2) Interject reality when appropriate.
      3) Get to client's feeling level.
      4) Discuss topics other than delusions.
   b. Aggression and hostility
      1) Help client express self verbally.
      2) Set limits and offer alternatives.
      3) Keep at a safe distance.
      4) Do not respond with aggression; use calm, controlled tone.
      5) Use direct, simple statements.
      6) Keep other clients away.
      7) Decrease stimulation with time out.
      8) Have back up and use speed when restraining.
      9) Seclude as last resort.
      10) Provide outlet for aggression.
      11) Monitor client.
   c. Fear of being poisoned
      1) Serve food in containers.
      2) Medications should be wrapped or in containers.
      3) Do not covertly put medications in juice.
      4) Open medications in presence of client.
   d. Attempt to de-escalate client's aggression; allow opportunity to gain control.
   e. Avoid verbal and nonverbal communication that could be interpreted as a threat.
   f. Respect the client's personal space, and avoid touching as client may strike out in response to fear and anxiety.
   g. Maintain an attitude of superiority.
      1) Small groups, ratio of one nurse to one client
      2) Activities that ensure success
      3) Limits without judging
      4) Increase self-esteem
      5) Encourage client to verbalize feelings

E. Pervasive Developmental Disorders (usually seen in children)
   1. Autistic disorders
      a. Characteristics
         1) Lack of interest in human contact
         2) Compulsive need for following routines; distressed by slight environmental changes
         3) Abnormal or no social play
         4) Autoerotic behavior (e.g., rocking, excessive masturbation)
         5) Abnormal nonverbal communication
         6) Self-mutilation (e.g., head banging)
         7) Impaired ability to form peer relationships
         8) Abnormal production of speech and content
         9) Obsessional attachments to inanimate objects
         10) Impaired ability to form peer relationships
       b. **NURSING INTERVENTIONS**
         1) Assess social and physical aspects of client.
         2) Assess family understanding and coping.
         3) Facilitate communication (verbal and/or nonverbal).
         4) Maintain optimum level of functioning and prevent regression.
   2. Attention deficit hyperactivity disorder (ADHD)
      a. Characteristics
         1) Fails to complete task
         2) Easily distracted
         3) Difficulty concentrating
         4) Acts before thinking, impulsive
         5) Has difficulty sitting still
       b. **NURSING INTERVENTIONS**
         1) Assist to communicate effectively.
         2) Set stage for improving ego function.
         3) Help learn more adaptive coping behaviors.
         4) Initiate supportive and educative methods for assisting parent and child.
         5) Promote client safety when head banging or other self-destructive behaviors are exhibited.
         6) Techniques to use:
            a) Play therapy
            b) Cognitive-behavioral therapy
            c) Family therapy
            d) Medication Therapy
               (1) Methylphenidate hydrochloride (*Ritalin*)
               (2) Amphetamine sulfate (*Adderall*)
               (3) Dextroamphetamine sulfate (*Dexedrine*)
               (4) Pemoline (*Cylert*)
               (5) Atomoxetine (*Strattera*)

TABLE II-7
ANTIPSYCHOTIC AGENTS AND ADVERSE REACTIONS

CHEMICAL CLASS	GENERIC NAME	TRADE NAME	MEDICATION ALERT
Phenothiazine, aliphatic	chlorpromazine	Thorazine	- Photosensitivity - Orthostatic hypotension
Phenothiazine, piperidine	- thioridazine - mesoridazine	- Mellaril - Serentil	
Phenothiazine, piperazine	- fluphenazine - perphenazine - trifluoperazine	- Prolixin - Trilafon - Stelazine	- High potency - Risk for extrapyramidal effects (EPS)
Thioxanthene, piperazine	thiothixene	Navane	
Butyrophenone	haloperidol	Haldol	
Dibenzoxazepine	- clozapine	- Clozaril	- Can cause agranulocytosis - Weekly CBCs required - Effective in treating clients not responding to other neuroleptics
Thienobenzodiazepine	- olanzapine - quetiapine - sertindole	- Zyprexa - Seroquel - Serlect	- Mirrored after Clozaril - Does not require weekly CBCs - Can cause significant weight gain
Benzisoxazole	risperidone ziprasidone aripiprazole	Risperdal Geodon Abilify	- Less risk of EPS - Targets both positive and negative symptoms - Can be used safely in older adult clients

ADVERSE REACTIONS	NURSING INTERVENTIONS	MEDICATION ALERT
Sedation	Most common in low-potency antipsychotics; ask primary care provider if entire dose can be given at bedtime	Sedation is common in Thorazine and Mellaril.
Extrapyramidal effects (EPS): parkinsonian symptoms (for example: fine hand tremors, pill rolling, drooling, muscle stiffness)	Report to the primary care provider; specific medication may be changed; antiparkinsonian medication is given to control manifestations.	EPS is usually associated with high potency (Stelazine, Navane, Haldol, and Loxitane); least likely to have EPS with Mellaril
Dystonia: muscle spasm of the face and neck; eyes rolling back in head	Report to primary care provider; usually an antiparkinsonian medication is given and the antipsychotic medication is changed.	Dystonia is most common in males taking Haldol, Prolixin, Stelazine.
Akathisia: restlessness, inability to sit still	Call primary care provider; if treated with antiparkinsonian medications, may need to change antipsychotic medication	
Tardive dyskinesia: lip smacking, sucking, tongue protrusion, jerking of the head and neck, extension and flexion of the fingers, back and forth movement of spine, movement of the arms	Careful observation in early steps of treatment; discontinue medication at first sign to prevent permanent disability; abnormal involuntary movement scale (AIMS) is used to assess clients for permanent adverse reactions	

TABLE II-7
ANTIPSYCHOTIC AGENTS AND ADVERSE REACTIONS (CONTINUED)

ADVERSE REACTIONS	NURSING INTERVENTIONS	MEDICATION ALERT
Anticholinergic - Dry mouth - Constipation - Urinary retention - Blurred vision - Nasal congestion - Orthostatic hypotension caution client to stand up slowly	- Provide candies, fluids. - Provide laxatives; modify diet. - Monitor I&O. - Client teaching: effects transient and disappear in a week. - Increase humidity (Use showers.). - Monitor BP frequently, sitting and standing.	Thorazine, Mellaril, Risperdal, and Zyprexa have potential to cause orthostatic hypotension, especially in older adults.
Hypotension	Monitor BP frequently, sitting and standing; caution client to stand up slowly	
Photosensitivity	Sunscreen; cover up with clothing	Thorazine: exposure to sun causes dark purplish pigmentation of skin.
Agranulocytosis	Observe for signs of infection or nosebleeds and report immediately if present; discontinue medication; monitor weekly CBCs.	Most often seen with Clozaril
Retinopathy	Sunglasses	Thorazine and Mellaril may cause retinopathy.
Neuroleptic malignant syndrome (NMS) (Can be fatal)	Discontinue medication and report immediately if manifestations occur (altered consciousness, unstable BP and pulse, fever, muscle rigidity, diaphoresis, and tremors) (extrapyramidal effects with fever)	All neuroleptics can cause NMS, an extreme emergency situation.
Endocrine - Breast enlargement	- Yearly breast exams	- Neuroendocrine effects are most often seen with Mellaril; these symptoms are related to decreased hypothalamic function.
- Decreased libido; ejaculatory incompetence	- Decrease dose or change to high-potency medications.	
- Appetite increase, weight gain	- Exercise/diet regimen	- Most common adverse effect of Zyprexa is weight gain; Seroquel is an alternative medication to use if client has extreme weight gain.

DRUG INTERACTIONS
- MAOIs
- Anticonvulsants

F. Medications: antipsychotics (for schizophrenic and paranoid behavior patterns); compliance is a problem secondary to adverse reactions.

1. Blocking dopamine receptors
   a. Target positive manifestations
      1) Negativism
      2) Combativeness
      3) Disorganization
      4) Hallucinations, delusions
      5) Flat affect
      6) Suspiciousness
      7) Seclusiveness
      8) Self-care deficits
   b. Negative manifestations not affected
      1) Apathy
      2) Withdrawal
      3) Insight
      4) Lack of interest
      5) Blunted affect
      6) Judgment
2. Antipsychotic agents (major tranquilizers or neuroleptic agents) (See Table II-7.)
3. Medications to control extrapyramidal reactions (CNS)
   a. Commonly used
      1) Trihexyphenidyl (*Artane*)
      2) Benztropine mesylate (*Cogentin*)
      3) Diphenhydramine (*Benadryl*)
   b. Adverse reactions: anticholinergic
      1) Blurred vision
      2) Dry mouth
      3) Constipation
      4) Urinary retention
      5) Drowsiness
      6) Nervousness
      7) Photosensitivity
      8) Hypotension
4. Medication abuse potential with benztropine mesylate (*Cogentin*) and antihistamines
5. Benztropine mesylate (*Cogentin*) contraindicated for clients with narrow angle glaucoma

MOOD DISORDERS AND ASSOCIATED BEHAVIORS

A. Depression and Elation

1. Definition
   a. Depression: mood state of gloom, despondency, and dejection, accompanying physical, cognitive, and behavioral responses
   b. Mania: predominant mood is elevated; great amount of activity
2. Continuum of emotional responses (See Table II-8.)
3. Range and severity of moods
   a. Grief: average duration is 24 months; known as dysfunctional grief when the client is unable to accept loss after 24-month period
      1) Precipitating factors
         a) Death in family
         b) Separation
         c) Divorce
         d) Physical illness
         e) Work failure
         f) Disappointment
      2) Stages (Kübler-Ross)
         a) Denial
         b) Anger
         c) Bargaining
         d) Depression
         e) Acceptance
       3) **NURSING INTERVENTIONS**
         a) Accept client's stage.
         b) Encourage expression of feelings.
         c) Help through stages by providing anticipatory guidance.

KEY INFORMATION
 4) Unresolved grief produces psychotic and neurotic manifestations such as chronic depression, psychosomatic disorders, acting-out behavior

TABLE II-8
CONTINUUM OF EMOTIONAL RESPONSES

ADAPTIVE RESPONSES		MALADAPTIVE RESPONSES
- Sadness - Grief	- Dysthymic - Cyclothymic - Reactive - Exogenous	- Major depression - Bipolar disorder - Endogenous
No treatment ⟶ Psychotherapy ⟵⟶ Medications		
Duration of illness increases ⟶		

b. Moderate mood disorders
  1) Types
     a) Dysthymia: chronically depressed mood
     b) Cyclothymic: cycles of depression and hypomania (not as severe as mania)
  2) Characteristics: depression (dysthymia)
     a) Pessimism
     b) Insomnia or hypersomnia
     c) Social withdrawal
     d) Feelings of worthlessness, not caring, little pressure, irritability
     e) Low energy
c. Severe mood disorders
  1) Major depression
     a) Weight gain or loss of more than 10 lb
     b) Sleep disturbances
     c) Loss of pleasure or interest in usual activities, including sex
     d) Low energy, fatigue
     e) Feelings of helplessness and hopelessness
     f) Decreased concentration
     g) Psychomotor retardation or agitation
     h) Anger turned inward
     i) Inability to make decisions
     j) Suicidal ideation
     k) Delusional about guilt, unworthiness, sin
     l) Social withdrawal
     m) Persistent physical manifestations such as headaches, digestive disorders, chronic pain
     n) Lack of self-care
  2) Characteristics of mania
     a) Extroversion
     b) Flight of ideas
     c) Accelerated speech
     d) Accelerated motor activity
     e) Anger turned outward
     f) Impulsivity
     g) Arrogant, demanding, controlling behavior with underlying feelings of vulnerability and inadequacy
     h) Delusions of grandeur
  3) Bipolar: alternate periods of depression and mania with a short period of "normalcy" in between
     a) Manic periods decrease over time.
     b) Depressive periods increase.
     c) Suicide potential is greatest during period of "normalcy."
 d. **NURSING INTERVENTIONS**
  1) Depression
     a) Structure environment and time.

Promote client's physical well-being.
     b) Initiate suicide precautions.
     c) Communicate with client to decrease loneliness.
     d) Build trust, and arrange for short, frequent visits.
     e) Encourage client to focus on strengths and promote ADLs.
     f) Schedule nonintellectual activities such as leatherwork, sanding.
     g) Encourage goal setting to provide success.
  2) Mania
     a) Provide for physical welfare.
     b) Provide frequent, small feedings using finger foods.
     c) Protect client from impulsive activity to promote safety.
     d) Reduce external stimuli (Client responds to environment).
     e) Communicate calmly to client.
     f) Initiate milieu activities such as walks, ball tossing, creative writing, and drawing; avoid competitive games.
  3) Interventions are specific to client behavior. For example:
     a) Depression: lack of sleep; re-establish sleep patterns.
     b) Mania: weight loss; re-establish eating patterns (finger foods, decrease stimuli).
  4) Priority nursing care is given to client who is suicidal (frequent interactions and monitoring).
  5) Clients are most at-risk for suicide between depressive and manic episodes.
e. Suicide
  1) Definition: self-imposed death stemming from depression, especially hopelessness and negative feelings about the future
  2) High-risk groups: depressed, hallucinating, delusional, organic mental disorders, substance abusers, adolescents, chronic or painful illness, older adults, sexual identity conflicts
  3) Danger signs
     a) Specific plan (Ask client for specifics.)
     b) Giving away personal items, completing wills, finalizing personal or business matters
     c) Making amends
     d) Change in behavior in a depressed client
     e) Gesture or history of attempt

TABLE II-9
ANTIDEPRESSANT AGENTS

CHEMICAL CLASS	GENERIC NAME	TRADE NAME	MEDICATION ALERTS
Tricyclic antidepressants (more adverse reactions)	- imipramine - desipramine - amitriptyline - nortriptyline - protriptyline - doxepin - amoxapine	- Tofranil - Norpramin - Elavil - Aventyl - Vivactil - Sinequan - Asendin	- Tricyclic antidepressants (TCAs) inhibit serotonin uptake from synaptic gap.
Tetracyclic antidepressant	- maprotiline - mirtazapine	- Ludiomil - Remeron	
Selective serotonin reuptake inhibitors (SSRIs)	- fluvoxamine - fluoxetine - sertraline - paroxetine - escitalopram - citalopram	- Luvox - Prozac - Zoloft - Paxil - Lexapro - Celexa	- SSRIs act to inhibit the reuptake of serotonin into the CNS neurons - SSRIs have fewer adverse effects and can be used safely in older adults
Serotonin norepinephrine Reuptake Inhibitor (SNRI)	- duloxetine	- Cymbalta	- Also used in treating diabetic neuropathy
Newer antidepressants	- trazodone - nefazodone - bupropion HCL - venlafaxine HCL	- Desyrel - Serzone - Wellbutrin/Zyban - Effexor	- Effective in the treatment of depression - Wellbutrin should not be double-dosed and must be tapered off slowly to prevent seizures. -Wellbutrin must not be given at the same time as Zyban (Both are different trade names for bupropion.).

ADVERSE REACTIONS	NURSING INTERVENTIONS	MEDICATION ALERTS
Anticholinergic effects (can be treated – usually clear in 1 week) - Dry mouth - Constipation - Urinary retention - Blurred vision - Aggravated glaucoma	- Increasing fluids, good oral hygiene - Bulk, diet, exercise, stool softeners - Urecholine, monitoring I&O - Corrective lenses or pilocarpine drops, large print - Ophthalmologist consult	All tricyclic and tetracyclic medications can cause dry mouth, constipation, blurred vision, drowsiness, and hypotension.
Cardiovascular effects - Postural hypotension - Direct effects on the heart: tachycardia, arrhythmia, conduction defects - Fluid retention: can lead to heart failure	- Take BP regularly, sitting and standing to monitor cardiovascular effects - Use smaller divided doses in clients with known heart disease; avoid in those with cardiac conduction defects or recent myocardial infarction. - Check vital signs regularly; weigh client daily; check for fluid retention.	Tricyclic antidepressants are potentially lethal in cases of overdose.
Allergic reactions - Rashes	- Observe and report to primary care provider.	- Prozac most commonly causes skin rash.

TABLE II-9
ANTIDEPRESSANT AGENTS (CONTINUED)

ADVERSE REACTIONS	NURSING INTERVENTIONS	MEDICATION ALERTS
- Photosensitivity	- Provide sunscreen, protect skin with clothing, observe carefully.	
- Insomnia	- Single morning dose	- Insomnia is common with Prozac.
- Tremors and seizures	- Observe carefully; advise client to avoid caffeine.	- Wellbutrin or Celexa should not be taken if there is a history of seizure disorder; do not double dose if a dose is missed; luvox, used to treat OCD, can also induce seizures and induction of a manic episode.
- Excessive perspiration	- Observe, report, provide comfort measures.	
- Erection/orgasm difficulty (may cause noncompliance)	- Switch to a lower dose or to a less anticholinergic preparation	
- Anxiety, restlessness	- Observe, report, may have to discontinue	

MEDICATION INTERACTIONS	ADVERSE REACTIONS	MEDICATION ALERTS
MAO inhibitors	14-day waiting period before changing from MAOI to antidepressant or vice versa	Do not use tricyclic or SSRIs concurrently with MAOIs
Antihypertensives and heart medications	Causes hypotension or hypertension	
Antacids	Inhibits absorption	
Antipsychotics	Potentiates anticholinergic effects	
CNS depressants/alcohol	Potentiated effects	

TABLE II-10
ANTIDEPRESSANT AGENTS: MAOIS

CHEMICAL CLASS	GENERIC NAME	TRADE NAME
MAOIs	- isocarboxazid - phenelzine - tranylcypromine	- *Marplan* - *Nardil* - *Parnate*

ADVERSE REACTIONS	NURSING INTERVENTIONS	MEDICATION ALERTS
Hypertensive crisis: elevated BP, palpitations, diaphoresis, chest pain, and headache that can lead to intracranial hemorrhage and death	Teach clients to avoid foods with high tyramine content such as aged cheeses, fermented foods, chocolate, liver, bean pods, yeast, sausage and bologna, beer, Chianti and vermouth wines; limit amounts of ETOH, sour cream, yogurt, raisins, soy sauce; teach clients to avoid OTC and prescription medications such as antidepressants, sedatives, cough and cold preparations, which interact to produce hypertensive crisis.	Monitor client's blood pressure and assess for report of headache.

TABLE II-10
ANTIDEPRESSANT AGENTS: MAOIS (CONTINUED)

ADVERSE REACTIONS	NURSING INTERVENTIONS	MEDICATION ALERTS
Anticholinergic disturbances: dry mouth, constipation	Increase fluids, bulk in diet, and exercise.	
CNS effects: drowsiness, fatigue, headache, restlessness	Some can be expected to last for a short period; increase activity, short afternoon nap.	
Orthostatic hypotension (drop in BP due to change in position)	Monitor BP frequently: lying, sitting, standing; teach to rise slowly.	
Delay in ejaculation/orgasm	Take dose in morning if sexual activity is in evening.	
Insomnia	Give single morning dose; relax several hours before bedtime.	

MEDICATION INTERACTIONS	ADVERSE REACTIONS	MEDICATION ALERTS
Tricyclic antidepressants	Hypertensive crisis	Must wait 2 weeks before changing to a different antidepressant medication
CNS depressants	Decrease liver function	
Dibenzoxazepines	Hypertensive crisis	
Amphetamines	Potentiate action	
Antihypertensives (diuretics)	Decrease action	

TABLE II-11
ANTIMANIA AGENTS AND MOOD STABILIZERS

CHEMICAL CLASS	GENERIC NAME	TRADE NAME	MEDICATION ALERTS

Lithium
- Blood level
  - .8 to 1.2 mEq/L: therapeutic
  - Above 1.5 mEq/L: toxic
  - 2.0 mEq/L: lethal
	- lithium	- *Eskalith*
		- *Lithonate*
		- *Lithotabs*
		- *Lithobid*
			- A client who is to start lithium therapy should be ruled out for thyroid, cardiac, and renal problems before initial therapy; lithium should be discontinued prior to surgery, ECT, and during pregnancy; it is essential to monitor lithium levels routinely to maintain a therapeutic range.
			
			- ½ life to 24 hr

Anticonvulsants	- valproic acid	- *Depakote*	- Depakote should not be used in clients with liver or hepatic disease; must monitor LFTs, CBCs.

TABLE II-11
ANTIMANIA AGENTS AND MOOD STABILIZERS (CONTINUED)

CHEMICAL CLASS	GENERIC NAME	TRADE NAME	MEDICATION ALERTS
Anticonvulsants (continued)	- gabapentin - carbamazepine - lamotrigine	- *Neurontin* - *Tegretol* - *Lamictal*	- Do not stop anticonvulsant medications suddenly, may have seizures. - Anticonvulsants are used in the maintenance treatment of bipolar disorder to act as a mood stabilizer.

ADVERSE REACTIONS	NURSING INTERVENTIONS	MEDICATION ALERTS

- Initial effects of lithium	- Interventions for all adverse reactions:
	  - Instruct client of short duration.
	  - Observe client carefully for changes in manifestations.
	  - Lithium work-up: renal, thyroid, ECG.
	  - Check blood levels.
	  - Regular physicals.
	  - Lower doses in older adult clients.
		Teach client that initial adverse reactions are common.

- Fine tremor	- Eliminate caffeine; adjust dose.	
- Transient nausea	- Use side rails; assist when up.	
- Drowsiness, lethargy	- Avoid using machinery.	
- Loose stools, abdominal discomfort	- Take with meals; change to slower release form.	
- Polyuria		
- Thirst		
- Weight gain, fatigue		
- Toxic levels of lithium - Causes: Elevated doses of medication, low sodium levels, prolonged vomiting or diarrhea	Carefully observe blood levels as sodium decreases and lithium levels increase; hold doses and obtain blood level; liver function/hematology levels need to be monitored with valproic acid.	- If lithium toxicity is suspected and blood levels exceed 2.0, discontinue medications and begin fluid and electrolyte therapy. - Discontinue lithium therapy 48 to 72 hr preoperatively; prolongs the action of Anectine

- Results:
    - Vomiting
    - Diarrhea
    - Lethargy
    - Muscle twitching
    - Ataxia
    - Slurred speech
    - Coma, seizure, cardiac arrest		

MEDICATION INTERACTIONS	ADVERSE REACTIONS	MEDICATION ALERTS
- Diuretics	- Increase risk of lithium toxicity, do not use with Haldol	Use cautiously with neuroleptics.
- Antipsychotics - Sodium bicarbonate	- Neurotoxicity, especially in older adult clients - Promote excretion, lowering serum level	
- ECT/surgery	- May cause neurotoxicity	
- Pregnancy	- Crosses placental barrier	

TABLE II-12
SLEEP AGENTS

CHEMICAL CLASS	GENERIC NAME	TRADE NAME	MEDICATION ALERT
Benzodiazepine	- flurazepam - temazepam - halcion - ativan	- *Dalmane* - *Restoril* - *Triazolam* - *Lorazepam*	- Intended for short-term use to treat insomnia - Dangerous in overdose and abrupt withdrawal - Can have paradoxical response, hyperactivity, especially in older adults and children
Newer sleep agents	- Zolpidem - eszopiclone	- *Ambien* - *Lunesta*	- Used for short-term treatment of insomnia

f) Client indicating that he/she "feels better" or "has everything figured out"

4) **NURSING INTERVENTIONS**
   a) Initiate crisis intervention.
   b) Take all gestures seriously.
   c) Initiate suicide precautions.
      (1) Stay with client.
      (2) Establish safety contract.
      (3) Remove sharp and harmful objects.
   d) Maintain personal contact providing care, concern, neutral tone, hope, and goals.
   e) Provide diversional activities with increasing numbers of people.
   f) Acknowledge that safety is always the first priority.

B. Treatments
1. Antidepressant agents (table II-9)
2. Antidepressant agents: MAOIs (See Table II-10.)
3. Antimanic agents and mood stabilizers (See Table II-11.)
4. Electroconvulsive therapy (ECT)
   a. Characteristics
      1) Used mainly with clients who are severely depressed
      2) Used after other methods have been tried and failed
      3) Grand-mal seizure induced by passing an electric current through the temporal lobes and hypothalamus for 0.1 to 1 second
      4) Slight grimace and/or plantar flexion and toe movement may be observable
      5) Dose: six to 20 treatments, three times a week
   b. Medications
      1) General anesthesia
      2) Muscle relaxant succinylcholine chloride (*Anectine*)
      3) Atropine sulfate: to dry secretions and block vagal reflexes

c. **NURSING INTERVENTIONS**
   1) Verify that informed consent has been obtained.
   2) Maintain NPO after midnight.
   3) Take baseline vital signs every 15 min postoperatively.
   4) Remove prostheses and jewelry.
   5) Empty bladder.
   6) Reassure client that memory loss is temporary for up to 2 months.
   7) Educate client and family for ECT as a treatment modality.
   8) Prepare client and family for the temporary memory loss post-treatment.
   9) Monitor client for decreased respirations as a potential adverse effect of Anectine.
d. Recovery period
   1) Monitor vital signs.
   2) Maintain a patent airway.
   3) Position on side to prevent aspiration.
   4) Provide reorientation to person, place, and time.
   5) Assist to ambulate.
   6) Resume ADLs as soon as possible.
   7) Provide symptomatic treatment of residual headache or nausea.

SECTION V

PERSONALITY DISORDERS

A. Definition: individual personality traits reflecting chronic, inflexible, and maladaptive patterns of behavior that impair social and occupational functions

B. Causes
1. Genetic abnormalities
2. Learned responses
3. Deficiencies in ego and superego development
4. Unresponsive, inappropriate parent-child relationship
5. Early separation

C. Manifestations

1. Antisocial: sociopathic/psychopathic (usually men)
   a. Superficial charm, wit, intelligence; manipulative, often seductive behavior
   b. Inability or refusal to accept responsibility for self-serving, destructive behavior
   c. Failure at school and work; delinquency, rule violations, inability to keep a job
   d. Repeated substance abuse
   e. Thefts, vandalism, multiple arrests
   f. Inability to function as a responsible person; no give or take
   g. Fights, assaults, abuse of others
   h. Impulsiveness, recklessness, inability to plan ahead
   i. Inappropriate affect: not sorry for violating others, no guilt
   j. Does not seek treatment
   k. Does not change with punishment
2. Borderline (usually women)
   a. Impulsive and unpredictable behavior in self-damaging areas: spending, sex, gambling
   b. Unstable and intense interpersonal relationships, rapid attitude shifts, idealization, devaluation
   c. Inappropriate, intense anger
   d. Manipulative, splitting behaviors
   e. Identity disturbance with uncertain self-image and imitative behavior
   f. Intolerance of being alone, chronic feelings of emptiness or boredom
   g. Unstable affect with mood swings
   h. Self-destructive behavior: suicidal gestures, self-mutilation, frequent accidents and fights

D. NURSING INTERVENTIONS

1. Be aware of own feelings.
2. Approach client directly; confront.
3. Reinforce appropriate behavior.
4. Set limits.
5. Protect other clients from verbal and physical abuse.
6. Set clear rules and regulations with consequences for rule violation.
7. Establish contract for behavioral changes.
8. Initiate group treatment, help identify manipulative behavior.
9. Recognize manipulative behaviors and be clear about boundaries and rules.
10. Hold frequent interdisciplinary meetings to address client behaviors and to provide consistency in treatment.
11. Encourage verbal expression of feelings.
12. Encourage responsibility and accountability.
13. Teach social skills.

CHEMICAL DEPENDENCE/ABUSE

A. Substance-Related Disorders

1. Definition
   a. Abuse: drug use leading to legal, social, and medical problems
   b. Addiction: refers to physical dependence
   c. Dependence: need resulting from continued use; results in mental and physical discomfort upon withdrawal of the substance
2. Contributing factors
   a. Genetic predisposition
   b. Peer pressure and social approval
   c. Low self-esteem
   d. Low frustration tolerance
   e. Availability
3. Defense mechanisms
   a. Denial
   b. Rationalization
   c. Intellectualization
   d. Projection
   e. Blaming
4. Behavioral effects
   a. Reduces anxiety
   b. Sense of well-being
   c. Inhibits self-control
   d. Dependence: physical and psychological addiction
   e. Tolerance: need for increasing amounts to achieve the same effect
5. Alcohol dependence and abuse
   a. General characteristics
      1) Abuse vs. dependence
      2) Central nervous system depressant with progression from relaxation to slurred speech and impaired motor activities to stupor and anesthesia
      3) Physical effects occurring in all systems
         a) Nervous system: psychosis, dementia, seizure disorders; Wernicke-Korsakoff's syndrome secondary to dementia; memory loss, ataxia, confusion (thiamine and niacin deficiency)
         b) Cardiac: arrhythmias, myopathy, hypertension
         c) Gastrointestinal: gastritis, cirrhosis, pancreatitis, hypoglycemia, ulcers, esophageal varices
         d) Respiratory: COPD, pneumonia, cancer

TABLE II-13
SUBSTANCE ABUSE

DRUG	MANIFESTATIONS OF INTOXICATION	WITHDRAWAL SYNDROME	METHOD OF DETOXIFICATION
Hallucinogens: psychedelics, LSD, mescaline peyote, marijuana "gateway drugs"	Flushing of skin, dilated pupils, transient increase in pulse rate and blood pressure, hallucinations, psychosis, marked anxiety, depression, suicidal thoughts, confusion, paranoia	None	None required; "bad trips" can be treated with diazepam (*Valium*) or more simply, by "talking down" through verbal reassurance and emotional support; flashbacks may occur for several months.
Phencyclidine (PCP, angel dust)	Vertical or horizontal nystagmus, increased BP and heart rate, ataxia, marked anxiety, emotional lability, dysarthria, euphoria, agitation, delusions, grandiosity, irrationality, violence, synthesis (seeing colors when loud sound is heard); sensation of slowed time; can lead to dangerous behavior	None	Minimize social stimulation and control environment; administer ascorbic acid (vitamin C tablets or cranberry juice); do not "talk down"; treat with diazepam if excited; if psychotic, admit to psychiatric unit and treat with antipsychotic medication.
Stimulants: amphetamines, amyl nitrate, cocaine (See separate category.)	Restlessness, irritability, anxiety, tachycardia, cardiac arrhythmia, paranoia, psychosis with clear sensorium, elation, grandiosity, psychotic behavior, perspiration or chills, nausea and vomiting; weight loss with prolonged use	- Use of high doses associated with a rapidly developing syndrome on withdrawal: - persecutory delusions - ideas of reference - aggressiveness and hostility - anxiety - psychomotor agitation - suicidal ideations - Prolonged, heavy use yields withdrawal syndrome after 2 to 4 days of depression and fatigue	None usually required; psychiatric hospitalization for severe withdrawal symptoms or addiction
- Cocaine/Crack: no longer a "rich man's drug" - Same dose consistently can cause an overdose	Same as amphetamines; overdose: syncope, chest pain, seizures, death may result from cardiac and respiratory failure; high dose use: visual and tactile hallucinations and "cocaine bugs"; a "rush" of increased self-confidence and well-being, confusion, anxiety, paranoia; headache, palpitations followed by "crashing"	- Sleepiness, depression, lack of energy or motivation, poor concentration, irritability, "cocaine craving," psychosis - Can cause a stroke in the fetus	Hospitalization for high-dose "crack" or freebase use or the polyaddicted; others treated in outpatient programs

TABLE II-13
SUBSTANCE ABUSE (CONTINUED)

DRUG	MANIFESTATIONS OF INTOXICATION	WITHDRAWAL SYNDROME	METHOD OF DETOXIFICATION
Opiates: heroin, morphine, Dilaudid, Demerol, Percodan, codeine, Opium, methadone	Mitosis, euphoria, drowsiness, dysphoria, apathy, psychomotor retardation, slurred speech, impaired attention or memory, impaired social judgment; chronic use can lead to malnourishment, criminal behavior, sexually transmitted disease, HIV/AIDS with IV drug use	Withdrawal begins after 8 to 12 hr and lasts 3 to 5 days; severity varies with extent of abuse; lacrimation, rhinorrhea, sweating, piloerection, diarrhea, yawning, mild hypertension, tachycardia, fever, insomnia, dilated pupils, restlessness, abdominal cramps, anxiety	Can be accomplished "cold turkey" or medically managed with antianxiety agents, methadone, or clonidine (Catapres)
Sedative-hypnotics: barbiturates, Equanil, Miltown, benzodiazepines, Ativan, Librium, Valium, Klonopin, Xanax	Mental impairment, confusion, nystagmus, and lack of motor coordination, ataxia, depression, dysarthria; frequently used by alternating with alcohol: which can lead to overdose	Weakness, insomnia, nausea, postural hypotension develop within first 48 hr and last 5 to 7 days; seizures may occur at any time, especially within first few days; delirium may develop between days 3 and 7 and last for 3 to 5 days.	Can be medical emergency; hospitalization required and pentobarbital or phenobarbital used to prevent precipitous withdrawal

e) Genitourinary system: fetal alcohol syndrome (There is no documented safe amount of alcohol in pregnant women.), decreased libido

f) Skin and skeletal: ulcers, spider angiomas, fractures

4) Psychological and social effects

    a) Erratic, impulsive, abusive behavior

    b) Poor judgment, loss of memory

    c) Family problems

    d) Depression, low self-esteem

    e) Suicide

    f) Job loss

b. Alcohol withdrawal syndrome

1) Definition: physical manifestations developing 6 to 8 hr after abstinence from alcohol

2) Manifestations (autonomic nervous system)

    a) Shakiness

    b) Anxiety

    c) Mood swings

    d) Insomnia

    e) Impaired appetite

    f) Some confusion

    g) Elevated vital signs

c. Alcohol withdrawal (delirium tremens)

1) Definition: acute withdrawal of alcohol 2 to 4 days after last drink; 72-hr period most dangerous and fatal if unmanaged medically

2) Manifestations

    a) Confusion

    b) Disorientation

    c) Visual and auditory hallucinations

    d) Convulsions

    e) All manifestations of withdrawal

d. Treatment

1) The best treatment for alcohol withdrawal is prevention or early detection and treatment.

2) Inpatient detoxification: 3 to 7 days; purpose is to medically manage withdrawal and prevent delirium tremens.

    a) Antianxiety medications

    b) Fluids and vitamins

    c) Antidiarrheal medications

    d) Symptomatic relief: analgesics, fluids, sleeping medications

    e) Seizure precautions: antiseizure medications, magnesium sulfate, and sedation

    f) Diet: high-protein, high-carbohydrate, low-fat foods

    g) Decreased stimuli

    h) No restraints

3) Delirium tremens

    a) Quiet moderately lit area

b) Decreased stimuli
c) Reality orientation

e. **NURSING INTERVENTIONS**
1) Administer medications and treatments as prescribed.
2) Observe for physical complications.
3) Provide rest and nutrition.
4) Observe for manifestations of depression and suicide.
5) Provide firm limits.
6) Be nonjudgmental.
7) Monitor visitors.
8) Assist in identifying use of defense mechanisms (denial).
9) Encourage rehabilitation programs and aftercare (e.g., Alcoholics Anonymous [AA]); alcoholism is characterized by periods of relapse and sobriety; prognosis: recovery, not cure.
10) Educate and support family; discuss support groups such as Al-Anon and Alateen.

f. Aftercare
1) AA: 12-step program of sobriety
2) Disulfiram (*Antabuse*): medication used to prevent use of alcohol; aversion therapy
   a) Sensitizes the client to alcohol
   b) If alcohol is used, client suffers headache, vomiting, nausea, flushing, hypotension, tachycardia, dyspnea, chest pain, palpitations, confusion, respiratory and circulatory collapse, convulsions, and possible death.
   c) Avoid drinking alcohol for 2 weeks after last dose.
   d) Warn client that alcohol is present in cough medication, rubbing compounds, vinegars, aftershave lotions, and some mouthwashes.
3) Naltrexone (*Trexan*): agent used for narcotic and alcohol addiction; reduces cravings
4) Catapres (*Clonidine*): reduces cravings in opioid withdrawal
5) Methadone (*Methadone*): maintenance therapy medication that blocks cravings in heroin addiction

Substance Abuse

A. **Definition:** Substance abuse is the term used to designate the use of psychoactive drugs, including alcohol, to the extent of significant interference with the user's physical, social, and or emotional well-being; it is characterized by preoccupation with the drug and loss of control over its use; if the quantity and duration of abuse is sufficient, physical dependence may develop with tolerance and risk of a withdrawal syndrome when drug use is terminated. (See Table II-13.)

B. **General characteristics**
1. Abuse vs. dependence
2. Effect on CNS depends on the type of substance.
3. Psychological and social effects
   a. Isolation and withdrawal
   b. Family and work problems
   c. Loss of property
   d. Incarceration
4. Physical effects
   a. Cardiac failure
   b. Liver failure
   c. Pulmonary emboli
   d. Gangrene
   e. Malnutrition
   f. Trauma
   g. Psychosis

C. **Common Drugs Abused** (See Table II-13.)

D. **Rehabilitation:** 30 days to 2 years; change lifestyle

E. **NURSING INTERVENTIONS**
1. Carry out medical regime.
2. Observe for manifestations of withdrawal.
3. Provide quiet, safe environment.
4. Monitor visitors.
5. Be nonjudgmental, accepting, firm attitude.
6. Set limits.
7. Monitor nutrition.
8. Promote sleep.
9. Refer for detoxification, rehabilitation, and aftercare.
10. Support family in seeking help (Al-Anon).

SECTION VII

ORGANIC MENTAL DISORDERS

A. **Normal Aging**
1. Life-cycle changes
   a. Physical health
   b. Emotional: integrity, despair
   c. Intellectual changes
   d. Social changes such as retirement, widowhood

B. **Organic Mental Disorders** (OMD): psychological and behavioral problems resulting from organic conditions; may be reversible or irreversible

1. Delirium: acute brain syndrome; decreased attention and level of awareness; usually temporary and reversible; rapid onset; identifiable stressor
   a. Disturbance
      1) Disturbances in sleep and wakefulness
      2) Attention: easily distracted, illusions
      3) Restless and disoriented
      4) Difficulty concentrating
      5) Disorganized speech
   b. Causes
      1) Medical
      2) Surgical
      3) Pharmacological
      4) Neurological
2. Dementias
   a. Definition: sustained and often progressive intellectual impairment
   b. General manifestations
      1) Lingering
      2) Gradual, progressive
      3) Language disorders (e.g., confabulation, blocking)
      4) Motor impairment (ataxia)
      5) Disintegrating personality and behavior
      6) Memory impairment (short-term)
      7) Judgment impairment
      8) Thinking impairment (abstract)
      9) Degeneration (1 to 15 years postonset)
   c. Types
      1) Wernicke-Korsakoff's syndrome (dementia associated with alcoholism)
         a) Memory (long or short term); impairment is predominant
         b) Confabulation
         c) Polyneuritis
         d) Flat affect
         e) Ataxia
         f) Confusion
         g) Learning impairment
      2) Alzheimer's disease (primary degenerative dementia)
         a) Onset: 45 years or older

         b) Gradually progressive and chronic
            (1) Orientation disturbance
            (2) Concentration decreases
            (3) Forget words
            (4) Denial
      3) Dementia
         a) Disorientation
         b) Anxiety, denial
         c) Delusions, hallucinations, paranoia
         d) Agitation
         e) Physical deterioration
      4) Multi-infarct dementia: difference from Alzheimer's is mainly its step-wise progression, rather than gradual decline; trauma induced (stroke, neurosurgery)
3. **NURSING INTERVENTIONS:** allow as much independence as possible
   a. Manage physical manifestations.
      1) Medical care: physical problems
      2) Adequate nutrition: provide finger foods, tolerate poor manners
      3) Exercise and rest: range of motion exercises, walks, naps, keep awake during the day
      4) Elimination: monitor I&O, diet, limit fluids at bedtime, use stool softeners, toilet at regular intervals
   b. Assist client with ADLs.
      1) Break down tasks into short simple steps.
      2) Provide clear expectations.
      3) Allow ample time.
      4) Remain with client.
      5) Assist with grooming and hygiene.
      6) Maintain matter of fact manner and avoid embarrassing client.
   c. Promote client safety. (Evaluate and implement as needed.)
   d. Optimize cognitive abilities.
      1) Eliminate multiple stimuli.
      2) Speak using short, simple sentences (slow, distinct, soft voice).
      3) Maintain consistency: establish routine, familiar caregivers.

TABLE II-14
MEDICATIONS USED IN THE TREATMENT OF ORGANIC MENTAL DISORDERS

GENERIC NAME	TRADE NAME	ACTIONS
Donepezil	Aricept	- Used in the treatment of Alzheimer's disease
Rivastigmine	Exelon	- Slows the disease progression
Galantamine	Reminyl	
Memantine	Namenda	

4) Orient client to person, place, and time.
5) Use visual cues such as pictures, labels, calendar, and/or clock.
e. Provide opportunities for socialization.
1) Provide human contact.
2) Allow children to interact.
3) Provide for alternatives therapies.
   a) Pet therapy
   b) Music therapy
   c) Reminiscence therapy
f. Families
1) Explain the disorder.
2) Explain regression and provide activities such as photo albums, music, games.
3) Provide resources: Alzheimer's Disease and Related Disorders, Inc.
4) Discuss need for family to obtain support, relief.
5) Understand that counseling is necessary at times.

KEY INFORMATION

 It is important to remember that the basic principle underlying all care for the cognitively impaired is to facilitate the highest level of functionality possible while fostering independence.

SECTION VIII

EATING DISORDERS

A. Anorexia/Bulimia
1. Definitions
   a. Anorexia: refusal to eat and relentless self-induced pursuit of thinness; up to 21% die
   b. Bulimia: binge-purge cycle of eating
2. Causes
   a. Adolescent struggle for independence and control
   b. Feelings of control are related to body
   c. Family problems: denial, conflict avoidance, enmeshment, chaotic home environment
   d. Society promotes thinness, dieting
3. Comparison (anorexia and bulimia) (See Table II-15.)
   a. Obedient, bright, ambitious
   b. Perfectionist, type-A personalities
   c. Low self-esteem
   d. Preoccupied with food
   e. Depression
   f. Manipulation
4. Effects
   a. Anorexia: holding in
      1) Skeletal muscle atrophy; emaciated, loss of fatty tissue, lanugo
      2) Hypotension
      3) Constipation

4) Susceptible to infections
5) Blotchy, sallow skin
6) Dryness and loss of hair
7) Amenorrhea
8) Electrolyte imbalance
9) Cause of death: cardiac dysrhythmia; arrest
   b. Bulimia: letting go
1) Electrolyte imbalance
2) Dental caries
3) Gingival infections, erosion of tooth enamel
4) Susceptible to infections
5) Binging
6) Vomiting
7) Use and abuse of laxatives and diuretics

 5. **NURSING INTERVENTIONS**
   a. Recognize need for hospitalization.
   b. Provide nutrition.
1) Monitor I&O.
2) Monitor 30 to 60 min after eating.
3) Help with relaxation prior to eating.
4) Enforce a behavior-modification plan.
5) Positively reinforce client for weight gain.
6) Administer parenteral feedings as needed.
   c. Teach coping skills.
1) Encourage recognition and verbalization. of feelings
2) Reinforce realistic perception of weight and appearance.
3) Promote acceptance of self-responsibility.
4) Provide limit setting and consistency.
   d. Family
1) Therapy
2) Education
   e. Refer to self-help groups.
1) American Anorexia/Bulimia Association, Inc.
2) Anorexia Nervosa and Associated Disorders (ANAD)

KEY INFORMATION

 Recognize that many clients with eating disorders are extremely resistant to change, and progress may be slow; remember the seriousness and life-threatening consequences of an eating disorder.

SECTION IX

DEVELOPMENTAL DISABILITIES

A. Definition: adaptive ability compromised by an alteration in the pattern or rate in stages of development during childhood: functional limitations in self-care, learning, mobility, self-direction, self-sufficiency in independent living; diagnosis based on IQ and socially adaptive behavior

TABLE 11-15
ANOREXIA/BULIMIA CONTRASTED

ANOREXIA	BULIMIA
- Younger (13 to 22)	- Older (20 to 30)
- Underweight	- Normal or slightly overweight
- Unable to maintain body weight at 85% of expected body weight	- Weight fluctuates considerably
- Introvert	- Extrovert
- Amenorrhea	- Amenorrhea
- Starvation	- Binge eating
- Don't admit abnormal eating patterns	- See patterns and fear loss of control
- Intense fear of becoming obese	- Hide food, hoard
- Prefers health foods	- Prefers high-calorie food
- Preoccupation with buying, planning, and preparing foods	- Repeated crash dieting, use of laxatives, diuretics, amphetamines
- Rigorous exercise	- Abuse of alcohol and/or drugs, petty crime, obsessive compulsive disorder
- Electrolyte imbalance	- Electrolyte imbalance
- Still views self as overweight	- Aware that behavior is abnormal
- Cardiac arrhythmias	- Excessive dental caries-secondary to vomiting

B. Causes
1. Genetic
   a. Chromosomal
      1) Down's syndrome (trisomy 21): congenital mental retardation with motor involvement
      2) Klinefelter's syndrome (XXY): gonadal defect with subnormal intelligence and social adaptation
   b. Errors of metabolism
      1) Phenylketonuria (PKU): accumulation of phenylalanine, which is toxic to the brain; retardation may be avoided by strict dietary avoidance of phenylalanine
      2) Tay-Sachs disease: inherited disorder of lipid metabolism causing mental retardation, blindness, and muscle weakness
2. Acquired
   a. Prenatal: viruses, toxins
   b. Perinatal: anoxia, injury, prematurity
   c. Postnatal: infections, poisons, trauma, deprivation

C. Levels of Mental Retardation: based on IQ level (normal range is 80 to 110)
1. Mild
   a. Social and communication skills
   b. Vocational skills, minimal self-support
   c. May be self-sufficient and independent as adult
   d. IQ range: 50 to 70
   e. Mental age of approximately 8 to 10 years
2. Moderate
   a. Can care for self
   b. Poor awareness of social conventions
   c. May learn to count
   d. May contribute to own support under close supervision
   e. IQ range: 35 to 49
   f. Mental age of approximately 5 to 6 years
3. Severe
   a. Poor motor and speech
   b. May learn simple work tasks
   c. IQ range: 20 to 34
   d. Mental age of a toddler
4. Profound
   a. Very limited, or no self-care ability
   b. IQ range: below 20
   c. Mental age of an infant

D. Emotions: client with a developmental disability has a full range of emotions and may be subjected to the full range of emotional illnesses

E. NURSING INTERVENTIONS

1. Know growth and development.
2. Assess physical status.
3. Perform Denver Developmental Screening Test.
    a. Gross motor
    b. Language
    c. Fine motor
    d. Personal, social
4. Help parents with grieving; suggest parent support groups.
5. Encourage early intervention programs.
6. Encourage parents to get help and rest through respite care; make sure parents know all available resources (e.g., medical, social, educational, legal, community).
7. Promote prevention.
    a. Health teaching such as nutrition, obstetrical care
    b. Immunizations
    c. Prenatal counseling and family planning
    d. Psychological needs

SECTION X

FAMILY VIOLENCE

(See also Unit IV, Section VI.)

A. Definition: abuse of a violent physical or verbal nature within a family, which crosses socioeconomic, religious, racial, and/or cultural lines

B. Types of Abuse
1. Physical: nonaccidental use of force that results in injury, pain, or impairment
2. Psychological: inflicting of mental anguish by threats, humiliation, or fear
3. Sexual: any kind of nonconsensual sexual contact
4. Neglect: failure of the caregiver to provide essential food, clothing, shelter or medical care; it may also include abandonment
5. Social: isolation
6. Material or financial (especially in older adults): may include theft or embezzlement of life savings

C. Abused Persons
1. Spouses
2. Children
3. Older adults

D. Risk Factors
1. Physical or cognitive impairment of the victim
2. Isolation of the victim
3. Caregiver stress
4. History of violence in the home
5. Pathology or mental incapacity of the abuser

E. Characteristics of Abuser
1. Low self-esteem
2. Substance abuser
3. Projects anger
4. Anxious
5. Depressed
6. Has come from an abusive household (victimization), was abused as child
7. Socially isolated
8. Impulsive, immature
9. Guilt ridden

F. Characteristics of Abused Persons
1. Adult victims often also were victims of child abuse
2. Accepts responsibility for others (codependency issues)
3. Helpless
4. Suicidal at times
5. Submissive
6. Frightened of being harmed or killed
7. Emotionally or physically dependent on abuser

G. General Manifestations of Abused Persons
1. Psychological manifestations
    a. Sleep disorders such as nightmares
    b. Headaches
    c. Anxiety or fear
    d. Depression
    e. Suicidal ideation
    f. Substance abuse
    g. Disruptive behavior at home, school, or work
    h. Runaway behavior
    i. Frequent emergency room visits
    j. Anger or agitation
    k. Personality changes
    l. Hesitation to talk openly
    m. Withdrawal or resignation
2. Physical manifestations
    a. Unexplained fractures (especially spiral), bruises or burns
    b. Hunger and dehydration
    c. Poor hygiene
    d. Inappropriate dress
    e. Difficulty walking or sitting
    f. Missing essential aid items such as glasses, dentures, hearing aids
    g. Venereal disease or genital infection
    h. Repetitive hospital admissions or missed medical appointments
3. Financial manifestations (especially among older adults)

TABLE II-16
MANIFESTATIONS OF ABUSE IN CHILDREN

TYPE	PHYSICAL	BEHAVIORAL
Physical abuse	- Multiple injuries and/or in various stages of healing - Unexplained bruises, burns, fractures or lacerations - Incongruence between explanation and injury - X-rays show numerous injuries	- Wary of strangers - Labile behavior - Depressed, frightened, stiff, rigid, distant, does not seek out parents - Nonverbal communication inconsistent with verbal communication
Physical neglect	- Appearance: poor hygiene and dress - Medical and physical problems unattended	- Fatigue - Withdrawal - Substance abuse
Sexual abuse	- Venereal disease - Pregnancy - Pain or itching in perineal area; difficulty walking or sitting	- Unusual sexual behavior or knowledge - Poor peer relations - Reports of sexual assault
Emotional abuse		- Decreased self-esteem - Lack of emotional response (no tears) - Hypochondriasis (vague complaints) - Slowed growth and development - Sleep disorders or neglect - Behavioral extremes - Delinquent (runs away)

a. Lack of knowledge about personal finances
b. Reluctance to discuss finances
c. Disparity between income and lifestyle
d. Financial deprivation for essentials (e.g., food, medical treatment, drugs, housing or clothing)
e. Sudden withdrawals or closing of bank accounts

H. NURSING INTERVENTIONS

1. Be aware of the signs of abuse in children, spouses, and older adults.
2. Recognize that many adult victims of abuse deny that it is occurring. They may be in denial due to isolation, shame, or fear of reprisal.
3. Be ready to listen.
4. Ask in detail about manifestations.
5. Build trust.
6. Be nonjudgmental.
7. Offer the victim support in seeking help (e.g., phone number of shelter).
8. Report suspected cases of child and older adult abuse to the proper authorities (legal responsibility).
9. Encourage adult victims to file for an "Order of Protection" when appropriate.
10. Assist to identify support system; identify resources for housing, money, legal aid, vocational counseling, crisis center for therapy.

SECTION XI

SEXUAL ASSAULT (RAPE)

A. Characteristics

1. Crime of violence: force, penetration, lack of consent
2. Motives: power, anger, intimidation
3. Myths
   a. Provoked by victim's actions or mode of dress
   b. Victim promiscuous
   c. Women can avoid rape; cannot be raped against their will
   d. Rape is an impulsive act
   e. Older adults are not raped
   f. Women frequently get revenge by accusing men of rape
   g. Only women can be raped

B. Post-Traumatic Stress Disorder

1. Disorganization
2. Reorganization
3. Physical, emotional, and behavioral stress

C. NURSING INTERVENTIONS

1. Crisis intervention: "Rape Trauma Syndrome"
   a. Use empathetic, understanding approach.

b. Provide safe and secure environment.

c. Encourage verbalization about feelings.

d. Clarify what happened.

e. Offer support and reassurance.

f. Provide referrals for ongoing counseling.

2. Emergency treatment

    a. Allow choices (loss of control).

    b. Have consent forms for evidence and treatment.

    c. Offer comfort and provide privacy.

    d. Take history: "What occurred?" Allow client to verbalize feelings.

    e. Perform physical examination. Do not undress client until the client agrees, preferably after law enforcement has arrived.

    f. Collect medical evidence (x-rays, specimens, photos) and assist law enforcement authorities (must follow legal "chain of evidence" for future potential court action).

    g. Provide emotional support.

    h. Arrange for medical follow-up for STDs, AIDS; Venereal Disease Research Laboratory test.

3. Help with psychological trauma

    a. Disrupted relationships

    b. Phobias

    c. Nightmares

    d. Flashbacks

    e. Family and sexual relations

    f. Talking and working through feelings

SECTION XII

LEGAL ASPECTS OF MENTAL HEALTH NURSING

A. Types of Admissions

1. Voluntary

    a. Client admits him/herself

    b. Client consents to all treatment

    c. Client can refuse treatment, including medications, unless danger to self or others

    d. Client can demand and receive discharge

2. Involuntary or judicial process

    a   Initiated when someone files a petition

    b. Certification of the likelihood of serious harm to self or others, or unable to care for self

    c. At end of statutory time must be released, put on voluntary status, or have a hearing

3. If client is under 18 years of age, parents can confine with confirmation by a neutral fact-finder

B. Judicial Precedents

1. Rights: unless incompetent, client maintains all previous rights

2. Right to treatment: efforts by staff consistent with medical knowledge

    a. Humane psychological and physical environment

    b. Qualified personnel and adequate nursing

    c. Individual treatment plan

3. Competency hearing

4. Least restrictive environment

C. Informed Consent Required

1. Electroclusive therapy

2. Medications

3. Seclusion

4. Restraint

D. Clients' Rights

1. Right to treatment (or to refuse treatment)

2. Access to stationery and postage

3. Access to unopened mail

4. Visits by primary care provider, attorney, clergy

5. Visits by other people (daily)

6. Keep personal possessions

7. Keep and spend money

8. Storage space for personal items

9. Telephone access

10. Hold property, vote, marry

11. Make wills, contracts

12. Educational resources

13. Sue, be sued

14. Challenge hospitalization

E. NURSING INTERVENTIONS: Promote and provide care to the mental health client in the least restrictive environment.

F. Insanity as a Defense

1. Insanity: determined in court; legal terminology

2. McNaughten rule: At the time of the crime, did the client know the nature and quality of the act, or did the client not know right from wrong?

3. Present

    a. Does client know right from wrong?

    b. Was client mentally ill at the time of the crime?

    c. Is client able to conform to the requirements of the law?

    d. Is the client able to assist in his/her defense?

TABLE II-17
MENTAL HEALTH TERMS

TERMS	DEFINITIONS
AFFECT:	Mood or feeling tone
AKATHISIA:	Regular restless movements or pacing
ANHEDONIA:	Inability to experience pleasure
APRAXIA:	Loss of purposeful motor movements
ASSOCIATIVE LOOSENESS:	Disturbance of thinking in which ideas shift from one subject to another in unrelated themes
BINGING:	Ingestion of large quantities of food in a short period of time
BLACKOUTS:	A person that drinks heavily and appears to function normally, but later is unable to recall prior events
CATATONIA:	State of psychological immobilization that can revert to episodes of extreme agitation
CLANG ASSOCIATION:	Meaningless rhyming of words
COMORBIDITY:	The presence of one or more disorders (or diseases) in addition to a primary disease or disorder; often used to identify when a client has manifestations of both physical illness and a psychiatric illness
COMPULSION:	Repetitive purposeless ritualistic behavior performed in accordance with specific rules or routine manner in an attempt to reduce anxiety
CONCRETE THINKING:	Thinking characterized by immediate experience rather than abstract thought
CONFABULATION:	A compensatory mechanism for memory loss; filling in the memory gaps with imaginary stories the teller believes to be true
COUNTER -TRANSFERENCE:	Experience where the therapist transfers his or her feelings for significant others onto the client
CRISIS:	A conflict that cannot readily be resolved by using usual coping mechanisms
DEFENSE MECHANISMS:	Mental strategies used to help cope with areas of conflict
DEINSTITUTION -ALIZATION:	Discharge of a large number of psychiatric clients from inpatient treatment centers to the community
DELUSION:	A fixed false belief held to be true even with evidence to the contrary
DENIAL:	Unconscious attempt to escape unpleasant realities by denying their existence
DESENSITIZATION:	Gradual systematic exposure of the client to feared situations under controlled conditions
DISSOCIATION:	Disturbance in the integrated organization of memory, identity, perception, or consciousness
DUAL DIAGNOSIS:	Having a chronic dependence on a drug or alcohol in addition to another mental health disorder
ECHOLALIA:	Repetition by one person of what is said by another
ECHOPRAXIA:	A meaningless imitation of movement
ENABLING:	Helping a chemically dependent person avoid experiencing the consequences of his or her drinking or drug use
EXTRAPYRAMIDAL REACTION:	A reversible side effect of some psychotropic drugs characterized by muscle rigidity, drooling, restlessness, shuffling gait, and blurred vision
FLIGHT OF IDEAS:	Rapid flow of speech in which the person jumps from one idea to another before the first idea had been concluded
GRANDIOSITY:	Exaggerated belief or claim about one's importance or identity
GRIEF:	An emotional response to a recognized loss
HALLUCINATION:	False sensory perception without external stimuli that can involve any of the senses
HYPOMANIA:	An elevated mood with symptoms less severe than those of mania
IDEAS OF REFERENCE:	False impressions that outside events have special meaning for oneself
ILLUSIONS:	Misinterpretation of a real, external sensory experience
INSIGHT:	Understanding and awareness of the reasons and meanings behind one's motives and behaviors
JUDGMENT:	The ability to make logical or rational decisions
LABILE:	Having rapidly shifting emotions
LEAST RESTRICTIVE:	Client right that mandates that the least drastic means are to be used to achieve a specific purpose

TABLE II-17
MENTAL HEALTH TERMS (CONTINUED)

TERMS	DEFINITIONS
LIMIT SETTING:	Clear statement of rules with consistent reinforcement
LOOSENESS OF ASSOCIATION:	Person's spoken words appear unrelated, illogical, and confused, and connections in thought are interrupted
MANIA:	Pervasive unstable elevated mood
MANIPULATION:	Behavior that is self-directed to get needs met at the expense of others
MILIEU THERAPY:	Management of the client's environment to promote a positive living experience and facilitate recovery
NARCISSISM:	Self-involvement with lack of empathy for others
NEOLOGISM:	Coined word with special meaning to the user
NEUROLEPTIC MALIGNANT SYNDROME:	A rare and sometimes fatal reaction to high potency antipsychotic medications. Symptoms include muscle rigidity, fever, and elevated WBC
OBSESSION:	Repetitive, uncontrollable thought
PARANOID:	Irritable suspicions of distrust that are defended without basis in reality
PERSEVERATION:	Involuntary repetition of the same thought, phrase, or motor response associated with alterations in brain activity
POVERTY OF SPEECH:	Speech that is brief, unclear, and uncommunicative
PREMORBID:	Occurring before development of a disease
PSYCHOSIS:	State in which there is impairment in a person's ability to recognize reality, communicate and relate to others appropriately
PURGING:	Purposeful vomiting or elimination of a substance that has been ingested
REFRAMING:	A technique that involves changing one's viewpoint of a situation and replacing it with another viewpoint that alters the entire meaning
SECONDARY GAINS:	Benefits from being ill, such as attention
SELF-ESTEEM:	The degree of feeling worthwhile or valued
SELF-IMAGE:	One's thoughts about one's own self
SOMATIZATION::	The expression of a psychological stress through physical symptoms
SPLITTING:	The tendency to label individuals into "all good" or "all bad" categories
TARDIVE DYSKINESIA:	Irreversible, involuntary tonic muscular spasms of the tongue, fingers, toes, neck, and pelvis that results from long-term use of antipsychotic medications
TRANSFERENCE:	Unconscious phenomenon in which feelings, attitudes, and wishes toward significant others in one's early life are linked to and projected onto others, usually a therapist in one's current life
WAXY FLEXIBILITY:	The extremities remain in a fixed position for a long period of time
WORD SALAD:	Spoken words and phrases having no apparent meaning or logic

UNIT THREE

MATERNAL NEWBORN NURSING

UNIT CONTENT

SYMBOLS

 Key Points

 Nursing Interventions

! Points to Remember

SECTION I

REVIEW OF FEMALE REPRODUCTIVE NURSING

Pregnancy

A. Anatomy and Physiology of the Female Reproductive Tract

1. External genitalia
   a. Mons pubis
   b. Labia majora
   c. Labia minora
   d. Clitoris
   e. Vestibule
      1) Urethral orifice
      2) Skene's glands
      3) Hymen and vaginal introitus
      4) Bartholin's glands
   f. Perineum
2. Internal genitalia
   a. Fallopian tubes
   b. Uterus
      1) Fundus
      2) Cervix
   c. Vagina
   d. Ovaries

B. Fertilization and Fetal Development

1. Conception (fertilization)
   a. Definition: union of sperm and ovum
   b. Conditions necessary for fertilization
      1) Maturity of egg and sperm
      2) Timing of deposit of sperm
         a) Lifetime of ovum is 24 hr
         b) Lifetime of sperm in the female genital tract is 72 hr
         c) Ideal time for fertilization is 48 hr before to 24 hr after ovulation
         d) Menstruation begins approximately 14 days after ovulation
      3) Climate of the female genital tract
         a) Vaginal and cervical secretions are less acidic during ovulation (sperm cannot survive in a highly acidic environment)
         b) Cervical secretions are thinner during ovulation (sperm can penetrate more easily)
   c. Process of fertilization (7 to 10 days)
      1) Ovulation occurs
      2) Ovum travels to fallopian tube
      3) Sperm travel to fallopian tube
      4) One sperm penetrates the ovum
      5) Zygote forms (fertilized egg)
      6) Zygote migrates to uterus
      7) Zygote implants in uterine wall
      8) Progesterone and estrogen are secreted by the corpus luteum to maintain the lining of the uterus and prevent menstruation until placenta starts producing these hormones; (note: progesterone is a thermogenic hormone that raises body temperature, an objective sign that ovulation has occurred)
   d. Placental development
      1) Chorionic villi develop that secrete human chorionic gonadotropin (HCG), which stimulates production of estrogen and progesterone from the corpus luteum (production of HCG begins on the day of implantation and can be detected by the 6th day)
      2) Chorionic villi burrow into endometrium, forming the placenta
      3) The placenta secretes HCG, human placental lactogen (HPL), and (by week 3) estrogen and progesterone
   e. Fetal membranes develop and surround the embryo, fetus
      1) Amnion: inner membrane
      2) Chorion: outer membrane
      3) Umbilical cord
         a) Two arteries carrying deoxygenated blood to placenta
         b) One vein carrying oxygenated blood to fetus
         c) No pain receptors
         d) Encased in Wharton's jelly
         e) Covered by chorionic membrane
   f. Amniotic fluid
      1) Production origins
         a) Maternal serum during early pregnancy
         b) Fetal urine in greater proportion during latter part of pregnancy
         c) Replaced every 3 hr
         d) 800 to 1,200 mL at end of pregnancy
      2) Functions
         a) Protection from trauma and heat loss
         b) Facilitates musculoskeletal development by allowing for movement of the fetus
         c) Facilitates symmetric growth and development
         d) Source of oral fluid for fetus
   g. Placental transfer of material to and from the fetus
      1) Diffusion across membrane (e.g., gases, water, electrolytes)
      2) Active transport via enzyme activity (e.g., glucose, amino acids, calcium, iron)

3) Pinocytosis: minute particles engulfed and carried across the cell (e.g., fats)
4) Leakage: small defects in the chorionic villi cause slight mixing of material and fetal blood cells
5) Nutrients and wastes are exchanged in the placenta, but the blood does not intermingle

C. Fetal Development
1. Pre-embryonic: first 2 weeks
2. Embryonic: 3 to 7 weeks
3. Fetal: 8 to 40 weeks
   a. Full term: between 37 and 42 weeks, or more than 2,500 grams
   b. Preterm: 20 to 37 weeks, or between 500 and 2,500 grams
   c. Post-term: more than 42 weeks

D. Terminology
1. Gravida
   a. Definition: number of times pregnant, including present pregnancy
   b. Variations: primigravida, multigravida
2. Para
   a. Definition: number of pregnancies delivered after the age of viability, whether born alive or dead
   b. Variations: nullipara, primipara, multipara
3. Five-digit system
   a. G: Gravida: number of pregnancies
   b. T: Term infants: number of deliveries after 37 weeks
   c. P: Preterm: number of preterm deliveries, or deliveries between 20 and 37 weeks
   d. A: Abortions: number of medical abortions before 20 weeks
   e. L: Living: number of living children (For GTPA count multiples as one number. For L count the number of living children.)

Signs of Pregnancy
A. Presumptive (subjective)
1. Amenorrhea: missed periods
2. Nausea and vomiting: morning sickness, probably due to HCG; usually lasts about 3 months
3. Fatigue: first trimester
4. Urinary frequency: caused by enlarging uterus pressing on bladder
5. Breast changes: tenderness and tingling, nipples pronounced, full feeling, increased size, areola darker
6. Quickening: mother's perception of fetal movement around 16 to 20 weeks; fluttering sensation

B. Probable (objective)
1. Chadwick's sign: bluish coloration of the mucous membranes of the cervix, vagina, and vulva
2. Goodell's sign: softening of cervix; occurs beginning of the third month
3. Hegar's sign: softening of the isthmus of the uterus, between the body of the uterus and cervix; occurs about the 6th week
4. Enlargement of abdomen: uterus just above symphysis at 8 to 10 weeks; at umbilicus at 20 to 22 weeks
5. Braxton-Hicks contractions: painless contractions occurring at irregular periods throughout pregnancy; felt most commonly after 28 weeks
6. Uterine souffle: soft blowing sound; blood flow to placenta same rate as maternal pulse
7. Pregnancy test positive: HCG in serum and urine
8. Ballottement: can push fetus and feel it rebound
9. Pigmentation changes: increased pigmentation, chloasma, linea nigra, and striae gravidarum

C. Positive
1. Fetal heartbeat: by Doppler at 8 to 10 weeks
2. Fetal movements: felt by examiner
3. Fetal outline: on sonogram

Assessment of Date of Delivery
A. Nägele's Rule: first day of last menstrual period (LMP) minus 3 months plus 7 days; in most cases, add 1 year

B. Other Parameters: fundal heights, quickening, sonograms

Physical Adaptations and Discomforts of Pregnancy
(See Table III-1.)

Teratogenic Effects on Fetal Development
A. Teratogen
1. Definition: nongenetic factor producing malformations of the fetus; greatest effect on those cells undergoing rapid growth, thus time is important
2. Types
   a. Chemical agents (e.g., insecticides)
   b. Radiation
   c. Drugs/Medications: alcohol, tetracycline (*Sumycin*), chemotherapeutic agents, phenytoin (*Dilantin*), narcotics, nicotine, megavitamins, warfarin (*Coumadin*), lead, lithium, carbamazepine (*Tegretol*), and mercury

TABLE III-1
ADAPTATIONS TO PREGNANCY

ADAPTATIONS TO PREGNANCY	TRIMESTER	NURSING INTERVENTIONS
Gastrointestinal: - Nausea/vomiting	1	- Small frequent meals; eat crackers or dry toast before getting up in the morning; eat dry meals; drink liquids between meals
- Constipation, flatulence and heartburn	2, 3	- Exercise; increase fluid and fiber in diet; stool softeners if recommended by provider
- Bleeding gums	2, 3	- Use soft toothbrush for dental care
- Gallstones	2, 3	- Avoid fatty foods
- Heartburn	2, 3	- Small frequent meals; avoid spicy, fatty foods; no sodium bicarbonate as antacid; antacids as recommended by provider
Urinary Tract: - Frequency during first and third trimester due to pressure on bladder	1, 3	- Void when first urge felt; wear a pad if leaking
- Glomerular filtration rate increases (glycosuria)		
- Increase in urinary infections	2, 3	- Increase fluid intake
Breasts: - Increase in size and nodularity, striae	1	
- Tenderness and tingling	1	- Wear supportive bra
- Hypertrophy of Montgomery tubercles	2	
- Darkening of areola	2	
- Colostrum secreted	2, 3	
Vagina: - Epithelium undergoes hypertrophy and hyperplasia		
- Increased vascularity		
- Increased pH: good for growth of Candida (thrush)	1, 2, 3	- Report itching and burning to provider
- Increase in discharge; leukorrhea is common	1	- Promote cleanliness by bathing daily; avoid douching; avoid nylon undergarments
Respiratory system: - Increase in volume of up to 40 to 50% between 16th to 34th week		
- Diaphragm is pushed upward; ribcage flares out; breathing changes from abdominal to chest		
- Increase in oxygen consumption by 15%		

TABLE III-1
ADAPTATIONS TO PREGNANCY (CONTINUED)

ADAPTATIONS TO PREGNANCY	TRIMESTER	NURSING INTERVENTIONS
Respiratory system (continued): - Stuffiness, epistaxis, and changes in voice occur as a result of increased estrogen levels	1	- Cool moist air may help; avoid over-the-counter decongestants and sprays
- Dyspnea	3	- Proper posture; sleep with head propped up
Skin: - Areola darkens - Abdominal striae, linea nigra - Diaphoresis - Chloasma: mask of pregnancy - Vascular spider nervi; chest, neck, arms, and legs	2, 3	Daily bathing; powder

Metabolism/Nutrition:
- Basal metabolic rate increased by 20%
 	
- Water retention: edema
 	
- Weight gain: 20 to 25 lb recommended by adding 300 to 500 calories per day
  - Adequate protein intake, especially for teens
  - Increase iron during last eight weeks
 	
- Pica: craving for non-nutritive substances
	2, 3
	
	2, 3
		- Elevate legs and feet when sitting; avoid prolonged standing; do not wear garters or clothing with restrictive bands around the legs; avoid crossing legs at knees
		
		- Eat a well-balanced diet

Perineum: - Increased vascularity - Venous congestion of the perineum	2, 3	Kegel exercises
Cardiovascular: - Cardiac output increases by 30% - Blood volume progressively increases and peaks around 30 to 40 weeks at 47% above prepregnant state - Plasma volume increases greater than RBC and Hgb, resulting in "pseudo anemia" - Pulse rate increases by 10 to 15/min; blood pressure drops slightly in second trimester due to peripheral dilatation effects of progesterone; returns to normal by third trimester		

TABLE III-1
ADAPTATIONS TO PREGNANCY (CONTINUED)

ADAPTATIONS TO PREGNANCY	TRIMESTER	NURSING INTERVENTIONS
Cardiovascular (continued): - Varicose veins may develop	2, 3	Elevate legs; avoid standing for long periods of time; avoid constrictive clothing
Uterus: - Growth is influenced by estrogen - 500 to 1,000-fold increase in capacity - Cervical secretions form mucus plug		
Endocrine: - Increase in size and activity of thyroid - Increase in size and activity of anterior lobe of pituitary - Increase in size and activity of adrenal cortex - Increase in production of relaxin causes joint and back pain	 2, 3	 Pelvic rock; good body mechanics; supportive shoes

d. Bacteria and viruses
   1) Syphilis
       a) Spirochete does not cross placenta until after 18th week; treat as soon as possible; can treat later since penicillin does not cross placenta
       b) Can cause late abortions, stillbirths, and congenitally infected infants
   2) Gonorrhea: causes injury to eyes at birth (ophthalmia neonatorum)
   3) TORCH syndrome – severe effects on the fetus
       a) Toxoplasmosis: protozoan contracted by ingesting raw meat or feces of infected animal (e.g., cats); pregnant women should not change cat litter boxes
       b) Rubella: first trimester most serious; causes congenital heart problems, cataracts, hearing loss; clients cannot receive the rubella vaccine during pregnancy as it is a live virus; if they receive the immunization in the postpartum period, they must understand that they should not become pregnant for at least 3 months
       c) Cytomegalovirus: member of the herpes family; causes congenital and acquired infection; principal organs affected: liver, brain, and blood; most common mode of transmission is respiratory droplet; employees in day care centers,

developmentally delayed, and health care settings are especially high risk
       d) Herpes simplex virus, Type 2 (HSV-2)
           (1) Transmitted to infant vaginally in intrauterine cavity or during delivery; do not deliver vaginally if active lesions are present
           (2) Affects blood, brain, liver, lungs, CNS, eyes, skin
           (3) Perinatal mortality: 96%; 50% of survivors have neurological or visual abnormalities
   4) Chlamydia: causes conjunctivitis and pneumonia in the newborn
   5) AIDS
       a) Transmitted via breast milk
       b) 30% chance of transmission in utero or during delivery
       c) Treatment of mother with zidovudine (*AZT*) while pregnant can reduce chance of transmission to fetus to approximately 8%

Emotional and Psychological Adaptations to Pregnancy

A. Stressors
   1. Circumstances of pregnancy
   2. Meaning of pregnancy to the couple
   3. Responsibilities associated with parenthood
   4. Resources available to family

B. Development Tasks of Pregnancy

1. First trimester: accept the biological fact of pregnancy; it is common to feel ambivalent early in pregnancy
2. Second trimester: accept growing fetus as a newborn to be nurtured
3. Third trimester: prepare for the birth and parenting of the newborn

C. Emotional Responses

1. Self-concept related to body image
2. Mood swings related to biophysical and social changes
3. Ambivalence related to fear and anxiety
4. Sexual concerns related to biophysical changes

Prenatal Care

A. Initial Assessment

1. Complete history
2. Baseline laboratory data: CBC, blood type and Rh-antibody, urinalysis, STD, group-B streptococcus, alpha fetoprotein, rubella titer, tuberculosis skin test, test offer of HIV.
3. Vital signs, weight, urine test for protein and glucose
4. Physical exam: fundal height, fetal heart rate (FHR), fetal activity
5. Internal exam
   a. Adequate pelvic outlet, signs of pregnancy (First visit)
   b. Cervical changes, especially in last weeks (e.g., "ripe cervix")
   c. Vaginal smear for *Neisseria gonorrhea*, chlamydia, group B strep, human papillomavirus (HPV) cultures, and pap test
6. Psychosocial assessment

B. Health Teaching

1. Nutrition
2. Expected discomforts
3. Danger signs (The nurse must be able to differentiate potential complications from the normal discomforts or physical adaptations of pregnancy.)
   a. Bleeding
   b. Rupture of membranes (ROM)
   c. Contractions (Braxton-Hicks contractions usually go away when position is changed)
   d. Signs of pregnancy-induced hypertension (PIH), toxemia
   e. Burning on urination
   f. Fever
   g. Significant decrease in fetal activity
4. Childbirth education
   a. Childbirth class instruction

1) Fetal growth and development
2) Breathing exercises
3) Position for comfort
4) Relaxation and comfort

5. Follow-up prenatal visits
   a. Every 4 weeks until 28 weeks of gestation
   b. Every 2 weeks until 28 to 36 weeks of gestation
   c. Every week until 36 of gestation to delivery

C. Ethical Issues

1. Rights of fetus
2. Fetal tissue or organs for transplants
3. In vitro fertilization
4. Fertility medications (multiple pregnancy)
5. Intrauterine surgery

SECTION II

REVIEW OF LABOR AND DELIVERY

Components of Labor

A. Power (Uterine Contractions)

1. Frequency: from the beginning of one contraction to the beginning of the next contraction
2. Duration: from the beginning of one contraction to the end of that same contraction
3. Intensity: strength of contraction, measured with fingertips lightly on the fundus (mild, moderate, and strong); accurate measurement can only be made with an internal monitor
4. Regularity: establish a pattern that increases in frequency and duration
5. Effacement: thinning of cervix, 0 to 100%
6. Dilatation: opening of cervix, 0 to 10 cm

B. Passenger (Fetus)

1. Lie: relationship of the cephalocaudal axis of the infant to the cephalocaudal axis of the mother
   a. Transverse lie
   b. Longitudinal lie
2. Presentation: body part of the passenger that enters the pelvic passageway first is called the "presenting part"
   a. Cephalic
      1) Vertex: occiput (most common)
      2) Brow: sinciput
      3) Face: mentum
   b. Breech
      1) Complete: sacrum
      2) Frank
      3) Footling
   c. Shoulder

3. Position: relationship of the landmark on the presenting fetal part to the front, sides, and back of the maternal pelvis
   a. Maternal pelvis includes left or right posterior, anterior, transverse aspects
   b. Fetal landmarks are: occiput (O), mentum (M), sacrum (S), and scapula (Sc)
   c. Most common is left occiput anterior (LOA)
4. Attitude or habitus: to the relationship of the fetal parts to one another, usual is "fetal position"
5. Station: the relationship between the presenting part and the ischial spines; O-station is engagement
6. Cardinal movements of descent
   a. Descent
   b. Flexion
   c. Internal rotation
   d. Extension
   e. External rotation or restitution

C. Passageway (Maternal pelvis)
1. False pelvis helps support pregnant uterus
2. True pelvis forms bony canal; inlet, pelvic cavity, outlet
3. Types
   a. Gynecoid: normal female (50%), best for delivery
   b. Android: normal male (20%), not favorable
   c. Platypelloid: flat female pelvis (5%), not favorable
   d. Anthropoid: apelike (25%), favorable
4. Cephalopelvic disproportion (CPD)

D. Psyche
1. Physical preparation for childbirth
2. Cultural heritage
3. Previous experience
4. Support systems
5. Self-esteem

Fetal Assessment

A. Sonogram
1. Purpose
   a. Locate placenta
   b. Diagnose multiple pregnancy
   c. Identify some congenital anomalies
   d. Determine gestational age

2. **NURSING INTERVENTIONS**
   a. Assure that client has a full bladder.
   b. Provide client education.

B. Fetal Monitoring
1. Purpose
   a. Determine FHR: normal is 120 to 160/min.
   b. Recognize periodic changes in FHR.
   c. Determine frequency and duration of contractions.

2. Types
   a. Auscultation with fetoscope; palpation
   b. External electronic monitoring
   c. Internal electronic monitoring
      1) Provides actual intrauterine pressures
      2) Provides beat-to-beat variability of the FHR, which is an indication of the sympathetic and parasympathetic nervous system status
3. Periodic changes
   a. Early decelerations: head compression
   b. Variable decelerations: cord compression
   c. Late decelerations: uteroplacental insufficiency
   d. Accelerations: usually a sign of fetal well-being
4. Variability
   a. Long term
   b. Short term

C. Kick Counts
1. Definition
   a. Maternal tracking and counting of fetal movement as a reliable screening of fetal well-being during the third trimester of both low- and high-risk pregnancies
   b. Types of fetal movement counted include kicks, turns, twists, swishes, rolls, and jabs
2. Parameters
   a. A healthy fetus should have 10 kicks in less than 2 hr
   b. Most fetuses will take less than 30 min to achieve 10 kicks

3. **NURSING INTERVENTIONS**
   a. Assess kick count daily.
   b. Select the time of day when the fetus is most active; after a meal, after an activity, or in the evening.
   c. Assess the kick count at the same time every day.
   d. Assess in lying or otherwise comfortable position. Encourage client to relax and recognize this as a special, precious moment.
   e. Write down the time of first and tenth kick.
   f. If the fetus is sleeping, awaken it with a glass of juice.

D. Nonstress Test (NST)
1. Purpose
   a. Assess fetal well-being.
   b. Look for increase in FHR (accelerations) with fetal activity (reactive NST)
2. A nonreactive, nonstress test is NOT reassuring

E. Contraction Stress Test
1. Types
   a. Oxytocin challenge test (OCT)
   b. Nipple stimulation test

2. Purpose
   a. Look for three contractions in 10 min
   b. No late decelerations determines fetal well-being
3. A negative CST IS reassuring

F. Biophysical Profile
1. Purpose
   a. Determine fetal well-being after questionable NST.
   b. Determine amount of amniotic fluid.

2. **NURSING INTERVENTIONS**
   a. Provide client education.
   b. Provide emotional support.

G. Amniocentesis (performed after 16th week)
1. Purpose
   a. Determine fetal anomalies, sex, fetal maturity
   b. Determine lecithin-sphingomyelin (L/S) ratio, bilirubin levels, creatine levels

2. **NURSING INTERVENTIONS**
   a. Provide client education.
   b. Assess for premature labor and hemorrhaging.
   c. Provide RhoGAM for client who is Rh-negative.

H. Chorionic Villi Sampling
1. Purpose
   a. Determine fetal anomalies, genetic defects
   b. Early test: 8 to 10 weeks

2. **NURSING INTERVENTIONS**
   a. Provide client education.
   b. Provide RhoGAM for client who is Rh-negative.

Signs of Impending Labor
A. Lightening
B. Braxton-Hicks Contractions
C. Weight Loss (1 to 3 lb)

TABLE III-2
STAGES OF LABOR

STAGES	CHARACTERISTICS	NURSING INTERVENTIONS
- **First Stage**: ("stage of dilatation") begins true labor; ends with complete cervical dilatation; composed of of three phases	- Duration: primigravida 3.3 to 19.7 hr; multigravida 0.1 to 14.3 hr	- Admission; assessment: medical and OB history, vital signs, FHR, signs of labor, weight, vaginal exam (if no active vaginal bleeding)
- Latent phase	- 0 to 4 cm dilatation; mild to moderate contractions every 15 to 20 min, lasting 10 to 30 seconds; backache, cramping, bloody show; mother talkative, cheerful, anxious	- Diversional activities; time contractions; assess maternal-fetal status; pelvic rock; promote hydration; use breathing patterns; evaluate labor progress
- Active phase	- 5 to 7 cm dilatation; strong contractions every 3 to 5 min, lasting 30 to 60 seconds	- Assess maternal-fetal status; backrubs; comfort measures; mother may feel apprehensive; provide encouragement; provide analgesia or anesthesia if requested and is appropriate; promote hydration and elimination; keep perineum clean; promote rest between contractions; evaluate labor progress
- Transitional phase	- 8 to 10 cm dilatation; strong contractions of 2 to 3 min, lasting 50 to 90 seconds; legs may cramp; nausea/vomiting, perspiration on forehead and upper lip; dark, profuse bloody show; mother may have amnesia between contractions, is irritable, anxious, and self-oriented	- Assess maternal-fetal status; provide much reassurance; provide comfort measures; pant/blow with pushing urges; be supportive and help mother maintain control with breathing; evaluate labor progress

TABLE III-2
STAGES OF LABOR (CONTINUED)

STAGES	CHARACTERISTICS	NURSING INTERVENTIONS
- Second stage: ("stage of delivery") begins with complete dilatation of the cervix and ends with delivery	- Duration: primigravida .3 to 1.9 hr; multigravida .9 to .69 hr; contractions 2 to 3 min, lasting 50 to 90 seconds; client has urge to push and is exhausted	- Assess maternal-fetal status; coach pushing; promote comfort; record time of delivery, episiotomy/lacerations, medications, or anesthetics; evaluate labor progress
- Third stage: ("placental stage") begins with delivery of newborn; ends with delivery of placenta	- Mild contractions continue until placenta expelled, normally within 30 min; client may have to push to help expel placenta	- Assess maternal status, blood loss; note time of placenta delivery; administer an oxytocic after placenta separation, if ordered; promote bonding
- Fourth stage: First 1 to 4 hr after delivery. Client usually remains in birthing unit until stable.	- Cramping uterine discomfort; rubra vaginal discharge with small clots; discomfort if episiotomy done; client feels happy, relieved, excited	- Assessment of vital sign, fundus, lochia, and perineum. Usual protocol is every 15 min for first hour; every 30 min for 2 hr; and every 60 min for 1 hr. Provide comfort measures and assist with initial breastfeeding.

D. Cervical Changes

E. Increase in Back Discomfort

F. Bloody Show

G. Rupture of Membranes

    1. Client should contact primary care provider

    2. **NURSING INTERVENTIONS**

        a. Monitor FHR.

        b. Check for prolapsed cord.

        c. Test vaginal secretions for alkalinity with Nitrazine paper.

        d. Watch for signs of infection/meconium.

H. Sudden Burst of Energy

Stages of Labor

Analgesia in Labor

It is important to make nursing assessments of the mother, fetus, and labor status before administering analgesia in labor; given too early, analgesia can slow down labor; given too close to delivery, analgesia can result in respiratory depression of the newborn; ideally, active labor (at least 4 cm) should be established before analgesics are administered

TABLE III-3
MEDICATIONS USED IN LABOR AND DELIVERY

NAME: GENERIC (TRADE)	USE
1. Oxytocin (Pitocin)	- Induces labor, stimulates labor, or contracts uterus after delivery
2. Methylergonovine maleate (Methergine)	- Contracts uterus after delivery
3. Ritodrine hydrochloride (Yutopar)	- Treats premature labor
4. Terbutaline sulfate (Brethine)	- Treats premature labor
5. Hydralazine hydrochloride (Apresoline)	- Treats high blood pressure
6. Magnesium sulfate	- Controls convulsions when used with PIH; treats premature labor
7. Calcium gluconate (generic only)	- Antidote for magnesium sulfate toxicity
8. Rh(D)immune globulin (RhoGAM)	- Prevents sensitization of Rh⁻ mother carrying Rh-positive fetus
9. Naloxone HCl (Narcan)	- Treats respiratory depression
10. Betamethasone (Celestone)	- Stimulates lung development in premature infant
11. Prostaglandin E₂ gel (Cervidil)	- Softens and thins cervix

TABLE III-4
ANALGESIA/ANESTHESIA FOR LABOR AND DELIVERY

A. **Analgesics**: butorphanol tartrate *(Stadol)*, nalbuphine hydrochloride *(Nubain)*, meperidine hydrochloride *(Demerol)*; often mixed with hydroxyzine HCl *(Vistaril)* or promethazine HCl *(Phenergan)* to potentiate; do not give if within 2 hr of delivery — infant may be depressed and require naloxone HCl *(Narcan)*

B. **Local anesthetic**: given locally into perineal tissue during second stage just prior to delivery

C. **Paracervical**: numbs cervix; good for 1st stage of labor; should not be given after dilation of 8 cm (danger of injecting fetal head); can cause fetal bradycardia

D. **Pudendal**: numbs vagina and perineum; good for 2nd stage, large episiotomy, or if anterior-posterior repair is to follow delivery

E. **Epidural**: may have in active phase, when 4 cm dilated or on oxytocin; numbs from the waist down
   1. Nursing interventions: take BP every 5 min until stable; assess bladder; assist in turning and pushing; hydrate client; assess fetal heart rate
   2. Complications: hypotension and fetal distress; turn client on side, increase IV rate, give oxygen

F. **Saddle (spinal)**: numbs from waist down
   1. Complications: headaches, may need blood patch
   2. Nursing interventions: use good body mechanics when moving client

G. **General**: used primarily for emergency cesarean birth

Complications During Labor and Delivery

A. Fetal Distress
1. Etiology
   a. Uteroplacental insufficiency
      1) Acute uteroplacental insufficiency
         a) Excessive uterine activity associated with oxytocin *(Pitocin)*
         b) Maternal hypotension: epidural, venacaval compression, supine position, internal hemorrhage
         c) Placental separation: abruptio, previa
      2) Chronic uteroplacental insufficiency
         a) Pregnancy-induced hypertension
         b) Diabetes mellitus
         c) Postmaturity
    b. **NURSING INTERVENTIONS**
      1) Stop oxytocin induction.
      2) Turn client on left side.
      3) Administer 8 to 10 L of oxygen via face mask.
      4) Increase IV fluids.
      5) Notify provider.

B. Premature Rupture of Membrane (PROM)
1. Etiology
   a. Infection
   b. Trauma

 2. **NURSING INTERVENTIONS**
   a. Assess FHR.
   b. Assess for infection.
   c. Assess for prolapsed cord.
   d. Give ampicillin 4 g IV load then 2 g every 4 hr.

C. Umbilical Cord Compression
1. Etiology
   a. Prolapsed cord
      1) Causes: abnormal presentation, inadequate pelvis, presenting part at high station, multiple gestation, prematurity, PROM, polyhydramnios
      2) Complications: fetal asphyxia
    3) **NURSING INTERVENTIONS**
      a) Place client in Trendelenburg or knee-chest position.
      b) Perform sterile vaginal exam to support presenting part and relieve cord pressure.
      c) Administer oxygen 8 to 10 L via face mask.
      d) Prepare for delivery.
   b. Nuchal cord (cord around neck)

D. Premature Labor
1. Etiology
   a. Chronic pyelonephritis
   b. Incompetent cervix
   c. Multiple pregnancy
   d. History of premature births

e. Sepsis

f. Placental disorders

2. **NURSING INTERVENTIONS**

a. Place client on bed rest.

b. Assess for signs of infection; monitor vital signs, and FHR.

c. Administer ritodrine HCl (*Yutopar*), terbutaline (*Brethine*), or magnesium sulfate as prescribed to stop premature labor.

d. Provide emotional support.

e. Administer betamethasone (*Celestone*) to promote fetal lung development.

f. Prepare for delivery if client is near term.

E. Emergency Childbirth

1. Have mother pant, unless breech.

2. Support perineum.

3. If membranes not ruptured, do so.

4. Feel for cord around infant's neck; gently slip over head.

5. Clear out mucus; keep infant dry and warm.

6. Do not cut cord.

7. Deliver placenta: expect gush of blood and lengthening of cord; save placenta.

8. Massage client's uterus to shrink it; place infant on client's breast.

F. Amniotic Fluid Emboli

1. Definition: amniotic fluid in bloodstream

2. Often happens at delivery

3. Emergency situation, often fatal

G. Dystocia

1. Definition: prolonged, difficult labor

2. Etiology

a. Dysfunction of uterine contractions

b. Abnormal position

c. Cephalopelvic disproportion

d. Maternal exhaustion

3. **NURSING INTERVENTIONS**

a. Prolonged labor varies depending on the cause.

b. Prolonged labor can vary from rest to cesarean birth.

Operative Obstetrics

A. Episiotomy

1. Definition: incision made into the perineum during delivery

2. Purpose

a. To spare muscles from overstretching/ lacerations; to avoid difficulty holding urine in later life

b. Limit pressure on infant's head

3. **NURSING INTERVENTIONS**

a. Assess for healing, infection, laceration of the anal sphincter (4th-degree tear), and hemorrhage.

b. Teach client Kegel exercises.

B. Forceps

1. Definition: obstetric instrument used to aid in delivery

2. Indications

a. Poor progress

b. Fetal distress

c. Persistent occiput posterior position

d. Exhaustion (maternal)

3. **NURSING INTERVENTIONS**

a. Assess infant for intracranial hemorrhage, facial bruising, and facial palsy.

b. Assist with delivery as needed.

c. Check FHR before traction is applied.

4. Complications

a. Lacerations to cervix or vagina

b. Rupture of the uterus

c. Compression of cord

C. Vacuum Extraction

1. Definition: an OB procedure using a suction cup to aid in delivery

2. Indications

a. Poor progress

b. Fetal distress

c. Occiput posterior/occiput transverse position

d. Exhaustion (maternal)

3. **NURSING INTERVENTIONS**

a. Assess FHR every 5 min.

b. Assess for cerebral trauma.

c. Inform parents that caput will disappear in a few hours.

D. Cesarean Birth

1. Definition: incision into abdominal wall and uterus to deliver fetus

2. Types

a. Low transverse: decrease chance of uterine rupture with future pregnancies; less bleeding after delivery

b. Classical: good for emergency delivery; provides more room

3. Indications

a. Fetal distress

b. Cephalopelvic disproportion

c. Placenta previa, abruptio

d. Uterine dysfunction

e. Prolapsed cord

f. Diabetes mellitus

g. Toxemia

h. Malpresentation

4. **NURSING INTERVENTIONS**
   a. Perform postoperative assessment.
   b. Perform postpartum assessment.
5. Vaginal birth after cesarean birth: current accepted standard of care

E. Induction of Labor

1. Definition: process of initiating labor
2. Indications
   a. Maternal disease: cardiac, PIH
   b. Placental malfunctions (e.g., partial previa)
   c. Fetal conditions (e.g., anomaly, death)
   d. Postmaturity
3. Method used to soften cervix; Cervidil placed in cervix then removed after 12 hr; start oxytocin 1 hr after removal
4. Methods used to initiate induction
   a. Oxytocin (*Pitocin*)
   b. Rupture of membranes (ROM) (amniotomy)
 5. **NURSING INTERVENTIONS**
   a. Assess FHR.
   b. Assess for prolapsed cord, ruptured uterus.
   c. Stop oxytocin (*Pitocin*) if contraction lasts longer than 90 seconds or at signs of fetal distress

SECTION III

REVIEW OF POSTPARTAL ADAPTATIONS AND NURSING ASSESSMENT

A. Postpartum Assessment

1. Breasts
2. Uterus
3. Bladder
4. Bowel
5. Lochia (rubra, serosa, alba)
6. Episiotomy
7. Deep vein thrombosis
8. Emotion

B. Puerperium

1. Definition: period of time during which the body adjusts and returns to a near prepregnancy state; usually lasts 6 weeks, can last up to 1 year
2. Uterus (involution)
   a. Fundus is at umbilicus after delivery; 1 finger-breadth above umbilicus 12 hr after delivery; decreases 1 fingerbreadth a day; by 10th day, is at symphysis pubis
   b. Fundus involutes faster if client breastfeeds infant
3. Lochia
   a. Definition: vaginal discharge following delivery

   b. Color
      1) Rubra (1 to 4 days)
      2) Serosa (4 to 7 days)
      3) Alba (7 days to 6 weeks)
   c. Odor: if foul smelling, may indicate infection
   d. Amount: moderate at first, will increase with activity
   e. Afterpains: due to involution of uterus; more severe with multiple births (e.g., twins), polyhydramnios; administration of oxytocin, breastfeeding
   f. Menstruation: resumes in about 6 to 8 weeks in non-nursing mothers; and can vary with nursing mothers
4. Breasts
   a. Engorgement
      1) Non breastfeeding: don't stimulate
         a) Ice
         b) Supportive bra
         c) Pain medication
      2) Breast feeding
         a) Frequent hot showers
         b) Frequent feedings
         c) Massage
5. Perineum
   a. Episiotomy or laceration
      1) Edema
      2) Pain
 b. **NURSING INTERVENTIONS**
      1) Take sitz baths.
      2) Use sprays or ointments.
      3) Perform Kegel exercises.
6. Gastrointestinal
   a. Sluggish bowels
   b. Increased appetite
   c. Hemorrhoids
 d. **NURSING INTERVENTIONS**
      1) Administer stool softeners.
      2) Instruct client to increase dietary fiber and fluids.
      3) Suggest sitz baths and/or witch hazel pads for comfort.
7. Urinary tract
   a. Lessened sensation of bladder fullness
   b. Urinary retention
   c. Difficulty urinating
8. Temperature
   a. First 24 hr, there can be an increase up to 38° C (100.4° F) due to dehydration; exhaustion
   b. WBC normally elevated
9. Skin diaphoresis
   a. Diuresis
   b. Night sweats
   c. Increased output
10. Postpartal chill
   a. Neurologic or vasomotor response to impending delivery

b. Normal immediately following delivery
11. Cardiac
    a. Tachycardia
    b. May occur in first 10 days of postpartum secondary to decreasing blood volume

Psychological Adaptation

A. Self-Concept
1. Body image
2. Fatigue
3. Discomfort

B. Maternal Role: Reva Rubin's stages
1. Taking-in phase: lasts about 2 days; mother focused on self; passive, dependent, fingertip touching
2. Taking-hold phase: increasing independence, ready to learn
3. Letting-go phase

C. Postpartum Depression
1. Mood swings, depression
2. Usually peaks on 5th day, if lasts longer than 10 days, notify primary care provider
3. Related to hormonal changes and fatigue; if continues, must seek professional help

Complications During the Postpartum Period

A. Hemorrhage
1. Definition: blood loss of more than 500 mL for normal spontaneous vaginal delivery, or blood loss of more than 1,000 mL for cesarean birth
2. Etiology
   a. Early: atony
   b. Late: retained placenta
   c. Lacerations, hematomas

3. **NURSING INTERVENTIONS**
   a. Atony: massage fundus first, assess bladder, administer oxytocic medications; (prostaglandin F2a) (carboprost tromethamine) may be prescribed if these measures don't stop the bleeding; do not give to clients with asthma; PID; cardiac, pulmonary, renal or hepatic conditions
   b. Retained placenta, lacerations and hematoma: surgery may be necessary

B. Thromboembolic Disease
1. Etiology
   a. Increased clotting factors postpartum
   b. Venous stasis
   c. History of heart disease, endometritis, and leg varicosities

2. **NURSING INTERVENTIONS**
   a. Assess temperature.

b. Have client ambulate to prevent stasis.
c. Elevate client's leg; provide heat, blood thinner, antibiotics; do not rub.

C. Infection (temperature greater than 38° C [100.4° F])

1. **NURSING INTERVENTIONS**
   a. Encourage early ambulation.
   b. Elevate the client's legs.
   c. Monitor clotting factors.
   d. Implement bleeding precautions when administering anticoagulant therapy.
2. Complications
   a. Pulmonary embolism
   b. Peritonitis
   c. Pelvic cellulitis

SECTION IV

REVIEW OF REPRODUCTIVE RISKS AND COMPLICATIONS

Pregnancy

A. High-Risk Pregnancy
1. Younger than 16 and older than 35 years of age
2. Above gravida 4
3. Over or underweight
4. Drug and alcohol abuse; smoking
5. Previous blood transfusions
6. Poverty income level
7. Less than high school education
8. Unmarried
9. Unwanted pregnancy
10. Little prenatal care
11. Difficulty conceiving
12. Medical problem or pregnancy-induced disease
13. Multiple pregnancy (the greater the number of fetuses, the greater the risk)

B. Medical Problems
1. Cardiac problems
   a. Pathophysiology
      1) Pregnancy expands plasma volume, which increases cardiac output and causes an increased work load on the heart
      2) Can result in heart failure or death
   b. Prognosis
      1) Occurs in 1% of all pregnant women
      2) Danger of maternal death
         a) When blood volume peaks at end of 2nd trimester (30 to 50% increase in volume)
         b) During labor: increase of up to 20% from "milking" effect of contractions

    c) During delivery: due to sudden increase in volume at birth when uterus contracts fully

  c. Prenatal care
    1) Prevent infection.
    2) Consume diet high in protein, restrict weight gain, and do not limit salt unless ordered.
    3) Monitor for anemia.
    4) Provide anticoagulant therapy: use heparin, NOT warfarin sodium (*Coumadin*).
    5) Decrease activity, encourage rest, and reduce stress.

  d. Labor and delivery
    1) Avoid frequent changes of position.
    2) Avoid pain by use of medication, epidural.
    3) Avoid cesarean birth; deliver vaginally with epidural and forceps.
    4) Have ECG, fetal heart monitor, and oxygen ready.
    5) Monitor IV carefully.
    6) Use oxytocin (*Pitocin*) with caution.

  e. Postpartum
    1) Observe the client for the first 48 hr after delivery (heart failure).
    2) Watch for hemorrhage if oxytocin not used.
    3) Monitor I&O (cardiac failure).
    4) Avoid stockings.
    5) Assess for infection: prophylactic antibiotics may be given (prevent endocarditis).
    6) Plan for discharge: client will need help; ability to breastfeed.

2. Diabetes mellitus
  a. Pathophysiology affecting pregnancy
    1) Maternal insulin: does not cross placenta; by 12 weeks fetus makes insulin, but this does not lower blood glucose level (maternal control)
    2) First trimester: fetus draws large amounts of glucose for growth, so maternal need goes way down; may not need any insulin
    3) Second trimester: human placental lactogen and other hormones secreted by the placenta after the 18th week of pregnancy have anti-insulin effect; need for insulin will increase

  b. Prenatal care
    1) Blood glucose control imperative for good outcome; assess maternal HbA1c
    2) High incidence of congenital anomalies and still births if client not in good glucose control

  c. Labor and delivery
    1) Assess infant for maturity and well-being by amniocentesis, stress and nonstress testing, and estriol levels.
    2) A cesarean birth after 37 weeks may be necessary if placenta deteriorates.

  d. Postpartum
    1) Client will need insulin drops rapidly after delivery of placenta.
    2) Assess infant for hypoglycemia.
    3) Assess client for infection.

  e. Complications
    1) Pregnancy-induced hypertension
    2) Polyhydramnios
    3) Hypo/hyperglycemia
    4) Fetal death
    5) Macrosomia (dystocia)
    6) Spontaneous abortion

3. Gestational diabetes (2nd to 3rd trimester)
  a. May be controlled by diet alone
  b. 10 to 15% of clients need insulin
  c. Normal after delivery; increased risk of being diabetic later in life

C. Hyperemesis Gravidarum
1. Definition: excessive vomiting
2. Etiology: may be hormonal or psychological
3. **NURSING INTERVENTIONS**
  a. Monitor I&O.
  b. Administer IV fluids.
  c. Introduce foods slowly.
  d. Decrease stress; psychiatric care if necessary
  e. Assess for metabolic alkalosis.

D. Polyhydramnios
1. Definition: excessive amniotic fluid
2. Etiology
  a. Maternal diseases (toxemia, diabetes mellitus)
  b. Fetal malformation (esophagus not complete)
  c. Erythroblastosis
  d. Multiple pregnancies
3. Treatment
  a. Relieve pressure by amniocentesis
  b. Delivery

E. Abortion
1. Definition: expulsion of the fetus, usually before 20 weeks gestation (spontaneous or induced)
2. Etiology
  a. Abnormal fetus
  b. Infection
  c. Anomaly of reproductive tract
  d. Injury
  e. Unwanted pregnancy
3. Terminology
  a. Spontaneous: miscarriage

b. Therapeutic: termination of a pregnancy by medical intervention

c. Criminal: abortion done outside medical facilities; against the law

4. **NURSING INTERVENTIONS**

a. Save all pads and any tissues passed.

b. Assess for shock, infection, disseminated intravascular coagulation, thrombophlebitis.

c. Administer RhoGAM if Rh-negative.

d. Provide emotional support: do not give false encouragement (grieving necessary).

F. Ectopic Pregnancy

1. Definition: pregnancy that occurs outside the uterus; usually in the fallopian tube, but can be on the ovary, abdomen or interligaments

2. Etiology

a. Malformation of tubes

b. Pelvic inflammatory disease (PID)

c. Tumors

d. Adhesions secondary to surgery or endometriosis

3. Manifestations

a. Sharp abdominal pain (rupture of tube)

b. Shock

c. Mild manifestations initially (little or no bleeding)

4. Diagnosis and treatment

a. Culdocentesis (blood doesn't clot)

b. Removal of tube; may need blood transfusion

5. **NURSING INTERVENTIONS**

a. Watch for shock.

b. Provide usual postoperative care.

c. Provide emotional support; fear of happening again (only one tube remains).

G. Hydatidiform Mole/Molar Pregnancy

1. Definition: abnormal degeneration of the products of conception

2. Possible etiology (actual cause is unknown)

a. Abnormal ova

b. Protein deficiency

3. Manifestations

a. Bleeding: spotting too profuse; pass tan-colored, grape-like clusters (anemia secondary to blood loss)

b. Severe nausea and vomiting

c. Increased levels of human chorionic gonadotropin (HCG) (continues to increase)

d. Signs of pregnancy induced hypertension (PIH) before 24th week

e. Uterus enlarges at a rapid rate

4. Diagnosis and treatment

a. Laboratory values for increased HCG

b. Sonogram

c. Products removed by dilatation and curettage (D&C) (do not induce labor)

d. Monitor client closely for possible cancer; discourage client from becoming pregnant until cancer is ruled out (at least 1 year)

5. **NURSING INTERVENTIONS**

a. Monitor for signs of hypertension and hemorrhage.

b. Reinforce follow-up care to screen for chorioncarcinoma.

c. Provide emotional support.

H. Incompetent Cervix

1. Definition: defect in the cervix that prevents carrying a pregnancy to term

2. Manifestation: client has repeated 2nd trimester spontaneous abortions

3. Treatment: surgical procedures to close cervix (Shirodkar or Cerclage)

4. Prior to delivery: suture removed

I. Pregnancy-Induced Hypertension (PIH)

1. Definition: hypertensive disorder of pregnancy occurring after the 20th week or early postpartum

2. Pathophysiology: increased sensitivity to angiotensin II causes cyclic vasospasms leading to vasoconstriction; this is responsible for most or all symptoms of PIH

3. Terminology

a. Pre-eclampsia: mild or severe depending upon degree of manifestations; IV hydralazine (*Apresoline*) is the medication of choice for pre-eclampsia

b. Eclampsia: convulsions occurs

4. Manifestations

a. Edema: mild to severe swelling of hands, face; pitting of legs (or sacrum)

b. Proteinuria: from 1 gm/24 hr to 5 gm or more/24 hr

c. Hypertension: from 140/90 (or increase of 30/15 above base) to 160/110 or increase in systolic of 50 above base

d. Decrease in urinary output (must have at least 30 mL/hr)

e. Weight gain from edema

f. Headaches, visual disturbances, vasospasm

g. Hemoconcentration

h. Epigastric pain

i. Hyper-reflexia

5. Occurrence

a. Primigravida with age extremes (< 16, > 40)

b. Any chronic medical condition that affects the vascular system (e.g., diabetes mellitus, chronic hypertension, kidney disease, cardiac disease)

c. Family history

d. Multiple pregnancies (e.g., twins, triplets)

e.   Dietary deficiencies, especially protein

 6.   **NURSING INTERVENTIONS** (depends upon degree of illness; status can change very quickly)
a.   Assess vital signs, weight, edema, and protein in urine.
b.   Provide diet high in protein, adequate fluid intake, and do not restrict salt unless ordered.
c.   Promote bed rest, controlled environment, and lying on left side.
d.   Monitor I&O.
e.   Institute seizure precautions (have suction and oxygen ready).
f.   May have to stabilize client and deliver newborn.
   1)   Check reflexes, then give magnesium sulfate (MgSO$_4$); have calcium gluconate at beside (must be given slowly).
   2)   Assess for precipitous delivery and abruptio placenta.
7.   Disseminated intravascular coagulopathy: dangerous disorder of clotting leads to hemorrhage.

J. Abruptio Placenta
1.   Definition: premature separation of the placenta from the uterus
2.   Etiology
a.   Trauma
b.   PIH
c.   Multiparity
d.   Cocaine use
3.   Manifestations
a.   Bleeding: either internal or external
b.   Board-like abdomen, severe pain, tenderness, lack of contractions
c.   Bradycardia or no fetal heart rate (uteroplacental insufficiency)
4.   Treatment
a.   Usually immediate cesarean birth
b.   Treat for blood loss
 5.   **NURSING INTERVENTIONS**
a.   Observe for shock.
b.   Monitor vital signs and FHR.
c.   Assess for diffuse intravascular coagulation (DIC), infection, and anemia.

K. Placenta Previa
1.   Definition: placenta attaches low in the uterus, either near or covering the cervical os
2.   Etiology
a.   Older mothers
b.   Multiparity
3.   Types
a.   Total: completely covers cervix
b.   Partial: partial covering of cervical os
c.   Low lying: near to cervical os
4.   Manifestations: painless, bright red bleeding after

the 7th month (bleeding may be intermittent)
 5.   **NURSING INTERVENTIONS** (depends on type, severity, and gestational age)
a.   Client may need blood and can vary from bed rest to immediate cesarean birth.
b.   Observe for hemorrhage; count pads; monitor vital signs and FHR; be prepared for emergency cesarean birth; provide emotional support.
c.   Do not perform vaginal exams.

SECTION V

NURSING CARE OF THE NEONATE

A. Initial Care of Newborn
1.   Maintain patent airway by suction, position.
2.   Maintain temperature: dry, place newborn on mother or under radiant heat source.
3.   APGAR score: performed at 1 and 5 min after birth.
a.   Five areas scored: heart rate, respiratory effort, muscle tone, reflex irritability, color
   1)   7 to 10: good
   2)   3 to 6: moderately depressed
   3)   0 to 2: severely depressed
4.   Eye prophylaxis: erythromycin, or tetracycline (protects against infections caused by chlamydia and gonorrhea)
5.   Identification
6.   Vitamin K (A*quaMEPHYTON*)

B. Vital Signs
1.   Temperature range is 97 to 99° F; if too high: dehydration, sepsis, brain damage, overheated; if too low: infection, brain stem injury, cold
2.   Heart rate range is 120 to 150/min, dependent upon state; murmur is common at first from transient patent ductus arteriosus
3.   Respirations
a.   30 to 50/min
b.   Distress: nasal flaring, intercostal or xiphoid retractions, expiratory grunt, tachypnea
4.   Blood pressure is 80/40 mm Hg at birth, and 100/50 mm Hg by the 10th day

C. Head
1.   Measure head circumference
2.   Assess fontanels
a.   Posterior: triangular shaped, closes at 8 to 12 weeks
b.   Anterior: diamond shaped, closes at 18 months
c.   Bulging: increased intracranial pressure; depressed: dehydration

3. Molding
4. Caput succedaneum (edema of soft scalp tissue)
5. Cephalohematoma (hematoma between periosteum and skull bone)

D. Eyes
1. Blue-gray color
2. Strabismus is common ("cross-eye")
3. Small hemorrhage (clears in a few weeks)
4. Cataracts

E. Ears
1. Low-set ears are associated with anomalies
2. Infants hear acutely as mucus is absorbed

F. Nose
1. Patency: infants are obligatory nose breathers; can smell
2. Symmetry

G. Mouth
1. Sucking reflex
2. Epstein pearls (small white epithelial cysts along midline of hard palate)
3. Thrush (white patches that adhere to tongue, palate, and buccal mucosa)
4. Palate intact

H. Breast
1. Engorgement
2. Amount of breast tissue

I. Abdomen
1. Measure abdominal circumference
2. Palpate for masses
3. Umbilical cord
   a. Three vessels (one vein, two arteries) "AVA"
   b. Will fall off in 10 days; assess for infection

J. Skin
1. Normal variations
   a. Acrocyanosis: immature circulation (cyanosis of hands and feet)
   b. Milia (tiny white papules on face, distended sebaceous glands)
   c. Toxic erythema (pink papular rash on trunk)
   d. Vernix (white, cheese-like substance)
   e. Mongolian spots: birth marks (irregular areas of pigmentation)
   f. Lanugo (fine, downy hair on forehead, shoulders, back)
2. Color

K. Skeletal
1. Clavicles
2. Hips (Check for congenital hip dysplasia; feel for "Ortolani click")

L. Genitals
1. Female
   a. Swollen
   b. Pseudo menstruation
   c. Vaginal tag
2. Male
   a. Swollen
   b. Hypospadias (opening on underside of penis)
   c. Phimosis (stenosis that prevents foreskin from being retracted back; leads to problems with urination; treatment: circumcision)
   d. Testicles

M. Elimination
1. Void in first 24 hr: pink stains from urates
2. Patent rectum: meconium during first 24 hr

Assessment for Gestational Age

A. Physical Assessment (first 24 hr): for full-term newborn
1. Resting posture
2. Vernix distribution (very little)
3. Skin
4. Nails
5. Lanugo (very sparse)
6. Sole creases (present at full term)
7. Skull firmness
8. Breast tissue
9. Ear formation and cartilage (firm; springs back)
10. Genitalia
11. Recoil

B. Neurological Exam (after 24 hr)
1. Ankle dorsiflexion
2. Square window sign
3. Popliteal angle
4. Heel-to-ear maneuver
5. Scarf sign (contraindicated if fractured clavicle is suspected)
6. Neck extensors
7. Neck flexors
8. Horizontal position
9. Major reflexes
   a. Sucking: response to nipple
   b. Rooting: touch cheek and neonate will turn head to that side
   c. Grasping: touch palm, fingers curl
   d. Moro: "startle" reflex
   e. Tonic neck: turn head to one side in supine position: arm and leg on that side will extend, but flex on opposite side

C. Care of Newborn

1. Weigh daily: initial loss of 10% is normal; newborns should regain birthweight by the 2-week visit.
2. Record daily intake and number of wet and dry diapers.
3. Regulate temperature.
4. For circumcision, discuss options with parents.
   a. Permit signed
   b. Assess for hemorrhage, infection
   c. Required or forbidden by some cultures, religions, or ethnic groups.
5. Perform tests.
   a. Phenylketonuria (PKU): lack of enzyme to convert phenylalanine to tyrosine, Guthrie test: 24 hr after first milk feeding, again in 4 to 6 weeks
   b. Dextrostix: assess blood glucose level
   c. Cultures: if possible infection
6. Educate parents on general care such as feeding, bathing, dressing, cord, and circumcision care.
7. Promote attachment.
8. Assess need for parental support after discharge.

SECTION VI

REVIEW OF HIGH-RISK NEWBORN

Premature Newborn

A. Definition: gestational age of less than 37 weeks, regardless of weight

B. Physical Adaptation

1. Respiratory
   a. May lack surfactants
   b. At risk for respiratory distress syndrome (RDS)
      1) Retractions
      2) Nasal flaring
      3) Expiratory grunt
      4) Tachypnea
      5) Needs mechanical ventilation, oxygen, continuous positive airway pressure (CPAP)
2. Nutrition (fluid and electrolyte)
   a. May lack gag and sucking reflex if under 34 weeks
   b. Fed by gavage or hyperalimentation
3. Circulatory
   a. Patent ductus arteriosus is common
   b. Persistent fetal circulation
4. Complications
   a. Hypothermia
   b. Hypocalcemia

c. Hypoglycemia
d. Hyperbilirubinemia
e. Birth trauma
f. Sepsis
g. Intracranial hemorrhage
h. Necrotizing enterocolitis
i. Apnea

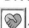 5. **NURSING INTERVENTIONS**
   a. Monitor vital signs.
   b. Maintain temperature.
   c. Assess hydration, nutrition.
   d. Promote attachment and bonding between parents and newborn.

Small for Gestational Age (SGA)

A. Definition: any newborn who falls below the 10th percentile on the growth chart at birth

B. Etiology

1. Placental insufficiency
2. Pregnancy-induced hypertension
3. Multiple pregnancy
4. Poor nutrition
5. Smoking, drugs, alcohol
6. Adolescent pregnancy

C. Complications

1. Perinatal asphyxia
2. Meconium aspiration syndrome
3. Hypoglycemia
4. Hypothermia
5. Infections

D. NURSING INTERVENTIONS

1. Support respirations.
2. Provide neutral thermal environment.
3. Provide adequate nutrition.
4. Observe for complications.
5. Protect from infection.
6. Support parents; promote bonding.

Large for Gestational Age (LGA)

A. Definition: newborn whose weight is at or above the 90th percentile (could still be premature)

B. Etiology

1. Diabetes mellitus
2. Genetic predisposition
3. Congenital defects

C. Complications

1. Birth trauma (e.g., fractured clavicle)
2. Hypoglycemia
3. Polycythemia
4. If mother diabetic, same risk and care as premature infant

D. NURSING INTERVENTIONS

1. Assess for trauma.
2. Assess for congenital abnormalities.
3. Assess for hypoglycemia, especially if infant of diabetic mother.

Postmature Infant

A. Definition: gestational age of over 42 weeks

B. Physical Findings
1. Dry, parchment-like skin
2. Longer, harder nails
3. Profuse scalp hair
4. Absent vernix
5. Hypoglycemia

C. Complications
1. Progressive aging of placenta
2. Difficult delivery
3. High perinatal mortality

Jaundice (Hyperbilirubinemia)

A. Causes
1. Physiological
   a. Never seen during first 24 hr; usually appears by third day
   b. Immature liver
2. Bruising
3. ABO incompatibility (Mother is O, newborn is A, B, or AB)
4. Rh incompatibility (erythroblastosis fetalis)
   a. Rh-negative mother and Rh-positive newborn
   b. Kernicterus (bilirubin encephalopathy) can lead to brain damage, anemia, and/or hepatosplenomegaly
   c. Treatment
      1) Phototherapy, sunlight, exchange transfusion
      2) RhoGAM administered at 28 weeks of gestation, and within 72 hr of delivery
      3) Note: RhoGAM also given to all Rh-negative mothers who abort after the 8th week of gestation
5. Breastfeeding

Substance Abuse and the Newborn

A. Drug Dependent
1. Manifestations of withdrawal
   a. Early manifestation: irritability
   b. Sneezing, nasal stuffiness
   c. High-pitched, weak cry
   d. Tremors
   e. Perspiration

   f. Feeding problems (weak suck)
   g. Transient tachypnea

2. **NURSING INTERVENTIONS**
   a. Prevent overstimulation to prevent possible seizures.
   b. Swaddle; hold infant firmly.
   c. Administer medications as prescribed.
   d. Provide small, frequent feedings (may need to gavage).

B. Fetal Alcohol Syndrome
1. Etiology: consumption of alcoholic beverages during pregnancy
2. Manifestations
   a. Feeding problems (weak suck)
   b. Distinctive facial features (microcephaly, small eyes, thin upper lip)
   c. CNS dysfunction (including mental retardation and seizures)
   d. Physical defects (limb anomalies, hyperactivity, cardiocirculatory defects, deafness)
   e. Withdrawal manifestations

3. **NURSING INTERVENTIONS**
   a. Protect infant from injury.
   b. Administer medications.
   c. Monitor fluid therapy.
   d. Decrease stimuli.
   e. Provide support to parents who may have to care for an infant who is difficult.
   f. Provide social service referral.

SECTION VII

NURSING CARE OF THE GYNECOLOGIC CLIENT

Vaginal Infections

A. Candidiasis (Yeast)
1. Manifestations
   a. Cheese-like discharge
   b. Itching
   c. Discomfort with urination and intercourse
2. Etiology and risk factors
   a. Diabetes mellitus, immunosuppressed
   b. Use of oral contraceptives or antibiotics, and frequent douching
3. **NURSING INTERVENTIONS**
   a. Administer miconazole (*Monistat*) or fluconazole (*Diflucan*).
   b. Discuss importance of cleanliness with client.
   c. Ensure that both partners are treated.

B. Trichomoniasis (sexually transmitted)
1. Manifestations
   a. Yellow, green, or gray discharge
   b. Discomfort with urination and intercourse
   c. Irritation and itching

2. **NURSING INTERVENTIONS**
   a. Administer metronidazole (*Flagyl*) unless client is in the first trimester of pregnancy.
   b. Treat both partners; abstain from sexual intercourse during treatment.

C. Condyloma (sexually transmitted)
1. Caused by human papillomavirus
2. Manifestations: presence of soft grayish-pink lesions on perineum (genital warts)

3. **NURSING INTERVENTIONS**
   a. Assist with application of podophyllum resin.
   b. Assist with cryosurgery with liquid nitrogen or laser (carbon dioxide laser) surgery.
   c. Educate client of increased risk for cervical cancer.
   d. Instruct client of need for close follow-up with pap smears.

Cancer

A. Cervical
1. Etiology: Human Papillomavirus (HPV) is responsible for most cervical cancer; half of cervical cancer cases occur between ages 35 and 55
2. Manifestations
   a. Heavy, foul-smelling blood during times other than menses
   b. Pelvic pain or pain during intercourse
3. Risk Factors
   a. Many partners with initial sex before age 18
   b. History of STDs
   c. Immunosuppressed
   d. Cigarette smoking
4. Screening
   a. Annual pap smear
   b. HPV DNA test
5. Treatment: conization, laser surgery, loop electrocautery excision procedure (LEEP), cryosurgery, hysterectomy, radiation, or chemotherapy
6. Prevention
   a. Delay initial intercourse.
   b. Avoid smoking.
   c. Have fewer sexual partners.
   d. Gardasil (Human Papillomavirus Quadrivalent) vaccine for ages 9 to 26

B. Endometrium
1. Manifestations
   a. Postmenopausal bleeding
   b. Abnormal bleeding
2. Treatment
   a. Radium
   b. X-ray therapy
   c. Hysterectomy

3. **NURSING INTERVENTIONS**
   a. Assess for grieving.
   b. Preoperative teaching.
   c. Provide postoperative care.
   d. Assess psychosexual needs.

C. Ovarian
1. Etiology: unknown, but high incidence with family history; ovarian cancer is the fifth leading cause of cancer death after lung, breast, colorectal, and pancreatic; mortality rates are greater in Caucasian women
2. Risk Factors
   a. Risk increases after age 50
   b. Risk increases if one or more relative has a history (mother, daughter, sister)
3. Screening
   a. CA 125 blood test
   b. Intravaginal ultrasound
   c. Pelvic exam

D. Breast
1. Warning Signs
   a. Lump in breast or armpit
   b. Thickening, dimpling, redness, pain, or asymmetry in breasts
   c. Pulling, discharge, or pain in nipple area
2. Risk Factors
   a. Initial menses before age 12, initial menopause after age 51
   b. First pregnancy after age 35
   c. Did not breastfeed
   d. Never been pregnant
   e. Family history of breast cancer
   f. Overweight and sedentary lifestyle
   g. Long-term use of hormone replacement therapy
   h. Use of oral contraceptives
   i. Alcohol use greater than one drink daily
3. Screening
   a. Mammogram: women 40 and older should get them every 1 to 2 years
   b. Clinical breast exam: women should receive this annually
   c. Breast self exam: women should perform this monthly 1 week after menses
4. Treatment: surgery, chemotherapy, radiation, or hormone therapy

Uterine Disorders

A. Myomas (Uterine Fibroids)
1. Definition: benign fibroid tumors of the uterine muscle
2. Etiology: African Americans over age 30 who have never been pregnant
3. Manifestations
   a. Pelvic pain or pressure
   b. Hypermenorrhea
4. Treatment: medication, surgery

B. Endometriosis
1. Definition: endometrial tissue located outside of uterus
2. Manifestations
   a. Severe dysmenorrhea
   b. Lower abdominal pain, pain during intercourse, back and rectal pain
   c. Abnormal bleeding
3. Treatment
   a. Oral contraceptives (hormone therapy)
   b. Surgery
   c. Pregnancy

Tubal Disorder

A. Pelvic Inflammatory Disease (PID)
1. Etiology
   a. Infections
   b. Venereal disease
2. Manifestations
   a. Vaginal discharge: foul smelling, purulent
   b. Pain in abdomen, lower back
   c. Elevated temperature, nausea, vomiting

3. **NURSING INTERVENTIONS**
   a. Administer antibiotic therapy.
   b. Educate client.

Menopause

A. Definition: complete cessation of menstruation for 1 year

B. Manifestations
1. Hot flashes
2. Palpitations
3. Diaphoresis
4. Osteoporosis

C. NURSING INTERVENTIONS

1. Assess psychosocial response.
2. Discuss merits of estrogen therapy, including prevention of osteoporosis, heart disease.
3. Use alternative therapies (diet, exercise, calcium supplements).

Infertility

A. Definition: decreased capacity to conceive

B. Etiology
1. Abnormal genitalia
2. Absence of ovulation
3. Blocked fallopian tubes
4. Altered vaginal pH
5. Sperm deficiency or decreased motility
6. Infection

C. Diagnosis
1. Examination of male reproductive organs
2. Examination of female reproductive organs

D. Management
1. Medication
   a. Clomiphene citrate (*Clomid*) or menotropins (*Pergonal*); associated with multiple births
   b. Hormone replacement
2. Artificial insemination
3. In vitro fertilization
4. Surrogate parenting

E. NURSING INTERVENTIONS

1. Provide emotional support.
2. Provide client education.

Contraception

A. Nursing Assessment

1. Determine client's knowledge about and previous experience with family planning.
2. Determine client's need for genetic counseling.
3. Identify infertility problems.
4. Assess risks to client's choice of contraceptive method.

B. Types
1. Natural (rhythm) method
   a. Use of calendar, basal body temperature, and cervical mucus methods.
   b. **NURSING INTERVENTION:** teach method

2. Oral contraceptives
   a. Side effects similar to pregnancy: initial discomforts, hypertension, clotting problems, fluid retention
   b. Contraindicated if client is:
      1) Over 35
      2) Hypertensive
      3) A smoker
      4) Has a history of clotting disorder

   c. **NURSING INTERVENTIONS**
      1) Teach method
      2) Assess for complications (increased blood pressure).

3. Injectable contraceptive: Medroxyprogesterone acetate (*Depo-Provera*)
   a. Side effects: irregular, unpredictable menses
   b. Administered every 3 months via IM injection
4. Ortho Evra Patch
   a. Skin patch worn on lower abdomen, buttocks, or upper body that releases progestin and estrogen
   b. Less effective in women weighing over 200 lb
   c. Worn for 3 weeks, removed for 1 week during menses
5. NuvaRing
   a. Flexible, 2-inch ring inserted into vagina, releases progestin and estrogen
   b. Can cause vaginal discharge, vaginitis, and irritation
   c. Worn for 3 weeks, removed for 1 week during menses
   d. If ring falls out for more than 3 hr, use back-up method until ring has been in place for 7 consecutive days
6. Intrauterine device (IUD)
   a. High risk of PID, ectopic pregnancy, perforation of uterus; periods may be heavy (anemia)
    b. **NURSING INTERVENTIONS**
      1) Instruct client in the need for follow up.
      2) Client should get regular pap tests.
      3) Teach client to feel for strings frequently.
7. Mechanical barriers
   a. Diaphragm
    1) **NURSING INTERVENTIONS**
      a) Teach client how to insert diaphragm.
      b) Teach client how to use spermicidal jelly with diaphragm.
      c) Teach client to leave in 6 to 8 hr after intercourse.
      d) Teach client to have diaphragm refitted if client gains or loses weight; after childbirth.
   b. Condom
    1) **NURSING INTERVENTIONS:** female condom (vaginal sheath)
      a) Teach client to use with spermicide.
      b) Protects against STDs, including HIV.
    2) **NURSING INTERVENTIONS:** male condom
      a) Teach client to leave space at end.
      b) Teach how to prevent slipping or tearing during removal.
      c) Protects against STDs, including HIV.
   c. Cervical cap: can be left in place up to 12 hr

8. Chemical barriers (spermicides)
    NURSING INTERVENTIONS
      a) Teach client about possible allergic reactions.
      b) Teach client how to clean equipment.
      c) Warn client not to douche for 6 to 8 hr after intercourse.
9. Sterilization
   a. Tubal ligation
    1) **NURSING INTERVENTIONS**
      a) Discuss permanency.
      b) Discuss methods of obstructing tubes.
    Vasectomy
   2) **NURSING INTERVENTIONS**
      a) Discuss permanency.
      b) Warn client of need for negative sperm count three times before attempting unprotected intercourse.
10. Unreliable methods
    a. Withdrawal/coitus interruptus
    b. Douching

UNIT FOUR

CHILD HEALTH
NURSING

UNIT CONTENT

SYMBOLS

 Key Points

 Nursing Interventions

 Points to Remember

SECTION I

GROWTH AND DEVELOPMENT

Characteristics of Development

A. Lifelong Process

B. Critical Periods

C. Proximodistal (development of fine motor skills)

D. Cephalocaudal ("head to tail" development)

Lifespan and Development of the Infant

Birth to 1 year

1. Physical characteristics
    a. Height: increases by 50% in first year
    b. Weight: birth weight doubles by 6 months; birth weight triples by 12 months
    c. Head: 70% of adult size at birth; 80% of adult size by end of first year
        1) Posterior fontanel: closes by 2 months of age
        2) Anterior fontanel: closes between 12 to 18 months of age
            a) Bulging: classic sign of increased intracranial pressure
            b) Sunken: classic sign of dehydration
    d. Dentition
        1) Drools at 4 months
        2) Primary teeth: by 12 months: six primary teeth (age of child in months minus 6 equals number of teeth) (See Table IV-1.)
         3) **NURSING INTERVENTIONS**
            a) Avoid medications that may stain teeth (e.g., tetracycline, iron).
            b) Avoid phenytoin (*Dilantin*): causes gingivitis and gingival hyperplasia.
            c) Teach parents that increased drooling, finger sucking, and biting on objects are all indicators of teething.
            d) Inform parents that cool or cold items (teething rings) are soothing.
            e) Use acetaminophen (*Tylenol*) for continued irritability.
            f) Educate parents that once dentition occurs, avoid nighttime bottle with juice or formula - it increases the incidence of dental caries ("bottle mouth" caries).
    e. Reflexes
        1) Rooting (disappears by 3 to 4 months)
        2) Tonic neck (disappears by 3 to 4 months)
        3) Palmar grasp (disappears by 3 to 4 months)
        4) Moro (disappears by 3 to 4 months)
        5) Sucking (continues through infancy)
        6) Stepping (disappears by 3 to 4 months)
    f. Vital signs
        1) Pulse ranges from 100 to 140/min, may even be as high as 160/min depending upon activity
        2) Respirations range from 30 to 40/min
        3) Immature thermoregulatory mechanisms
        4) Crying will increase all vital signs
2. Nutrition
    a. Infant feeding
        1) Allow infant to set own schedule.
        2) Breast or bottle feed infant depending upon mother's preference.
        3) Give vitamin supplements as prescribed; usually begun around 3 to 4 months (vitamin D and iron); fluoride supplements for infants who are breastfed.
        4) Have infant consume between 100 to 110 calories/kg/day.
    b. Introduction of solid foods
        1) Physiologic readiness
            a) Tongue extrusion reflex (fades by about 4 months)
            b) Digestive enzymes

TABLE IV-1
SCHEDULE OF PRIMARY TOOTH ERUPTION

ERUPTION	LOWER	UPPER
Central incisor	6 to 10 months	8 to 12 months
Lateral incisor	10 to 16 months	9 to 13 months
First molar	12 to 18 months	13 to 19 months
Cuspid	17 to 23 months	16 to 22 months
Second molar	23 to 31 months	25 to 33 months

     c) Motor skills: sit with support; head and neck control

     d) Interest in solid food

  2) Nutritional guidelines

     a) Introduce solids around 4 to 6 months.

     b) Introduce foods one at a time, at every 4 to 7 days (observe for allergy).

     c) Follow sequence food introduction at one-month intervals:

       (1) Rice cereal (good source of iron; no wheat)

       (2) Fruits and vegetables (yellow, then green)

       (3) Meats (begin with chicken, turkey)

       (4) Egg yolks (avoid egg whites)

     d) Begin table foods around 8 to 12 months.

       (1) No nuts, foods with seeds, raisins, popcorn, grapes (risk for aspiration)

       (2) Finger foods enhance thumb-finger apposition

     e) When switching from formula to cow's milk, avoid skim milk (not enough fat) because the infant needs whole milk.

     f) As amount of solids increases, reduce quantity of milk (no more than 30 oz/day).

     g) Never mix food or medication with formula.

     h) Avoid sweeteners such as honey or corn syrup (risk of botulism).

 c. Weaning

  1) Usually begins around 4 to 6 months with sips from a cup; can use training cup with sipper tube and/or handles

  2) Cup introduced gradually

  3) Bottle or breastfeeding removed one at a time; remove nighttime feeding last

  4) By 12 to 14 months, infant should be able to drink from a cup

 d. Nutritional concerns

  1) Colic

     a) Seen in infants younger than 3 months

     b) Paroxysmal abdominal pain associated with crying and accumulation of gas

     c) Associated with overfeeding, air swallowing, maternal insecurity

      d) **NURSING INTERVENTIONS**

       (1) Feed infant slowly with frequent burping.

       (2) Avoid excessive feedings.

       (3) Increase bonding between mother and infant.

       (4) Teach mother various feeding and holding techniques.

  2) Iron deficiency anemia

     a) Result of poor diet or low-iron stores in the newborn

     b) Seldom seen in first 6 months due to iron stores inherited from mother

     c) Most frequently seen in infants between 6 months and 1 year who ingest large quantities of milk

     d) RBCs appear microcytic and hypochromic

     e) Prevention: use of an iron-fortified formula and/or cereal

     f) Ferrous sulfate (*Feosol*) is the medication of choice

      g) **NURSING INTERVENTIONS**:

       (1) Administer medication between meals.

       (2) Administer with citrus juice for greater iron absorption.

       (3) Teach parents that liquid preparations may stain teeth.

       (4) Inform parents that iron may cause tarry stools.

3. Activity/rest

 a. Normal infants sleep 14 to 16 hr a day

 b. Nocturnal pattern of sleep develops by 3 to 4 months

4. Motor skills

 a. 2 months

  1) Smiles socially

  2) Demonstrates differentiated cry

  3) Turns head from side to side

 b. 3 months

  1) Follows object 180° horizontal and vertical (20/100 visual acuity at birth)

  2) Discovers hands

  3) Reaches for object

  4) Lifts head off bed; bears weight on forearms

 c. 4 months

  1) Recognizes familiar objects; moves extremities in response

  2) Sits with support

  3) Reaches for object

  4) Laughs aloud

  5) Begins to recognize parent

  6) Rolls back to side

  7) Exhibits almost no head lag

    d. 5 to 6 months
        1) Rolls over completely
        2) Bangs with object held in hand
        3) Vocalizes displeasure when object taken away
        4) Rakes object
        5) Exhibits no head lag
    e. 6 to 8 months
        1) Holds own bottle (6 months)
        2) Transfers toy (7 months)
        3) Begins pincer grasp (8 months)
        4) Shows a fear of strangers: "stranger anxiety"
        5) Sits alone (8 months)
    f. 9 to 12 months
        1) Pulls self to feet (9 months)
        2) Stands alone
        3) Walks with help
        4) Uses spoon, with spilling
        5) Cruises (9 months); crawls well (10 months)
        6) Claps hands on request
        7) Imitates behavior
        8) Smiles at image in mirror
5. Language development
    a. Vocalizes (distinct from crying) by 3 to 4 months
    b. Recognizes "no" by 9 months; own name by 10 months
    c. Two to three words in addition to "mama," "dada" by 12 months
6. Developmental stages
    a. Psychosocial development (Erikson)
        1) Trust vs. mistrust
        2) Quality of caregiver/child relationship
    b. Cognitive development (Piaget)
        1) Sensorimotor phase
            a) Reflexive
            b) Imitates and recognizes new experiences
        2) Object permanence
            a) Understands that self and object are separate (10 months)
            b) Will search for lost object (12 months)
            c) Separation anxiety (8 to 12 months)
7. Play
    a. Solitary
    b. Characteristics
        1) 1 to 3 months: verbal, visual, tactile stimuli
            a) Toys should be brightly colored, washable, of various sizes, shapes, and textures
            b) Enhance eye-hand coordination
                (1) Mobiles, cradle gyms
                (2) Busy box, toys with faces

            c) Stimulate auditory senses (e.g., rattles, music box)
        2) 4 to 6 months: initiates, recognizes new experiences
            a) Mobility increasing
            b) Hand coordination increasing
            c) Memory beginning
            d) Types of toys
                (1) Mirrors to see image
                (2) Chewable, large toys
                (3) Brightly colored rattles, beads
                (4) Squeeze toys, teething rings
                (5) Remove cradle gym to avoid accidents
        3) 6 to 12 months
            a) Increasing self-awareness
            b) Repeats pleasurable activities
            c) Object permanence
            d) Imitates behavior at 10 months; "peek-a-boo"
            e) Increased desire to explore
            f) Types of toys
                (1) Large boxes, kitchen utensils
                (2) Water play with supervision
                (3) Texture play: sand, dirt
                (4) Pouring, filling, dumping
                (5) Playing with food (beginning of self-feeding)
    c. Safety measures
        1) Toys should be large; short strings
        2) Constructed of nontoxic materials
        3) Always supervise
        4) Inspect toys for problems
            a) Rough edges
            b) Parts that can be pulled off and swallowed or aspirated
8. Health maintenance
    a. Safety
        1) Avoid overstimulation, rough handling.
        2) Limit-setting should involve redirecting behaviors to safer activities.
    b. Immunizations
        1) Schedule determined by Center for Disease Control and Prevention (CDC); recommendation published annually
        2) Protects infants and children from fourteen diseases by building immunity
            a) Diphtheria
            b) Hepatitis A
            c) Hepatitis B
            d) Haemophilus influenzae type B
            e) Influenza
            f) Measles
            g) Mumps
            h) Pertussis
            i) Meningococcal
            j) Polio

k) Rubella
l) Tetanus
m) Chickenpox
n) Rotavirus

c. Infant restraints
1) Use a semi-reclining infant car seat that faces rear until 10 kg (20 lb).
2) Use a car seat-belt to anchor restraint.
3) Middle of car's back seat is the safest area for the infant.
4) Infant seats should not be used in front seat because of passenger-side airbags.

d. Aspiration of foreign objects
1) Common problems include food, buttons from clothing, baby powder, and small-piece toys
2) Emergency measures for choking infant
a) Five back blows, five chest thrusts (repeat until successful)
b) No blind finger sweep

9. Health deviations
a. Accidents (leading cause of death over 1 year of age)
1) Falls (depth perception develops by 7 to 9 months)
2) Suffocation/aspiration/drowning
3) Burns

b. Caregiver education
1) Childproof environment
2) Constant supervision
3) Anticipatory guidance
a) Provide appropriate car seat restraint.
b) Assess temperature of bath water, formula, and food.
c) Do not prop bottle during feeding or at sleep time.
d) Supervise during bath time, changing table, and play time.
e) Select age-appropriate toys.
f) Turn handles of pots/pans away from reach.
g) Keep side rails up during sleep time.

c. SIDS (Sudden Infant Death Syndrome)
1) Cause unknown; multiple theories
2) Infants at risk
a) Mostly males, ages 2 to 4 months
b) Preterm infants with apnea problems
c) Multiple births
3) Occurs during sleep, usually in winter months
4) Caregiver education
a) Infant should sleep in supine or side lying position, not prone
b) Firm mattress, no pillow; avoid overheating during sleep
c) Lower incidence if breastfed

Lifespan and Development of the Toddler

12 months to 3 years

1. Physical characteristics
a. Large abdomen, long legged, clumsy
b. Slowing rate of growth for height and weight (adult height = approximately double height at 2 years)
c. Dentition
1) By 2 ½ years: all 20 primary teeth
2) Adult should brush child's teeth by age 2
3) First visit to dentist by age 2
d. Vital signs
1) Pulse: ranges from 80 to 110/min
2) Respirations: range from 25 to 35/min
3) Blood pressure: average is 100/70 mm Hg

2. Nutrition
a. Growth lag (80 calories/kg)
b. Expresses independence through food preferences; food fads are common
c. Wants to feed self; very ritualistic, messy
d. Space meals with frequent nutritious snacks (cheese, peanut butter and jelly sandwiches)
e. Small portions (physiologic anorexia)
f. Fluid requirements: 115 mL/kg/day (3 cups whole milk/day)

3. Activity/rest
a. Sleeps 10 to 12 hr with naps
b. Routines and rituals are reassuring
c. Nightmares and night terrors are possible

4. Motor skills
a. 13 to 16 months
1) Uses spoon and cup, but will spill
2) Walks without help (since about 13 months)
3) Climbs up and down stairs on buttocks
4) Mimics housework
5) Stacks 2 to 3 blocks (15 months)
6) Throws and drops things (15 months)
7) Loves containers of all kinds
b. 16 to 18 months
1) Runs clumsily; falls often
2) Throws ball overhand
3) Pulls and pushes toys
4) Uses spoon and cup without spilling
5) Removes clothes (shoes, socks)
6) Jumps in place
7) Kicks small ball
c. 2 years
1) Walks up and down stairs
2) Runs well
3) Turns knobs to open doors; unscrews lids
4) Dresses self in simple clothing
5) Builds tower of 5 blocks
6) Turns pages of a book
7) Climbs

d. 2 ½ to 3 years
    1) Holds crayon with fingers
    2) May have daytime bowel and bladder control
    3) Strings beads

5. Language development
  a. Ten words by 18 months
  b. May say "no" when agreeing (means "yes")
  c. Uses two-to three-word phrases by 2 years; vocabulary of 300 words; verbalizes needs (toileting, food, drink); uses pronouns
  d. Gives first and last name by 2 ½ years

6. Developmental stages
  a. Psychosocial development (Erikson)
    1) Autonomy vs. shame and doubt (1 to 3 years)
      a) Egocentric
      b) Negativism and temper tantrums
      c) Uninhibited at showing independence
    2) Gains control over bodily functions
  b. Cognitive development (Piaget)
    1) Sensorimotor (12 to 24 months)
      a) Objects are cause of action
      b) Separation anxiety
    2) Preoperational (24 months to 4 years)
      a) Concrete thinking begins
      b) Egocentric
      c) Symbolic play

7. Play
  a. Parallel play
    1) No sharing
    2) Ownership determined by possession of object
    3) Short attention span
  b. Types of activities
    1) Gross motor
      a) Jungle gym
      b) Push-pull toys
      c) Tricycle (2 ½ to 3 years)
    2) Fine motor
      a) Crayons, paints, paper
      b) Building blocks
      c) Musical toys
    3) Enjoys being read to

8. Health maintenance
  a. Toilet training (18 months to 2 years)
    1) Physiologic readiness (sphincter control at approximately 18 months)
    2) Imitation; potty chair
    3) May not be complete until 4 to 5 years of age (nocturnal control often delayed)
  b. Discipline
    1) Toddlers are negative and ritualistic
    2) Limits must be simple and consistent

  c. Safety
    1) Precautions
      a) Childproof the environment
      b) Supervise at all times
      c) Child restraints (may switch to forward-facing car seat when child weighs approximately 10 kg [20 lb])
    2) Immunizations
      a) MMR: 15 months
      b) HIB: 15 months
      c) DTaP, IPV: 18 months
      d) Varicella zoster (chickenpox): after 12 months

9. Health deviations
  a. Accidents
    1) Motor vehicles: passengers, pedestrians
    2) Burns
    3) Drowning/suffocation/aspiration
    4) Falls
    5) Ingestions
      a) Have phone number for poison control and emergency department posted by telephone.
      b) Lock up all medications and potentially toxic substances.
      c) Use child resistant caps appropriately.
      d) Never refer to medication as candy.
      e) Never transfer potentially toxic solutions from original containers.
  b. Anticipatory guidance
    1) Supervise toddler closely near water.
    2) Store flammables and lighters out of reach.
    3) Use child restraints in vehicles.
    4) Avoid easily aspirated foods such as grapes, hot dogs, popcorn, round candy, and nuts.

Lifespan and Development of the Preschooler

3 to 5 years

1. Physical characteristics: average 4 year old is 101 cm (40 inches) and 18 kg (40 lb)
2. Nutrition
  a. Growth lag (70 kcal/kg)
  b. Encourage finger foods (cheese, fruit)
  c. Food fads are common
3. Activity/rest
  a. May give up nap, but needs quiet time
  b. Peak time for sleep disturbances
    1) Refusal to go to bed
      a) Child resists bedtime; comes out of room frequently

b) **NURSING INTERVENTIONS**
   (1) Stress need for a consistent bedtime.
   (2) Help parent's identify strategies to ignore attention-seeking behaviors.
   (3) Suggest that the parents avoid bringing child into their bed (consider client's culture).
   (4) Promote use of a transitional object (blanket, toy).

2) Nighttime fears
   a) Child resists bed because of fears (dark, monsters)
    b) **NURSING INTERVENTIONS**
     (1) Tell parents to reassure child calmly.
     (2) Suggest that parents use a night-light for child.
     (3) Suggest that parents monitor bedtime TV viewing.

4. Motor skills
  a. 3 years
   1) Dresses with supervision; needs help with buttons
   2) Rides tricycle
   3) Climbs stairs with alternate feet
   4) Pours fluid from a pitcher
  b. 4 years
   1) Hops and skips on one foot
   2) Walks upstairs without use of handrail; alternates feet walking downstairs
   3) Uses scissors
   4) Laces shoes but cannot tie
  c. 5 years
   1) Hops and skips on alternate feet
   2) Walks backwards
   3) Can master two-wheel bike/roller skates
   4) Uses simple tools, prints name
   5) May master tying shoes

5. Language development
  a. 3 years
   1) Vocabulary of 900 words
   2) Talks constantly regardless of whether anyone is listening
   3) Complete sentences
  b. 4 years
   1) Vocabulary of 1,500 words
   2) Questions constantly
   3) Exaggerates; tells "tall tales"
   4) May stutter
   5) May pick up profanity
  c. 5 years
   1) Vocabulary of 2,000 words
   2) Uses all parts of speech

3) Speech 100% intelligible to others although some sounds may still be imperfect

6. Developmental stages
  a. Psychosocial development (Erikson)
   1) Initiative vs. guilt (3 to 5 years)
    a) Vigorous behavior
    b) Limit testing
   2) Child develops a conscience
  b. Cognitive development (Piaget)
   1) Preoperational (2 to 7 years)
    a) Egocentric in thought and behavior
    b) Concrete, tangible thinking
    c) Vivid imagination
     (1) Magical thinking (thoughts can cause events)
     (2) Peak age for fears
  c. Socialization
   1) 3 years
    a) May have an imaginary friend
    b) Increased ability to separate from parents
   2) 4 years
    a) May be bossy and impatient
    b) Privacy and independence become important
   3) 5 years
    a) Less rebellious; more responsible
    b) Cares for self and hygiene needs with minimal supervision
  d. Sexuality
   1) Knows own sex and sex of others by 3 years
   2) Masturbation is normal, healthy expression, if not excessive
   3) Sexual exploration demonstrated in playing doctor
   4) Answer questions honestly and simply

7. Play
  a. Cooperative play beginning
   1) Enjoys loud, physical activities
   2) More socialization during play
   3) Self-criticism or boasting evident
  b. Purposes of play
   1) Increase coordination
   2) Decrease tension, anxiety
   3) Deal with fantasies
   4) Enhance self-esteem
   5) Sense of power, control
   6) Increase knowledge of self
  c. Materials
   1) Physical: bat, ball, sand box, sled, bike, puzzles
   2) Dramatic: dress-up clothes, dolls, costumes; imitate adult behavior

3) Creative: pens, paper, crayons, paint, scissors, playdough, chalk
8. Health maintenance
   a. Safety
      1) Car seats
         a) Forward-facing seats for children weighing 40 to 80 lb
         b) Parents are encouraged to follow manufacturer's recommendation for height and weight
      2) Maintain immunization schedule
      3) Anticipatory guidance
         a) Traffic safety
         b) Water safety
         c) Personal safety; preventing abduction

Lifespan and Development of the School-Age Child

5 to 12 years

1. Physical characteristics
   a. Grows 2.5 to 5 cm/year (1 to 2 inches/year)
   b. Gains 1 to 3 kg/year (3 to 7 lb/year)
   c. Pubescent changes may begin to appear
      1) Girls: by approximately 10 to 12 years
      2) Boys: by approximately 12 to 14 years
   d. Vital signs approach adult normals
      1) Pulse: ranges from 60 to 80/min

TABLE IV-2
SCHEDULE OF PERMANENT TOOTH ERUPTION

ERUPTION	AGE
First molar	5 1/2 to 6 years
Medial incisor	6 to 7 years
Lateral incisor	7 to 8 years
Cuspid	10 to 12 years
Bicuspid	10 to 11 years
Bicuspid	11 to 12 years
Second molar	12 to 13 years

      2) Respirations: range from 18 to 20/min
      3) Blood pressure: averages 90 to 110/55 to 60 mm Hg
   e. Dentition
      1) Permanent teeth begin erupting at about 6 years (see table IV-2)
      2) 32 permanent teeth by 18 years of age
      3) May wear braces (orthodontia)
2. Nutrition
   a. Influenced by peers, mass media in food selections

   b. Junk and fast food preferred (empty calories); encourage nutritious snacks
   c. Obesity possible if inadequate exercise
3. Activity/rest
   a. Sleeps 8 to 10 hr/day with vivid dreams
   b. Somnambulism (sleep walking) is common
4. Motor skills
   a. Gross-motor skills
      1) Rollerskates/bicycles/skateboards/scooters
      2) Competitive sports
      3) Swimming
   b. Fine-motor skills
      1) Cursive writing
      2) Musical instruments
      3) Arts and crafts
      4) Keyboarding skills
5. Language development
   a. Masters all sounds by 7 ½ to 8 years
   b. Uses telephone and computer to communicate with peers
   c. Reads and writes
6. Developmental stages
   a. Psychosocial development (Erikson)
      1) Industry vs. inferiority (6 to 12 years)
         a) Primary tasks relate to learning skills, activities
         b) Afraid of failure; embarrassed by poor grades
      2) Child develops self-esteem
   b. Cognitive development (Piaget)
      1) Concrete operations (7 to 11 years)
         a) Classifies and sorts; enjoys collecting
         b) Concrete logic and problem solving
         c) Less egocentric
      2) Inductive thinking
   c. Socialization
      1) Prefers peers of same age and sex
      2) Responds positively to rewards
      3) Belonging is important: enjoys scouts, clubs, team sports; may join a gang
      4) Cliques may become evident (9 to 10 years)
      5) May be left alone for short periods (10 to 12 years); depends on maturity of child
   d. Sexuality
      1) Preadolescents need specific, age-appropriate information about puberty, physical changes (10 to 12 years)
      2) Answer questions openly and honestly
      3) Develops interest in opposite sex (10 to 12 years)
7. Play
   a. Cooperative
   b. Characteristics
      1) Clubs or gangs (8 to 12 years)
      2) Best friends (9 to 10 years)
      3) Secrets

c. Suggested play activities
      1) Table games
      2) Collections
      3) Computer or video games
      4) Community sports/group activities
      5) Creative: dance, art, music
8. Health maintenance
   a. Safety
      1) Prevention
         a) Focus on teaching child to be safe
         b) No longer under parental supervision at all times
      2) Recommended immunizations for 11 to 12 year old
         a) Tetanus, diphtheria, pertussis
         b) Human papillomavirus
         c) Meningococcal
   b. Common problems
      1) Swearing
      2) Lying
      3) Cheating
      4) Stealing
      5) Nail biting
      6) Sibling rivalry
         a) Often jealous of younger/older sibling
         b) Encourage parent not to become involved except in case of physical/emotional harm
   c. Discipline
      1) No punitive measures
      2) Consistency
      3) Withdrawal of privileges
      4) Time out
   d. Stress and coping
      1) School-age children face enormous societal pressures
      2) Do not have cognitive skills to deal with these pressures
      3) Professionals need to be aware that sleep problems, enuresis, changes in appetite, or behavioral problems may be indicative of inadequate coping
9. Health deviations
   a. Accidents
      1) Motor vehicles (use seat belts)
      2) Fractures due to increased activity (use helmets and other protective gear)
      3) Firearms
         a) Make sure firearms are always kept locked up and out of reach of children (these accidents are increasing in frequency)
      4) Drowning
   b. School phobia
      1) Fear or dread of school

      2) Manifestations
         a) Nausea, vomiting, and/or abdominal pain on school mornings
         b) Abrupt onset
         c) Manifestations subside when child is at home
      3) Etiology
         a) Teacher/child mismatch
         b) Fear of failure
         c) Bully
      4) Treatment
         a) Identify the child's cause for concern.
         b) Support child in attending school daily.
         c) Seek professional (psychiatric) help in severe cases.

Lifespan and Development of the Adolescent

12 to 20 years

1. Physical characteristics
   a. Very individualized
   b. By 17 years, 100% of adult stature
   c. Vital signs reach adult norms
   d. Dentition
      1) Third molars (wisdom teeth) by approximately 18 years
      2) Orthodontia in progress or completed
   e. Sexual maturation/puberty
      1) Female
         a) Breast enlargement (approximately 11 years)
         b) Pubic hair
         c) Growth spurt
         d) Menarche (onset of menstruation)
            (1) Approximately 11 years of age
            (2) Ovulation approximately 6 months to 1 year after menarche
      2) Male
         a) Body hair growth
         b) Growth of external genitalia
         c) Growth spurt/increased muscle mass
         d) Voice changes
         e) Ejaculation/nocturnal emission
2. Nutrition
   a. Growth spurt
   b. Increased protein, iron, and calcium needs
3. Activity/rest
   a. Sleep needs increase due to growth demands
   b. Tires easily
4. Motor skills
   a. Risk takers
   b. Sense of indestructibility
   c. General increase in physical and psychomotor skills enhances self-esteem

5. Language development
  a. Sophisticated ability to communicate via verbal and written means
  b. Use of slang prominent
6. Developmental stages
  a. Psychosocial development (Erikson)
    1) Identify formation vs. identify diffusion (12 to 18 years)
      a) Identify future career goals
      b) Incorporate physical changes into identity
  b. Cognitive development (Piaget)
    1) Formal operations (11+ years)
    2) Abstract thinking (ability to hypothesize)
  c. Socialization
    1) Emancipation from family
    2) Peer group major influence; has strong need to belong
    3) Employment
    4) Less adult supervision
  d. Sexuality
    1) Establishes sexual identity and orientation
    2) Experiments with intimate relationships
    3) Common issues
      a) Sexually transmitted diseases
      b) Human immunodeficiency virus (HIV)
      c) Adolescent pregnancy
7. Recreation
  a. Reflects psychosocial needs
  b. Group activities with mixed sexes
  c. May include dating, sports
  d. Suggested recreational activities for adolescent who is hospitalized
    1) Computer or video games
    2) Cards
    3) Portable CD player
8. Health maintenance
  a. Safety
    1) Accident prevention
      a) Focus on educating adolescent to make safe choices
      b) Be alert to signs of depression, substance abuse
    2) Immunizations
      a) Tetanus-diphtheria (Td) needed every 10 years
      b) Hepatitis B series if not previously administered
  b. Discipline
    1) Increased independence
    2) Consistency
  c. Stress and coping
    1) Faced with enormous societal pressures
    2) Feels pressure to belong, conform, and achieve
    3) Common reactions to stress

a) Early adolescent: mood swings and self-focused
b) Middle adolescent: increased rebellious behavior
c) Later adolescent: better coping skills
    4) Common problems
      a) Runaways
      b) Eating disorders
      c) Substance abuse
        (1) Nonprescription, illicit, or street drugs
        (2) Alcohol
        (3) Tobacco
9. Health deviations
  a. Crashes
    1) Motor vehicles
      a) Driver's education
      b) Drunk driving
    2) Firearms
    3) Spinal cord injuries
    4) Drowning
  b. Homicide
  c. Suicide

SECTION II

THE HOSPITALIZED CHILD

Stress of Hospitalization

A. Potential Regression
1. Children usually adapt well to hospitalization.
2. Respect child's use of this defense mechanism.
3. Assist child to achieve past developmental levels.

B. Child's Reaction to Hospitalization (Age/developmental specific)
1. Protest: strong, conscious need for parent; may be confused, frightened, crying
2. Despair: mourning period; may be withdrawn, apathetic
3. Denial: represses true feelings; feels parent has failed; interested in surroundings, but not parent

C. Developmental Influences on Stress of Hospitalization
1. Infant: trust vs. mistrust
  a. 0 to 6 months: loss of consistent caregiver
  b. 6 to 12 months: strong need for parent; separation anxiety
2. Toddler: autonomy vs. shame and doubt
  a. Separation anxiety, loss of significant other, inconsistency
  b. Loss of mobility due to restraints, crib

3. Preschooler: initiative vs. guilt
   a. Separation anxiety
   b. Threats to body integrity may cause increased aggression
   c. Concept of illness
      1) Magical thinking (believes that feelings and thoughts can cause illness)
      2) May believe illness or hospitalization is punishment
4. School-age child: industry vs. inferiority
   a. Loss of control
   b. Separation from: peers, school, and after-school activities
   c. Concept of illness
      1) Perceives an external cause for illness
      2) May view illness as a result of "doing something wrong"
      3) Understands difference between acute and chronic illness
5. Adolescent: identity vs. role diffusion
   a. Threats to body image
   b. Loss of control
   c. Separation from peers, school, and activities
   d. Concept of illness
      1) Believes self to be invulnerable
      2) Understands internal cause of disease
      3) Best cooperates with treatment plan if understands immediate benefits

D. Stress of Hospitalization on Family
1. Shock and Denial
   a. Allow verbalization of feelings; recognize and accept defense mechanisms.
   b. Enhance coping strategies.
   c. Allow family to stay with child as much as possible; open visitation policy.
   d. Explain that regressive behavior is normal and expected.
   e. Explain that separation anxiety is normal and expected.
2. Adjustment
   a. Encourage communication between family and medical personnel.
   b. Encourage family participation in decision making and care giving.

E. Reaction to Pain
1. Rule of thumb: assume that if a procedure would be painful for an adult, it is also painful for a child
 2. **NURSING INTERVENTIONS** (strategies for pain management)
   a. Age-appropriate assessment
      1) Ask child with age-appropriate language.
      2) Use pain-rating tool (e.g., Baker-Wong, Faces).

      3) Conduct developmental pain assessment
         a) Infant
            (1) Generalized body response of rigidity, thrashing
            (2) Loud crying, facial expression
            (3) May sleep to avoid pain experience
         b) Toddler
            (1) Localized response: will withdraw from pain
            (2) Physical resistance after painful stimulation
         c) Preschooler
            (1) Verbalizes pain
            (2) Attempts to avoid painful stimulus
            (3) May view pain as punishment
         d) School-age child
            (1) Verbalizes pain
            (2) Stalling behavior; vocal protest
            (3) Recognizes physical cause of pain
         e) Adolescent
            (1) Sophisticated verbal expression of pain
            (2) Less resistance offered: physical, vocal
            (3) Understands physical and psychological pain
   b. Use of pharmacologic control methods
      1) Weight-appropriate (kg/lb) dosages
      2) Oral and IV routes preferred over IM; child will avoid shot and not be medicated
      3) Conscious sedation: midazolam (*Versed*), fentanyl citrate (*Sublimaze*) for painful procedures
      4) PCA appropriate for children who understand cause and effect (approximately 7 years)
      5) Eutectic mixture of local anesthetics (*EMLA*) cream is a topical anesthetic that can be applied as a thick dollop and covered with a transparent dressing approximately 1 to 2 hr prior to a procedure (venipuncture, injection) to lessen the pain
   c. Use of nonpharmacologic control methods
      1) Distraction
      2) Relaxation
      3) Kinesthetic (rocking) stimulation

F. Strategies for Stress Reduction
1. Prehospital preparation, preoperative teaching, and tour
2. Specially trained pediatric staff

3. Use of outpatient facilities eliminates need for overnight hospitalization and separation
4. Therapeutic play
   a. Purposes
      1) Mastery of situation
      2) Ego strengthening
      3) Deal with fears, anxiety, and the unknown
    b. **NURSING INTERVENTIONS**
      1) Play with the child based on his developmental level and illness.
      2) Allow child to set the pace of play.
      3) Provide a variety of play materials.
      4) Reflect back the child's feelings.
5. Communication strategies
   a. Appropriate for situation
   b. Clear and consistent
   c. Communicate in an age-appropriate manner with the child
      1) Verbal
      2) Nonverbal

SECTION III

NURSING CARE OF THE CHILD WITH CONGENITAL HEART DEFECTS

Congenital Heart Defects

A. Hemodynamics of Fetal Circulation
1. Ductus venosus: carries oxygenated blood from placenta to inferior vena cava; partially bypasses liver; closes by approximately 8th week of life
2. Ductus arteriosus: bypasses flow of blood through lungs by shunting oxygenated and unoxygenated blood from pulmonary artery to aorta; closes by 7 to 10 days after birth
3. Foramen ovale: connects right and left atria; allows blood to flow from right atrium to left atrium, thereby bypassing the right ventricle and pulmonary circuit; closes by 2 to 3 months
4. Transition to newborn circulation
   a. At first breath, lungs expand, which increases blood flow to pulmonary system
   b. Pulmonary vascular resistance is decreased and systemic vascular resistance increases
   c. These changes lead to the closure of the ductus venosus, ductus arteriosus, and foramen ovale

B. Characteristics
1. Unknown etiology (always consider genetic factors in addition to intrauterine infection, radiation, or medications)

2. Incidence is 1 in 1,000 live births (accounts for 50% of all deaths in first year of life); may be associated with other birth defects, syndromes
3. May not be diagnosed while hospitalized in newborn nursery
4. Clinical signs include:
   a. Neonate and newborn
      1) Cyanosis: especially circumoral and acrocyanosis; cyanosis on exertion (feeding, crying)
      2) Dyspnea: especially on exertion
      3) Failure to thrive
      4) Frequent upper respiratory infections
      5) Feeding difficulty
      6) Weak or muffled cry
   b. Older child
      1) Cyanosis and dyspnea (as above)
      2) Impaired growth
      3) Fatigue
      4) Digital clubbing
      5) Squatting
      6) Polycythemia: increased RBC count to compensate for impaired gas exchange; increases oxygen-carrying capacity of blood
   c. Heart failure
      1) Tachypnea, dyspnea
      2) Exercise intolerance
      3) Tachycardia (above 160/min)
      4) Diaphoresis
      5) Hepatomegaly and edema (late signs)
5. Increased risk of bacterial endocarditis

C. Diagnosis
1. Cardiac catheterization
2. Echocardiography

D. Comparison of Acyanotic and Cyanotic Defects
(See Tables IV-3 and IV-4.)

E. NURSING INTERVENTIONS
 1. Correct knowledge deficit related to:
   a. Cardiac catheterization
      1) Consider developmental level of child when planning teaching strategies.
      2) Explain to parents that procedure is done under conscious sedation.
      3) Be alert to postprocedural concerns (same as adult).
   b. Anticoagulant therapy
      1) Explain why this is necessary for children who have prosthetic valves or increased blood viscosity.
      2) Instruct parents to be alert for signs of increased bleeding: excessive bruising, epistaxis, hematuria, and bloody stools.

TABLE IV-3
REVIEW OF ACYANOTIC CONGENITAL HEART DEFECTS

ANOMALY	HEMODYNAMICS	CLINICAL MANIFESTATIONS	TREATMENT
Patent Ductus Arteriosus A vascular channel between the left main pulmonary artery and the descending aorta, as a result of failure of the fetal ductus arteriosus to close	- Shunt of oxygenated blood from the aorta into the pulmonary artery - Increased left ventricular output and work load	- Usually asymptomatic, but frequent impairment of growth or heart failure - "Machinery murmur" - Wide pulse pressure	- Medical: administration of indomethacin (*Indocin*) (prostaglandin inhibitor) is effective in some newborns and premature newborns - Surgical: ligation of patent ductus (in infancy)
Ventricular Septal Defect Defect is in membranous muscular portion of the ventricular septum; may vary from small to large defect	- Shunt of oxygenated blood from left to right ventricle - Leads to right ventricular hypertrophy - Needs surgical repair - Bidirectional shunting may occur with very large defect (Eisenmenger's complex)	- May be asymptomatic - Heart murmur is heard in first week of life (systolic) - Growth failure, feeding problems during first year of life; failure to thrive; frequent respiratory infections - Heart failure is common	- Some small defects may close spontaneously - Open heart: direct closure suturing with plastic prosthesis (usually preschooler; may be done earlier in infancy for large defects)
Atrial Septal Defect Malfunctioning foremen ovale; or abnormal opening between the atria	- Shunting of oxygenated blood from left to right atrium - Increased right ventricular output and work load - May develop pulmonary hypertension (in adulthood, if not surgically treated in childhood)	- Acyanotic; asymptomatic - Soft blowing, systolic murmur - Thin and asthenic - Frequent episodes of pulmonary inflammatory diseases - Poor exercise tolerance	Open heart with direct closure or suturing with plastic prosthesis (usually preschooler)
Coarctation of aorta: - Preductal constriction of the aorta between subclavian artery and ductus arteriosus - Postductal constriction of aorta directly beyond the ductus	- Obstruction of the flow of blood through the constricted segments - Increased left ventricular pressure and work load - Extensive collateral circulation bypasses coarctated area to supply lower extremities with blood	- Hypertension in upper extremities with decreased BP in lower extremities - Weak or absent pulsations in lower extremities - Heart failure - May be asymptomatic; occasionally fatigue, headaches, leg cramps, epistaxis	- Surgical resection of coarctate area with direct anastomosis or use of a graft - Correction usually done by 2 years of age to prevent permanent hypertension

TABLE IV-4
REVIEW OF CYANOTIC CONGENITAL HEART DEFECTS

ANOMALY	HEMODYNAMICS	CLINICAL MANIFESTATIONS	TREATMENT
Tetralogy of Fallot: combination of four defects: 1) Pulmonary stenosis 2) Ventricular septal defect (VSD) 3) Overriding aorta 4) Hypertrophy of R ventricle	- Obstruction to outflow of blood from R ventricle into pulmonary circuit and increased pressure in the R ventricle leads to R to L shunting of unoxygenated blood thru the VSD directly into the aorta - Severity of defect depends on degree of pulmonary stenosis and size of VSD	- Acute cyanosis at birth - Cyanosis developing during early months that increases with physical exertion - Clubbing of fingers and toes - Systolic murmur - Acute episodes of cyanosis and hypoxia called "tet spells" or hypercyanotic episodes occur if oxygen supply cannot meet demand (e.g., with crying, exertion, exercise, feeding) - Squatting - Growth retardation	- Surgical: Blalock-Taussig procedures - provides blood flow to pulmonary arteries from the L or R subclavian artery - Repair: open heart closure of VSD and resection of stenosis Usually performed in first 2 years of life

Transposition of Great Vessels (TGV): the aorta originates from the R ventricle and the pulmonary artery from the L ventricle	- Two separate circulations without mixture of oxygenated and unoxygen-ated blood except through shunts
	
	- Mixture of blood may occur through one or more septal defects:
	  - Ventricular septal defect (VSD)
	  - Atrial septal defect (ASD)
	  - Patent ductus arteriosus (PDA)
		- Usually deep cyanosis shortly after birth or after closing of ductus
		
		- Early clubbing of toes and fingers
		
		- Poor growth and develop-ment, failure to thrive
		
		- Rapid respirations; fatigue
		
		- Heart failure
			- Prostaglandin medications are given to keep ductus arteriosus open until surgery. Prostaglandin inhibitors are given to close duct.
			- Repair: arterial switch is treatment of choice; must be done within first few days of life; great vessels reimplanted under complete circulatory arrest
			
			- Several other types of repair are all multiple stage approaches

3) Explain need for bleeding precautions.
c. Preoperative preparation
　1) Promote parental involvement to decrease anxiety.
　2) Include description of what child will feel during procedure, surgery (base on developmental level).
2. Diminished cardiac output related to failure of the myocardium to meet the demands of the body
　a. Promote reduced energy expenditures by providing adequate rest periods, planning care to reduce interruptions, and recognizing signs of fatigue; infant seat very helpful; avoid temperature extremes.

b. Administer and monitor medications that will promote cardiac function.
　1) Digoxin (*Lanoxin*) (same as adult) except:
　　a) Check apical heart rate 1 full min prior to administering - hold digitalis if heart rate is below: 100/min for infants; 80/min for toddlers and preschoolers; 60/min for school-age children and adolescents.
　　b) Administer medication on an empty stomach; do not give with food or juice; do not repeat dose if child vomits.

      c)   Digoxin therapeutic level is 0.8 to 2.0 mcg/dL

    2) Diuretics: furosemide (*Lasix*), chlorothiazide (*Diuril*), ethacrynic acid (*Edecrin*)

      a)   Monitor potassium levels and supplement losses; observe for hypokalemia - increases risk of digitalis toxicity.

      b)   Include daily weights, I&O, and respiratory assessment in daily care.

3.   Feeding challenges: less than body requirements, related to heart failure; "Cardiac" infants usually have a weak suck, become cyanotic during feedings, tire easily, and may fall asleep while feeding

   a.   Give small, frequent feedings using a soft nipple with a large hole.

   b.   Administer 24 kcal/oz formula to increase caloric intake.

   c.   Limit oral feedings to 20 min; gavage feed the remainder.

4.   Parental coping and support

   a.   Discipline is the most difficult area of parenting due to feelings of guilt and powerlessness.

   b.   Parents need help remembering child should be treated as normally as possible.

   c.   Counsel family regarding possibility of developmental delays; include infant stimulation in teaching.

   d.   Assist with potential grieving: loss of "perfect" infant.

Neurologic Defects

A. Hydrocephalus

1.   Characteristics

   a.   Definition: imbalance in either absorption or production of cerebrospinal fluid within intracranial cavity

   b.   Classification: either congenital or acquired

   c.   Usually diagnosed at birth or within 2 to 4 months of life

   d.   Often associated with other neural tube defect (myelomeningocele)

   e.   Clinical manifestations (categorized by age)

    1) Infant: increased head circumference, tense bulging anterior fontanel, distended scalp veins, high-pitched cry, irritability, feeding problems, discomfort when held

    2) Older child: headache, vomiting (especially in the morning), diplopia, blurred vision, behavioral changes, decreased motor function, decreased level of consciousness, seizures

2.   Diagnosis

   a.   May be detected on prenatal sonogram

   b.   Clinical signs

    1) Increasing intracranial pressure

    2) Increasing head circumference

   c.   Computed tomography or magnetic resonance imaging scan confirms diagnosis; shows excessive fluid in ventricles

3.   Treatment

   a.   Pressure relieved by surgical insertion of a shunting device

   b.   Components of a shunt include: catheter, reservoir, pumping device with one-way valve, and distal tubing with regulator valve

   c.   Most common type of shunt is ventriculoperitoneal

   d.   Complications include shunt failure and infection

   e.   Shunt will require revision (lengthening of tubing) as child grows

   f.   Early treatment necessary to prevent progressive mental retardation

 4.   **NURSING INTERVENTIONS**

   a.   Implement care that decreases ICP.

    1) Preoperatively measure head circumference by obtaining occipito-frontal measurement.

    2) Postoperatively

      a)   Perform frequent neurologic assessment with daily head circumference.

      b)   Position on nonoperative site; check anterior fontanel to determine positioning of the head; do not pump shunt without order.

      c)   Monitor for signs and symptoms of shunt failure: lethargy, vomiting, and irritability.

      d)   Institute seizure precautions.

   b.   Decrease infection

    1) Monitor for signs of shunt infection: elevated vital signs, decreased level of consciousness, vomiting, feeding problems

    2) Assess incision site frequently for manifestations of inflammation or leakage.

   c.   Implement care to meet physiologic and developmental needs.

B. Myelomeningocele: most common type of neural tube defect

1.   Definition: type of spina bifida, a fissure in spinal column leaving meninges and spinal cord exposed

2. Characteristics
   a. Failure of posterior laminae to fuse with herniation of saclike cyst of meninges, cerebrospinal fluid, and spinal nerves
   b. Usually associated with other neurologic defects (hydrocephalus)
   c. Unknown etiology
   d. May be prevented by folic acid supplementation by women of childbearing age prior to conception and through first trimester
3. Pathology
   a. Partial to complete paralysis determined by location of defect (usually lumbosacral)
   b. Musculoskeletal problems such as clubfoot, scoliosis, congenital hip dysplasia
   c. Sensory disturbances parallel motor dysfunction
   d. Bowel and bladder problems including constipation, incontinence, and neurogenic bladder
4. Diagnosis
   a. Amniocentesis: 98% accurate; elevated alpha fetoprotein, confirmed by prenatal sonogram
   b. Apparent at birth: visible sac
5. Treatment
   a. Decision to correct the defect or not is difficult as well as controversial
   b. Early surgical closure is advocated to preserve neural function, reduce risk of infection, and control hydrocephalus

 6. **NURSING INTERVENTIONS**
   a. Prevent infection
      1) Preoperatively; priority of care is to preserve integrity of sac
         a) Keep infant in prone position.
         b) Cover sac with 4 x 4 gauze moistened with sterile saline.
         c) Check sac for tears or cracks.
         d) Do not cover sac with clothing or diapers (places pressure on the sac).
         e) Perform perineal care to prevent contamination of sac.
         f) Monitor for manifestations of meningitis (irritability, anorexia, fever, seizures).
      2) Postoperatively; priority of care is to promote healing and preserve neurologic integrity
         a) Place infant in prone position with head slightly lower than body.
         b) Place protective barrier across incision to prevent contamination.
         c) Be aware of long-term problems of infection related to urinary retention, reflux, and chronic urinary tract infections.
            (1) Teach parents the Credé maneuver.
            (2) Encourage independent intermittent self-catheterization (can be performed as early as 5 to 6 years of age).
            (3) Stress hydration and early recognition of urinary tract infections.
            (4) Explain to parents that urinary diversion procedures are often required.
   b. Prevent injury
      1) Perform neurologic checks with daily head circumference.
      2) Monitor for manifestations of increased intracranial pressure.
   c. Promote effective coping strategies
      1) Parents will need help dealing with the issue of "chronic sorrow" as well as the long-term aspects of the condition.
      2) Remember that every family's method of coping is different. Offer options in nonjudgmental manner and provide for a supportive environment that will help families make the most appropriate choices.
   d. Increased risk for latex allergy: recognize that children with neural tube defects are at increased risk for latex allergy and that exposure to common medical (or other) products containing latex should be avoided (e.g., vinyl gloves, balloons)

C. Cerebral Palsy
1. Characteristics
   a. Early onset, permanent, nonprogressive disability
   b. Impaired movement and posture with abnormal muscle tone and coordination
   c. May be accompanied by language and cognitive deficits
   d. Causes undetermined; may be related to prenatal, perinatal, or postnatal factors
   e. Increased risk in neonates with an Apgar score of 5 or less
2. Diagnosis
   a. Classified by nature and distribution of neuromuscular dysfunction
   b. May not be diagnosed until child is several months old
   c. Confirmed by physical evaluation, or supplemental tests (e.g., electroencephalogram test, tomography, or metabolic screening)
   d. Early clinical signs
      1) Persistent primitive reflexes
      2) Hyper or hypotonicity (stiff or floppy arms and legs)

3) Poor hand control, body control
4) Feeding difficulties
5) Irritability
6) Delayed attainment of developmental milestones

3. Treatment (based on degree of disability)
   a. Physical therapy (active and passive)
   b. Anticonvulsants: phenobarbital or phenytoin (*Dilantin*)
   c. Modified toys or equipment to enhance development
   d. Surgery (to correct contractures or spastic deformities)

 4. **NURSING INTERVENTIONS**
   a. Prevent injury.
      1) Teach family and child safe use of adaptive devices.
      2) Modify environment to enhance safety.
      3) Institute seizure precautions if appropriate.
      4) Encourage physical safety techniques (aspiration precautions, adequate rest).
   b. Promote self care and independence.
      1) Encourage self-care activities to foster independence and confidence.
      2) Modify environment, devices to enhance development and increase functional abilities.
   c. Promote communication.
      1) Refer to occupational and speech therapy for evaluation and development of verbal and nonverbal communication skills.
      2) Teach caregivers alternative communication methods to facilitate positive adjustments of child and family.

Musculoskeletal Defects

A. Congenital Dysplasia of the Hip

1. Characteristics
   a. Refers to imperfect development of the hip of varying degrees
   b. Etiology unknown; familial tendency; females are eight times more likely to develop
   c. Manifestations: shortening of affected leg, asymmetrical gluteal folds, limited abduction, Ortolani's sign (audible "click" as examiner slips femoral head forward)
   d. Early detection critical: if untreated will lead to lordosis, scoliosis, "duck waddle"

2. Pathology
   a. The head of the femur must be properly located within the acetabulum for correct development of the hip joint
   b. As ossification proceeds, correcting the hip defect becomes more difficult

c. Once child begins to walk, prognosis becomes questionable
d. Most common type is subluxation (incomplete dislocation of hip)

3. Diagnosis
   a. Assessment techniques with newborn (Ortolani's "click")
   b. X-rays are difficult to read in early infancy because ossification of femoral head does not occur until 3 to 6 months of life

4. Treatment
   a. If diagnosed within first 2 to 3 months of life, the hip joint abduction is maintained via double diapering, Frejka pillow, splint, or Pavlik harness
   b. Once adductor muscles contract, traction and/or casting may be used; usually by 6 months (once the child is standing and walking) both methods are used in conjunction with surgery (Bryant's traction if below 2 years)

 5. **NURSING INTERVENTIONS**
   a. Promote neurovascular integrity.
      1) Conduct frequent neurovascular checks: CMS (circulation, motion, sensation).
      2) Provide routine cast care. If hip spica cast is used, teach parents not to use abductor stabilizer bar as a "handle" when moving child.
      3) Use Bryant's traction, where child's legs are elevated at 90° angle to body. The child's weight provides countertraction, and the correct amount of traction is applied if child's buttocks are elevated slightly above bed.
   b. Maintain skin integrity.
   c. Promote mobility.

B. Congenital Clubfoot (Talipes Equinovarus)

1. Characteristics
   a. Forefoot adducted, heel tilted inward (varus), plantar flexion at ankle
   b. Important to differentiate between positional and true clubfoot (true clubfoot cannot be positioned in normal alignment with range of motion)

2. Diagnosis and treatment
   a. Apparent at birth; longer treatment postponed, more soft tissue changes occur and correction more difficult.
   b. Serial casting is employed to gradually manipulate the foot into normal position; casts are changed at weekly intervals; as each new cast is applied, the foot is remanipulated and recasted.
   c. Dennis-Brown splint may be used to maintain position once casting is completed.

3. **NURSING INTERVENTIONS**
   a. Teach parents range-of-motion exercises and neurovascular assessments.
   b. Monitor for infection.
   c. Maintain skin integrity around cast edges.
   d. Promote developmental activities.

Gastrointestinal Defects

A. Cleft Lip
1. Characteristics
   a. Definition: failure of the maxillary processes to fuse with the nasal processes (may be unilateral or bilateral)
   b. Etiology: unknown, but strong genetic or environmental factors
   c. More common in males
   d. May or may not be accompanied by cleft palate
2. Pathology
   a. Prone to ear, nose, and throat infection
   b. Long-term problems include speech, hearing, and dentition problems
3. Diagnosis and treatment
   a. Defect apparent at birth
   b. Surgical repair initiated within first 3 months of life
   c. Staggered z-shaped suture line used to minimize scarring

4. **NURSING INTERVENTIONS**
   a. Preoperative nursing care
      1) Follow precautions during feedings.
      2) Assess strength of sucking reflex.
      3) Encourage parents to express concerns.
   b. Postoperative nursing care
      1) Monitor for respiratory distress.
      2) Maintain suture integrity.
      3) Provide age-appropriate activities.
   c. Preserve suture line
      1) Restrain elbows.
      2) Avoid sucking.
      3) Cleanse suture after each feeding.
   d. Maintain airway and prevent aspiration.
   e. Provide support to parents.

B. Cleft Palate
1. Characteristics
   a. Failure of palatine processes to fuse
   b. More common among females
   c. Defect may include both hard and soft palate
   d. Major problems are similar to cleft lip: feeding; aspiration; ear, nose, and throat infections
   e. May or may not be associated with cleft lip
2. Diagnosis and treatment
   a. Repair usually completed by 12 to 18 months of age to prevent speech problems

   b. Surgery may be performed in stages

3. **NURSING INTERVENTIONS**
   a. (See interventions for cleft lip.)

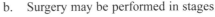

SECTION IV

NURSING CARE OF THE CHILD WITH AN ACUTE ILLNESS

Common Problems Associated with Acute Illness

A. Fever
1. Characteristics
   a. Classified as temperature in excess of 38° C (100.4° F)
   b. Not always related to severity of illness; varies from child to child
   c. Always consider
      1) Age of child: below 6 months is more serious concern
      2) If child is immunosuppressed or receiving chemotherapy
   d. Most fevers in children are viral, self-limiting; may play a role in recovery from infection
2. Diagnosis
   a. Feeling a child's skin for warmth is not an accurate indicator
   b. Always investigate family epidemiology and take a careful history for exposure to communicable diseases.
   c. Remember that diet, activity level, and behavioral changes are subtle diagnostic clues.
   d. Laboratory tests may include CBC, urinalysis, chest film, and blood cultures. A "septic work-up" includes all of the above with the addition of a lumbar puncture and urine culture.
3. Treatment
   a. Fever management is questionable because fever is considered a part of the body's defense mechanism.
   b. Antipyretics, such as acetaminophen (*Tylenol*) or ibuprofen (*Motrin*), should be given in weight-appropriate dose.
   c. No aspirin.

4. **NURSING INTERVENTIONS**
   a. Febrile seizures
      1) Usually seen in children between 6 months and 3 years old; related to sudden rise of temperature (above 38.9° C [102° F]); child usually has a respiratory or gastrointestinal infection
      2) Therapeutic treatment includes diazepam (*Valium*) and/or antipyretics.

3) Provide safe care during febrile seizure.
   a) Maintain airway.
   b) Prevent aspiration and injury.
   c) Observe the seizure.
b. Maintain fluid and electrolyte balance.
   1) Assess for signs of dehydration.
   2) Provide IV fluids.
   3) Monitor renal function.
c. Maintain afebrile status.
   1) Frequently assess temperature.
   2) Encourage clear liquids.
   3) Expose skin and avoid excessive clothing.
d. Knowledge deficit related to home care
   1) Educate parents regarding seizure precautions, methods to control fever, and how to prevent dehydration.
   2) Address parental fears about fevers.

B. Vomiting

1. Characteristics
   a. Assessment includes: amount, color, consistency, time of day emesis occurs, and relationship to eating
   b. Vomiting causes a loss of hydrochloric acid, which leads to metabolic alkalosis
2. Diagnosis
   a. Child is dehydrated and appears emaciated
   b. Diagnostic procedures for prolonged or unusual emesis may include: upper gastrointestinal series, barium enema, abdominal ultrasound, CT scan of abdomen, pH probe, esophagoscopy
   c. If metabolic alkalosis, may appear lethargic, poorly perfused, hyperventilating
3. Treatment
   a. It is essential to correct both the fluid and acid-base imbalance.
   b. If the vomiting is predictable and of brief duration, antiemetics may be prescribed to depress the vomiting center (e.g., promethazine HCl [*Phenergan*], chlorpromazine HCl [Thorazine], metoclopramide HCl [*Reglan*], trimethobenzamide [*Tigan*])
   c. Gastroesophageal reflux is treated with medications that promote gastric mobility and emptying, such as metoclopramide (*Reglan*) or omeprazole (*Prilosec*); take gastroesophageal reflux precautions (e.g., positioning with the head of the bed elevated, especially after meals or feeding)
 4. **NURSING INTERVENTIONS**
   a. Assess for signs of dehydration.
   b. Maintain fluid and electrolytes.
   c. Adhere to strict I&O and daily weights.
   d. Remain NPO status until asymptomatic.
   e. Introduce clear liquids slowly and frequently.

f. Administer antiemetics as prescribed.
g. Monitor for metabolic alkalosis.

C. Gastroenteritis (Diarrhea)

1. Characteristics
   a. Defined as an increase in fluid, frequency and volume of stool; usually results from increased rate of peristalsis; stools are watery, acidic, green in color, expelled forcefully; Na^+, K^+, and bicarbonate are also lost via the stool
   b. Diarrhea is serious in young children because:
      1) The extracellular space is larger, so greater amounts of fluid will be lost
      2) Younger children have a greater body surface area and gastrointestinal surface areas in relation to body weight
      3) Younger children have a higher basal metabolic rate, so the fluid and electrolyte balance is unstable
   c. Weight is a critical indicator of fluid loss in young children; 1 g of weight equals 1 mL of body fluid, a weight loss or gain of 1 kg in a 24-hr period represents a fluid shift of 1,000 mL; the loss of fluid and electrolytes in the diarrhea stool results in dehydration and electrolyte depletion
   d. Causative factors: bacteria (*salmonella, shigella*), viral (rotavirus), allergies, emotional disturbances, dietary and malabsorption problems
   e. Chronic nonspecific diarrhea or irritable bowel syndrome is the most common form of chronic diarrhea in children:
      1) Diarrhea persists longer than 3 weeks
      2) Normal growth and development
      3) No evidence of enteric pathogens
2. Diagnosis
   a. Serum electrolytes, CBC, and blood cultures may be prescribed.
   b. Antibiotic therapy is a common cause of diarrhea.
   c. Obtain a thorough history including dietary habits, family history, recent travel, or exposures to contagious illness.
3. Treatment
   a. Mild dehydration (2 to 9%) without hypernatremia; generally treated with oral rehydrating solutions; critical behaviors that demand immediate attention are persistent diarrhea, weight loss, bloody stools, or physiological changes such as deep breathing, listlessness, or reduced urinary output
   b. A secondary lactose intolerance may occur following gastroenteritis; child may be maintained temporarily on a lactose-free diet

c. Severe dehydration (greater than 10% weight loss) is an acute medical emergency; the child is NPO (12 to 48 hr), parenteral fluids are administered

 4. **NURSING INTERVENTIONS**
   a. Assess for signs of dehydration and skin integrity.
   b. Maintain fluid and electrolyte balance.
   c. Maintain daily weights and strict I&O.
   d. Apply skin barrier (zinc products).
   e. Monitor for metabolic acidosis.
   f. Remain NPO until asymptomatic.
   g. Introduce clear liquids slowly and frequently (avoid apple juice).
   h. Administer antidiarrheals as prescribed.

D. Respiratory Infections

1. Acute otitis media (most prevalent childhood disease)
   a. Characteristics
      1) Middle ear infections are common in children under age 5: (breastfed infants have decreased incidence)
         a) Eustachian tube is shorter, wider, and straighter
         b) Organisms from nasopharynx have easier access to middle ear
         c) Tonsils and adenoids are usually enlarged
         d) Young children have poorly developed immune mechanisms
         e) Infants and toddlers are supine a large portion of the day
      2) Usually follows an upper respiratory infection during which the swollen mucosa close off the eustachian tube; the growth of the organism along with the fluid retention in the ear combine to cause the infection
      3) Most frequently seen bacterial infection in young children; most serious long-term problem associated with otitis is conductive hearing loss, tinnitus or vertigo
      4) Clinical manifestations: fever; irritability; pulling, tugging or rubbing the affected ear; anorexia; signs of a upper respiratory infection; older children may report earache or pain when chewing or sucking; purulent discharge may be present
   b. Diagnosis
      1) Otitis media: otoscopy reveals an intact tympanic membrane that appears inflamed, bulging, and without a light reflex
      2) Chronic otitis media: otoscopy reveals dull, gray membrane with visible fluid behind eardrum
   c. Treatment
      1) Oral antibiotics; therapy should last 10 to 14 days
      2) Oral decongestants such as sympathomimetics (vasoconstriction) or antihistamines (reduce congestion) may be used; analgesics may be prescribed to reduce pain, discomfort
      3) Following completion of the antibiotic regimen, treatment effectiveness should be evaluated.
      4) Children with recurrent otitis media should be tested for hearing loss.
      5) Myringotomy (surgical incision of the ear drum) and insertion of pressure-equalizing (PE) tubes may be ordered in cases of recurrent chronic otitis media.

 d. **NURSING INTERVENTIONS**
      1) Pain
         a) Administer analgesics such as acetaminophen (*Tylenol*) as needed; apply warm compresses to affected ear; avoid foods that require chewing.
         b) Assess for nonverbal signs of discomfort; changes in behavior can be an early indicator of pain; humidity, clear PO fluids may also be helpful.
      2) Client teaching
         a) Instruct parents regarding the importance of antibiotic compliance; medication should be taken for 10 to 14 days (even after manifestations have gone away).
         b) Instruct parents in feeding techniques to reduce the incidence of ear infection: upright when feeding; breastfeeding offers protection against pathogens.
         c) Eliminate tobacco smoke and known or potential allergens from environment.
         d) Educate parents following myringotomy and PE tubes insertion, that some drainage from the ears is expected; report obvious bleeding and an abrupt rise in temperature; the ear should be kept dry; avoid activities that require submerging the head in water (use ear plugs for bathing).

2. Epiglottitis
   a. Characteristics
      1) Definition: acute bacterial infection of the supraglottic structures resulting in obstructive airway problems
      2) Seen primarily in children 2 to 8 years of age; considered a medical emergency, immediate treatment must be initiated
      3) Most common causative organism: H. influenza, type B
      4) Clinical manifestations: abrupt onset with rapid progression to severe respiratory distress, sore throat, stridor, high fever (38.9 to 40° C [102 to 104° F]), drooling, dysphagia, muffled voice; tripod position (sit upright, lean forward with mouth open and tongue protruding)
   b. Diagnosis
      1) Throat is red, inflamed with a cherry-red epiglottis; under no circumstance should an inspection of the throat be initiated unless emergency equipment is available (e.g., trach setup, ET tube); do not take a throat culture
      2) Lateral neck film (e.g., soft-tissue x-ray) reveals swollen epiglottis
   c. Treatment
      1) Parenteral therapy with IV antibiotics is begun immediately; PO antibiotics for 10 to 14 days following IV therapy
      2) Steroid therapy: frequently used for anti-inflammatory effects
      3) Intubation or tracheostomy usually necessary to prevent obstruction; extubation may occur within 3 to 4 days
      4) Vaccine prevention: H. influenza type B conjugate vaccine effective against H. influenza epiglottitis (See prevention column under communicable diseases, Table IV-10.)
    d. **NURSING INTERVENTIONS**
      1) Frequent assessment respiratory distress
      2) Available oxygen, suction, emergency
      3) Maintain NPO status.
      4) Do not leave child unattended.
      5) Give medications as prescribed:
         a) Humidified oxygen
         b) Bronchodilators
         c) Steroids
         d) Antibiotics
         e) Antipyretics
3. Laryngotracheobronchitis (croup)
   a. Characteristics:
      1) Most common form of croup; peak age is below 5 years; because of smaller airway diameter, child is more prone to significant airway narrowing
      2) May begin as an upper respiratory infection that proceeds to lower respiratory structures
      3) Most common causative organisms: parainfluenza viruses
      4) Clinical manifestations are the result of inflammation and subsequent narrowing of airway: hoarseness, barking or "seal-like" cough, inspiratory stridor, increasing respiratory distress
   b. Diagnosis
      1) Clinical manifestations are diagnostic
      2) Lateral or soft-tissue x-rays of neck may be ordered
   c. Treatment
      1) Humidity with cool mist provides relief by reducing inflamed mucosa
      2) Aerosol epinephrine (*Racepinephrine*) may also be used if child is hospitalized
      3) Corticosteroids may be used for their anti-inflammatory effects.
    d. **NURSING INTERVENTIONS**
      1) Monitor the child's respiratory status frequently.
      2) Provide humidified oxygen.
      3) Encourage fluids.
      4) Keep environment quiet and calm.
      5) Have suction and emergency intubation equipment available at the bedside.
      6) Assess parental anxiety.
      7) Medications
         a) Humidified oxygen
         b) Bronchodilators
         c) Steroids
4. Bronchiolitis
   a. Characteristics
      1) Acute viral infection that primarily affects bronchioles; most commonly seen in infants between 1 to 18 months of age; occurs in winter and spring months
      2) Respiratory syncytial virus (RSV) is responsible for half of the documented cases of bronchiolitis; mode of transmission is hand to nose, droplet infections; reinfection common in all ages
      3) Bronchiolar obstruction leads to hyperinflation and air trapping

4) The younger the child, the greater the chance of severe lower respiratory disease requiring hospitalization; infants at high risk for severe RSV infection include: premature infants, infants with underlying cardiac or respiratory conditions, infants with immune deficit

5) Clinical manifestations: initial manifestations of upper respiratory infection that progress to tachypnea; paroxysmal coughing, increased restlessness; nasal flaring, fever, cyanosis intercostal and substernal retractions, wheezing, and decreased breath sounds indicate severe lower-respiratory tract disease

b. Diagnosis
1) Manifestations are clinically diagnostic.
2) RSV is diagnosed using enzyme linked immunosorbent assay (ELIZA) from nasal secretions.
3) Chest film will reveal areas of consolidation that are difficult to differentiate from bacterial pneumonia; areas of hyperinflation

c. Treatment
1) Treated symptomatically; humidity, rest, adequate hydration are main therapeutic interventions; can be successfully treated at home in most cases
2) Rationale for hospitalization: tachypnea (> 70 breaths/min), severe retractions, change in behavior, hydration problems; at-risk children with chronic or debilitating diseases should be hospitalized
3) In serious cases, steroids and inhaled bronchodilators will be administered.
4) With severe RSV infection, ribavirin (*Virazole*), an antiviral aerosol, may be administered via oxygen tent or hood; teratogenic effects have been reported, so pregnant caregivers are at-risk, strict guidelines exist for use
5) Palivizumab (*Synagis*) immunization is given to at-risk infants during their first winter. (This includes infants born at less than 32 weeks gestation, a large number of those born between 32 and 35 weeks gestation, and children with chronic lung or heart disease.)

 d. **NURSING INTERVENTIONS**
1) Monitor respiratory status frequently.
2) Assess oxygen saturation levels and ABGs.
3) Maintain fluid and electrolyte balance.
4) Maintain isolation precautions.

5) Medications:
a) Bronchodilators
b) Steroids
c) Ribavirin (Virazole)
6) Provide teaching for parents.
a) Prevent recurring infection under children who are age 2 with the use of palivizumab (Synagis) or IV immunoglobulin.
b) Use a bulb syringe or humidifier.
c) Wash hands frequently.
d) Observe for signs of dehydration.

SECTION V

NURSING CARE OF THE SURGICAL CHILD

A. Preoperative Preparation (see also Unit I, Section III)
1. Assess parents' and child's level of understanding.
2. Teach based on developmental level of child.
3. Involve parents and allow discussion.
4. Gather baseline data.

B. Common Surgical Problems
1. Tonsillectomy and adenoidectomy (T&A)
a. Tonsils help protect body from infections; typically enlarged in children
b. Rationale for surgery
1) Chronic tonsillitis (controversial)
2) Massive hypertrophy that interferes with breathing (obstructive apnea)
c. Preoperative care
1) Assess bleeding and coagulation time.
2) Confirm child is free from current infection.
3) Prepare the child.
d. **NURSING INTERVENTIONS** (postoperative)
1) Hemorrhage: greatest risk first 48 hr, then to 7 days later; manifestations: frequent swallowing or clearing of throat, bright red emesis, oozing from capillary bed, shock (late sign, indicates significant blood loss); prevention: avoid coughing, sneezing, sucking on straw
2) Avoid red-colored foods. Offer cool fluids; ice pops to decrease edema and to relieve pain. Avoid pretzels, crackers, chips, and dairy products.
3) Pain: administer analgesics regularly first 24 hr – acetaminophen (*Tylenol*); may require rectal or parenteral route due to throat pain; may return to school in 1 to 2 weeks

2. Pyloric stenosis
   a. Congenital hypertrophy of pyloric sphincter
   b. Clinical manifestations
      1) Insidious vomiting occurring 2 to 3 weeks after birth, increasing in intensity until forceful and projectile (no bile) by about 6 weeks of age
      2) Small, olive-size mass in right-upper quadrant
      3) Weight loss, dehydration
      4) Chronic hunger
   c. Diagnosis
      1) History and physical signs
      2) Upper gastrointestinal series
      3) Barium swallow under fluoroscopy
   d. Treatment
      1) Correct dehydration, metabolic alkalosis
      2) Pylorus resected
    e. **NURSING INTERVENTIONS**
      1) Preoperative: NPO; daily weights; NG tube for gastric decompression; monitor I&O and specific gravity; monitor emesis
      2) Postoperative: position on right side to prevent aspiration; begin oral feedings 4 to 6 hr postoperatively after bowel sounds return; maintain in upright position after feeding in infant seat; start with small, frequent feedings of oral rehydration solution (*Pedialyte*); monitor for emesis; advance feeding as tolerated
3. Appendicitis
   a. Inflammation of vermiform appendix
   b. Problem in school-age children
   c. Characteristics
      1) Periumbilical pain radiating to right-lower quadrant; rebound tenderness
      2) Low-grade temperature
      3) Nausea and vomiting
      4) Elevated WBC count: 15,000 to 20,000 mm^3
      5) May perforate and lead to peritonitis; sudden relief of pain followed by increased pain and rigid abdomen; high fever
    d. **NURSING INTERVENTIONS**
      1) Preoperative nursing care
         a) Provide pain relief.
         b) Place in right side-lying position.
         c) Perform abdominal assessment frequently.
         d) Maintain NPO status.
         e) Provide fluid and electrolyte balance.
      2) Postoperative nursing care
         a) Assess vital signs and perform abdominal assessment frequently.
         b) Monitor for signs of infection.
         c) Promote mobility.
         d) Promote respiratory toileting.
         e) Provide pain management as ordered.
4. Intussusception
   a. Telescoping of the bowel
   b. Characterized by
      1) Colicky pain with knees drawn up
      2) Currant jelly stools
   c. Treatment
      1) Barium enema: diagnostic; may reduce intussusception by hydrostatic pressure
      2) Bowel resection if barium enema does not reduce
    d. **NURSING INTERVENTIONS**
      1) Prepare for procedure.
      2) Provide routine postoperative abdominal surgical care.
5. Hirschsprung's disease (megacolon)
   a. Congenital absence of parasympathetic ganglion in distal colon
   b. Bowel proximal to a ganglionic section becomes enlarged
   c. Characterized by
      1) In newborn: failure to pass meconium within 24 hr after birth
      2) In older child: recurrent abdominal distension; chronic constipation with ribbon-like stools; diarrhea; bile-stained emesis
   d. Treatment
      1) Cleansing enemas with antibiotics preoperatively
      2) Temporary colostomy
      3) Bowel resection to remove aganglionic portion
    e. **NURSING INTERVENTIONS**
      1) Colostomy care: same as adult
         a) Check stoma for color.
         b) Change dressings frequently (abdominal, perineal).
         c) Monitor accurate I&O.
         d) Avoid incision irritation (keep diapers low).
      2) Parent and child instruction
         a) Encourage independence based on age of child.
         b) Discuss diet and hydration.
6. Hernias
   a. Most common: inguinal and umbilical
   b. Always consider developmental level (e.g., mutilation fears) when preparing child
   c. Usually repaired in ambulatory surgery setting
   d. **NURSING INTERVENTIONS:** instruct parents:
      1) Care for surgical site.
      2) Note manifestations of an infection.

SECTION VI

NURSING CARE FOR CHILDHOOD ACCIDENTS

A. Ingestions
1. General information
   a. Provide emergency care: ABCs.
   b. Identify substance, save evidence of poison.
   c. Call poison control center for treatment advice.
   d. Remove substance.
      1) Activated charcoal
      2) Gastric lavage
      3) Specific antidote
   e. Provide supportive therapy.
   f. Educate parents about childproof environment.
   g. Provide anticipatory guidance.
      1) Infants and toddlers: at risk because everything goes into the mouth
      2) Adolescents: at risk for intentional ingestion
2. Types of ingestions (See table IV-5.)

B. Pediatric Medication Administration
1. General information
   a. Consider age and developmental level of child.
   b. Identify any contraindications to oral route (e.g., poor swallow, no gag reflex, oral surgery).
   c. Evaluate child's ability to cooperate and understand.
2. Preparation
   a. Use caution with calculation and administration; especially IV medications.
   b. Nearly all medications are administered to children by calculating the desired amount of medication according to the child's weight (mg per kg).
   c. Use vastus lateralis for IM injections.
   d. Place medication in, or on nipple, and allow infants to suck.
   e. If administering via oral syringe, never squirt directly into back of throat.

C. Burns (See also Unit I, Section XIII.)
1. Characteristics of burns in children
   a. Due to the difference in proportions of head, trunk and limbs, burn percentages are rated differently for children.
   b. Due to the high percentage of extracellular fluids in the child, fluid loss can quickly lead to hypovolemic shock.

2. Treatment
   a. Similar to adult
   b. Children are likely to resist eating enough calories to sustain healing and growth needs. Parenteral or enteral feedings are usually necessary.
3. Rehabilitation
   a. Incorporate play into the physical or occupational therapy regimens for improved success.
   b. Consider psychosocial needs of the child.
   c. Adjustment and transition back to school may be very difficult for the child who has sustained a disfiguring burn.

D. Fractures (See also Page 37.)
1. Characteristics of fractures in children
   a. Due to immaturity of bones and incomplete ossification, greenstick (incomplete) fractures are commonly seen
   b. Fractures to the epiphysis (growth plate) are of greater concern as growth in limb can be stunted depending on the amount of injury
2. Treatment
   a. Similar to adult, although pediatric fractures often have shorter healing times
   b. May use cast (plaster or, more commonly, fiberglass) soft splint, traction, or bracing

E. Child Abuse (See also page 114.)
1. Types
   a. Physical neglect: failure to provide necessities of life
   b. Physical abuse: deliberate infliction of injury
   c. Emotional neglect: failure to provide emotional nurturing
   d. Emotional abuse: deliberate assault on child's self-esteem
   e. Sexual abuse: use of child to meet adult's sexual needs
   f. Munchausen syndrome by proxy (MSBP): a disorder when a caregiver (usually parent) falsely reports or intentionally causes symptoms in their own child to seek attention
2. Risk factors
   a. Parental
      1) Poor self-esteem
      2) Abused as a child
      3) Lack of knowledge
      4) Lack of support system, poor coping skills
   b. Child
      1) Unwanted pregnancy or sex
      2) Difficult temperament, hyperactive
   c. Environment
      1) Chronic stress
      2) Socioeconomic factors

3. Recognition of abuse and neglect
   a. Physical neglect
      1) Failure to thrive: disruption in maternal-infant bonding; poor feeding behaviors; mother does not respond to infant's cues; weight less than 5th percentile; developmental delay
      2) Poor health care, lack of immunizations
      3) Failure to meet basic needs: malnutrition, poor hygiene
   b. Physical abuse
      1) Bruises: not on bony prominences, in varying degrees of healing; with patterns
      2) Burns: with immersion lines, in patterns
      3) Fractures: spiral, twisting
      4) Shaken baby: unconscious infant with retinal hemorrhage and no external signs of trauma
      5) Conflicting stories given by parents, child or others
      6) History incompatible with physical findings or developmentally improbable
      7) Delay in seeking medical attention
   c. Emotional neglect and abuse
      1) Extremes of behavior
      2) Poor self-esteem
   d. Sexual abuse
      1) Bruising of the genitalia
      2) STD
      3) Sudden change in behavior, regressive behavior
   e. Munchausen syndrome by proxy
      1) Victims usually under age 6
      2) May have lasting emotional impact
      3) Increased risk for child to develop Munchausen syndrome as adult
      4) Parent well versed in medical knowledge

 4. **NURSING INTERVENTIONS**
   a. Document suspected findings.
   b. Do not leave child unattended.
   c. Refer psychiatric consult.
   d. Establish trust with child.

SECTION VII

NURSING CARE OF THE CHILD WITH CHRONIC OR LONG-TERM PROBLEMS

A. Immune Disorders
1. Eczema
   a. Known as atopic dermatitis
   b. May be associated with bronchial asthma; often family history of asthma or atopy

   c. Due to hypersensitivity to:
      1) Food (e.g., milk, egg white)
      2) Pollen
      3) Environmental
      4) Psychological (element of anxiety)
   d. Characteristics
      1) Papules are red and oozing; predominantly on face and extensor surfaces in infants, flexural areas in children (e.g., knees, wrists, antecubital fossa)
      2) Lesions eventually become scaly
      3) Pruritus may lead to secondary infection
   e. Treatment
      1) Topical steroids: triamcinolone (*Kenalog*); avoid chronic use
      2) Diphenhydramine HCl (*Benadryl*) or hydroxyzine HCl (*Atarax*): reduces itching
      3) Elimination diet (e.g., milk, eggs, chocolate, wheat)
      4) Antibiotics if secondary infection occurs
    f. **NURSING INTERVENTIONS**
      1) Maintain skin integrity:
         a) Educate parents in methods to control dry skin to minimize itching.
            (1) Use nonsoap cleanser.
            (2) Apply lubricating creams.
         b) Advise parents that the child may be more comfortable in cotton, long-sleeved clothing.
         c) Instruct parents to launder with a nonsoap or hypoallergenic cleanser.
         d) Fingernails and toenails should be kept short to prevent scratching.
      2) Assess developmental needs.
      3) Provide a hypoallergenic diet.
      4) Provide parental support and education.
2. Bronchial asthma (See also Unit I, Section II.)
   a. Also known as reactive airway disease (RAD)
   b. Usually begins before 5 years of age
   c. Pathology and etiology
      1) Chronic condition with acute exacerbations
      2) In response to allergen or trigger, acute hyperactive changes occur in reactive (lower) airways
         a) Spasm of smooth muscle
         b) Edema of mucous membranes
         c) Thick, tenacious mucus
         d) Severe, sudden dyspnea
      3) Potential triggers
         a) Foods
         b) Inhalants (e.g., secondhand smoke)
         c) Infection
         d) Vigorous activity
         e) Stress, anxiety

f) Allergens (e.g., pet dander, dust)
g) Cold air
d. Characterized by
1) Paroxysmal, hacking nonproductive cough
2) Prolonged expiratory phase with expiratory wheeze
3) Respiratory distress, anxiety
e. Complications
1) Pneumonia
2) Atelectasis
f. Treatment
1) Chronic (home) management of child
a) Medications via nebulizer or metered-dose inhaler
(1) Bronchodilators: albuterol (*Proventil*) useful for acute attack; salmeterol (*Serevent*) for chronic daily use, not for acute attack
(2) Inhaled corticosteroids: effective in reducing airway hyper-reactivity; for chronic daily use, not acute attack; avoid chronic oral steroids since they can stunt growth

(3) Cromolyn sodium (*Intal*): mast-cell inhibitor; reduces allergic response; for chronic daily use, not acute attack
 b) **NURSING INTERVENTIONS**
(1) Avoid allergens and triggers.
(2) Teach correct use of metered-dose inhaler (with spacer device).
(3) Plan activities that require stop and start energy.
(4) Use of a peak-flow meter to monitor airway compliance
2) Status asthmaticus: severe respiratory distress requiring hospitalization
a) Bronchodilators
(1) Epinephrine (*Adrenalin*): subcutaneous
(2) Aminophylline (*Phyllocontin*): IV drip
b) Steroids: IV
c) Inhalants: bronchodilators - albuterol (*Proventil*), metaproterenol (*Alupent*)
d) Antibiotics: prophylactic
e) Hydration
f) Oxygen therapy

TABLE IV-5
OVERVIEW OF COMMON ACCIDENTAL INGESTION

INGESTION	CLINICAL MANIFESTATIONS	TREATMENT	NURSING INTERVENTIONS
Salicylate (*Aspirin*)	- Tinnitus - Hyperpyrexia - Seizures - Bleeding - Hyperventilation	- Emesis - Hydration - Vitamin K - Activated charcoal	- Anticipatory guidance - Bleeding precautions - Counseling if suicide attempt
Acetaminophen (*Tylenol*)	Liver necrosis in 2 to 5 days; nausea; vomiting; pain in right-upper quadrant; jaundice; coagulation abnormalities; hepatotoxic	- Emesis - Mucomyst (antidote)	- Counseling if suicide attempt - Liver assessment
Lead (paint, also in soil near heavily trafficked roadways, household dust)	- Developmental regression - Impaired growth (encephalopathy) - Irritability - Increased clumsiness	- Chelation therapy: to remove heavy metals - Promote hydration	- Neuro assessment - Diet high in calcium, iron - Educate parents to wash child's hands, toys, frequently to remove lead dust - Lead abatement
Hydrocarbons (kerosene, turpentine, gasoline)	- Burning in mouth - Choking and gagging - CNS depression	- DO NOT INDUCE EMESIS! - Activated charcoal - Gastric lavage	If vomiting, reduce aspiration.
Corrosives (drain or oven cleaner, chlorine bleach, battery acid)	- Burning in mouth - White, swollen mucus membranes - Violent vomiting	- DO NOT INDUCE EMESIS! - Dilute toxin with water - Activated charcoal	Keep warm and inactive.

3. Rheumatic fever: inflammatory disease affecting heart, joints, and CNS
  a. Characteristics
    1) Usually occurs 2 to 6 weeks after an upper-respiratory infection with group A beta-hemolytic strep
    2) Sequelae includes scarring and damage to mitral valve
  b. Diagnosis
    1) Elevated or rising antistreptolysin O (ASO) titer with elevated erythrocyte sedimentation rate (ESR)
    2) Jones Criteria (presence of two major, or one major and two minor manifestations)
    3) Manifestations include: arthralgia; fever; hot, red, swollen joints (polyarthritis); tachycardia with precordial friction rub; subcutaneous nodules; truncal rash (erythema marginatum)
  c. Treatment
    1) Medication therapy (penicillin, salicylates)
    2) Bed rest in the acute phase for cardiac rest
    3) Prophylactic antibiotics with all dental work
4. Chorea
  a. Sudden, involuntary movements with involuntary facial grimaces
  b. Muscle weakness and speech disturbances
  c. Is transitory; reassure parents that chorea will self-resolve

B. Musculoskeletal Disorders
1. Scoliosis
  a. Lateral curvature of the spine
  b. Most common form is idiopathic, seen (predominately) in adolescent females; unknown etiology
  c. Acquired scoliosis; associated with deformity resulting from other neuromuscular disorders
  d. Diagnosis
    1) Classic signs: truncal asymmetry; especially noted in hips and shoulders, posture
    2) Screening exam in school: child flexes at waist; one scapula more prominent
    3) Spinal x-ray
  e. Treatment
    1) Mild scoliosis (< 20° curvature): observation, encourage physical exercise
    2) Moderate scoliosis (20 to 40 degree curvature): fitted brace
      a) Goal is to prevent worsening of curve; not a cure

 b) **NURSING INTERVENTIONS**
  (1) Address developmental needs of client.
  (2) Client teaching; skin care, commitment of therapy, and fashion concerns
    3) Severe scoliosis (> 40° curvature): requires surgery
      a) Spinal fusion with instrumentation
      b) Requires prolonged immobilization in cast, brace, or body jacket
 c) **NURSING INTERVENTIONS**
  (1) Postoperative nursing care
    (a) Log roll for first 24 hr.
    (b) Perform neurovascular assessments frequently.
    (c) Promote pulmonary toileting.
    (d) Provide pain management.
    (e) Encourage age-appropriate activities.
2. Juvenile rheumatoid arthritis (JRA)
  a. Autoimmune, inflammatory disease of the joints
  b. Toddler and school-age child more commonly affected
  c. Etiology unknown
  d. Early diagnosis essential due to long-term complications (blindness, contracture); early onset often associated with spontaneous permanent remission
  e. Classification
    1) Systemic (fever, rash, and organomegaly in addition to joint involvement)
    2) Polyarticular (many joints)
    3) Pauciarticular (few joints)
  f. Characterized by:
    1) Swelling, thickening of joint
    2) Pain, stiffness, impaired range of motion
    3) Lethargy, weight loss
  g. Treatment
    1) Medications
      a) NSAIDs
      b) Methotrexate
      c) Corticosteroids
    2) Supportive treatment to maintain joint mobility
 h. **NURSING INTERVENTIONS**
    1) Promote mobility and range of motion.
    2) Encourage nutritional intake.
    3) Provide pain relief (medication, heat, and cold).
    4) Monitor for exacerbation of symptoms.

C. Endocrine Disorders

1. Type 1 diabetes mellitus
   (See also page 46.)
   a. Etiology
      1) May be autoimmune response to environmental factors
      2) Genetic component: inherit tendency, not disease
      3) School-age child (5 to 7 years or puberty)
   b. Characteristics
      1) Onset: rapid with progression to abrupt ketoacidosis
      2) Hypertrophy and hyperplasia of islet cells occur early
      3) Remission (honeymoon) phase
      4) Insulin replacement (cannot use oral hypoglycemics)
      5) Exercise lowers blood glucose
      6) Management difficult due to
         a) Immaturity of child
         b) Lack of insight
   c. Developmental needs
      1) Preschooler: biggest issues are the fear of injections and poor appetite (difficult to maintain diet); "free diet"
      2) School-age child: how will children maintain their regular activities (e.g., birthday parties, pizza after the soccer game)
      3) Adolescent: adolescents have difficulty complying; they are not interested in long-term effects; they want to be like their peers

D. Hematological Disorders

1. Hemophilia
   a. Characteristics
      1) Impaired coagulation: deficiency of clotting factors
      2) Sex-linked recessive trait more common in males
      3) Factor VIII and IX are most common deficiencies
      4) Hemarthrosis (bleeding into joint cavities), bruises easily
   b. Treatment
      1) Cryoprecipitate (transfusion that replaces missing clotting factor)
      2) Supportive therapy
    c. **NURSING INTERVENTIONS**
      1) Control bleeding.
         a) Immobilize joint.
         b) Provide ice packs.
         c) Administer cryoprecipitate.
            (1) Give prophylactic cryoprecipitate for invasive procedures.
            (2) Risk for AIDS and/or hepatitis is

decreased because of screening, but does still exist.
      2) Safety directed toward developmental level to prevent injury, bleeding
         a) Avoid contact sports (difficult for children).
         b) Childproof environment.
         c) Avoid aspirin.
      3) Provide parental support.
2. Sickle cell anemia (See also page 50.)
   a. Characteristics
      1) Presence of Hgb S, which accounts for elongated shape of RBCs
      2) Sickling occurs in response to
         a) Infection, stress
         b) Dehydration
         c) Decreased oxygen
         d) High altitude
      3) Sickling increases blood viscosity, which causes further sickling and RBC destruction
      4) Manifestations
         a) Severe pain
         b) Swelling
         c) Jaundice
      5) Types of crisis
         a) Vaso-occlusive: "hand-foot syndrome" caused by stasis of blood in capillaries; schema and infarction
         b) Sequestration: pooling of large amounts of blood in liver, spleen; hypovolemia and shock
   b. Treatment
      1) Eliminate cause of crisis
      2) Analgesics
      3) Blood transfusions
      4) Monitor complications
         a) Anemia
         b) Splenic sequestration
         c) Cerebrovascular accidents
    c. **NURSING INTERVENTIONS**
      1) Recognize crisis early.
         a) Increasing irritability
         b) Frequent infections
         c) Pallor
         d) Failure to thrive
      2) Provide hydration.
      3) Administer analgesics, antibiotics as prescribed.
      4) Provide oxygen.
      5) Reduce stress of hospitalization.
      6) Provide parental support.

E. Renal Disorders (See also Unit I, Section IX.)

1. Glomerulonephritis (See Table IV-7.)
2. Nephrotic syndrome (see Table IV-7.)

F. Metabolic Disorders
1. Cystic fibrosis (See Table IV-8.)
2. Celiac disease (See Table IV-8.)

SECTION VIII

NURSING CARE OF THE CHILD WITH AN ONCOLOGY DISORDER

A. Leukemia
1. Characteristics
   a. Most common childhood cancer
   b. Peak incidence: 3 to 5 years of age
   c. Etiology: unknown, may be related to environmental exposures (e.g., radiation)
   d. Characterized by proliferation of immature WBCs
2. Pathology
   a. Bone marrow failure secondary to invasion of cancer cells
      1) Temperature and infection from decreased (normal) WBCs
      2) Anemia, pallor, and fatigue from decreased RBCs
      3) Petechiae and epistaxis from decreased platelets
   b. Leukemic infiltrate
      1) Limb and joint pain
      2) Lymphadenopathy
      3) CNS involvement
      4) Hepatosplenomegaly/bleeding tendencies
3. Classification
   a. Acute lymphocytic (ALL)
   b. Acute nonlymphoid (ANLL)
   c. Acute myelogenous leukemia (AML)
4. Complications (secondary to bone marrow depression)
   a. Infection
   b. Intracranial hemorrhage
   c. Secondary cancer or relapse
5. Diagnosis: bone marrow aspiration reveals hypercellular marrow, abnormal cells
6. Treatments
   a. Terminology
      1) Induction, remission
      2) CNS prophylaxis, consolidation
      3) Maintenance
   b. Chemotherapy
      1) Purine antagonists: 6-mercaptopurine (*Purinethol*) (may affect kidneys)
      2) Alkylating agents: cyclophosphamide

(*Cytoxan*) (causes chemical cystitis)
      3) Folic acid antagonists: methotrexate (*Folex*)
      4) Plant alkaloid: vincristine sulfate (*Oncovin*) (neurotoxic)
      5) Steroids: prednisone (*Prelone*)
      6) Enzymes: L-asparaginase (*Elspar*)
   c. Radiation therapy for CNS involvement
 7. **NURSING INTERVENTIONS** (See Table IV-9.)

B. Nephroblastoma (Wilms' Tumor)
1. Characteristics
   a. Most frequent type of renal cancer
   b. Peak age is 3 years
   c. Most common clinical sign: swelling, mass within the abdomen
   d. May also see: anemia, hypertension, hematuria
2. Pathology
   a. Arises from embryonal tissue
   b. Encapsulated (do not biopsy, will "seed" tumor further)
3. Diagnosis
   a. IV pyelogram
   b. Computerized tomography
   c. Bone marrow to rule out metastasis
4. Treatment
   a. Nephrectomy and adrenalectomy
   b. Radiation and chemotherapy determined by staging
 5. **NURSING INTERVENTIONS**
   a. Preoperative care
      1) Begin treatment quickly, support parents, and keep explanations simple.
      2) Monitor blood pressure due to excess renin production.
      3) Prevent rupture of encapsulated tumor.
         a) Post sign on bed:
            DO NOT PALPATE ABDOMEN.
         b) Bathe and handle child gently.
   b. Postoperative care
      1) Problems related to radiation, chemotherapy (See Table IV-9.)
      2) Large surgical incision
         a) Pain management
         b) Gentle handling
         c) Prepare parents
      3) Protect remaining kidney
         a) Monitor blood pressure.
         b) Use dipstick urine for protein or blood.

C. Neuroblastoma
1. Characteristics
   a. Most frequently seen in children under 2

b. Frequently called "silent" tumor because by the time of diagnosis, metastasis has occurred
   c. Clinical signs include: abdominal mass, urinary retention and frequency, lymphadenopathy, generalized weakness, and malaise
   d. Primary site is abdomen, most often in flank area
2. Diagnosis
   a. Computerized tomography
   b. Bone marrow to determine metastasis
   c. Excessive catecholamine production
3. Treatment
   a. Surgery to remove as much of the tumor as possible and determine staging
   b. Chemotherapy and radiation determined by staging of tumor

 4. **NURSING INTERVENTIONS** (See Table IV-9.)

D. Hodgkin's Lymphoma
1. Characteristics
   a. Primarily affects adolescents and young adults
   b. Clinical signs include: painless enlargement of lymph nodes (cervical most common), metastasis related manifestations (persistent cough, abdominal pain), systemic problems (pruritus, night sweats, fever)
2. Pathology
   a. Malignancy originates in lymphoid system
   b. Metastasis may include spleen, liver, bone marrow, and/or lungs
3. Diagnosis
   a. Computerized axial tomography
   b. Lymph node biopsy, exploratory laparotomy (to stage)
4. Treatment
   a. Radiation and chemotherapy determined by clinical staging
   b. Surgical laparotomy
   c. Splenectomy

 5. **NURSING INTERVENTIONS**
   a. See Table IV-9.
   b. Instruct family on long-term care following splenectomy.
      1) Increased susceptibility to infection
      2) Prophylactic long-term antibiotic therapy is necessary (compliance issues)

TABLE IV-6
COMPARISON OF INSULIN SHOCK AND DIABETIC COMA GUIDE

	INSULIN SHOCK (HYPOGLYCEMIA)	**DIABETIC COMA (HYPERGLYCEMIA)**
Causes:	- Too much insulin - Not eating enough food - Engaging in unusual amounts of exercise - Delayed meals	- Too little insulin - Failure to follow diet - Infection, fever, emotional stress
Clinical Manifestations:	- Onset is abrupt, rapid - Skin is pale, moist - Vertigo (dizzy) - Urine is normal - Tachycardia - Hungry (polyphagia) - Normal urinary output - Normal thirst - Shallow respirations - Breath normal - Level of consciousness: inappropriate behavior, confused	- Onset is slow, insidious - Skin is hot, dry - No vertigo - Urine is positive for sugar and acetone - Normal pulse - Anorexia - Polyuria - Polydipsia - Deep, labored respirations - Acetone breath - Level of consciousness: lethargic, drowsy
What to do:	- Give fast-acting sugar (e.g., candy, orange juice). - Call provider. - Do not give insulin. - Glucagon if unconscious	- Call provider. - Encourage fluids without sugar. - Continue to check urine. - Give insulin as usual.

SECTION IX

NURSING CARE OF THE CHILD WITH AN INFECTIOUS DISEASE

A. Prevention

1. Immunizations
   a. Schedule recommendations established by CDC and reviewed by American Academy of Pediatrics.
   b. Contraindication with active illness and fever greater than 40° C (101° F)
   c. Precautions
      1) Hepatitis B - allergy to baker's yeast, liver disease
      2) DTaP - delay after 30 days after immunosuppression
      3) Hib - delay if child is ill
      4) MMR - do not administer if child is allergic to eggs, neomycin, gelatin. Also, do not give to pregnant women or those who expect to get pregnant in 3 months
      5) Varicella - do not administer if allergic to neomycin or gelatin
      6) Pneumococcal - sensitivity to diphtheria may cause anaphylaxis
      7) Influenza - do not administer if child is allergic to eggs; encourage those under going immunosuppressive therapy to receive a flu shot
      8) Meningococcal - unknown impact on pregnancy
2. Communicability
   a. Most communicable diseases are most contagious prior to the onset of manifestations or rash and in the early prodromal period
   b. Most require respiratory isolation precautions if the child requires hospitalization
   c. Most are preventable through immunization or other measures
3. Common childhood infections (See table IV-10.)

SECTION X

CPR GUIDELINES FOR CHILDREN AND INFANTS

A. Establish That the Victim Does Not Respond

B. Activate:

1. Unwitnessed event: activate the Emergency Response System (EMS) after performing five cycles of CPR
2. Sudden, witnessed event: activate EMS after verifying that the victim is unresponsive

C. Open the Airway

1. Use head tilt and chin lift unless trauma is suspected; when trauma is suspected, use jaw thrust

D. Rescue Breathing

1. Open the airway, look, listen, and feel. Take at least 5 seconds and no more than 10 seconds.
2. Give 2 breaths, each 1 second long. If unable to get chest to rise and fall, reposition and try again.
3. If chest is still not rising and falling, suspect obstructed airway and perform back blows and chest thrusts. Do not perform a blind finger sweep of the mouth. Only try to remove an object from the mouth that you can see.

E. Check Pulse

1. Child (ages 1 to 8): carotid pulse; if no pulse or if pulse is less than 60/min with signs of poor perfusion, start CPR
2. Infant (less than 1 year): Brachial pulse; if no pulse or if pulse is less than 60/min with signs of poor perfusion, start CPR

F. Start CPR

1. Compression location
   a. Child: center of breastbone between nipples
   b. Infant: just below nipple line on breastbone
2. Compression method
   a. Child: heel of one hand
   b. Infant: two fingers (two thumb-encircling hands for two-rescuer CPR)
3. Compression depth: ⅓ to ½ depth of chest
4. Compression rate: 100/min for infant and child
5. Compression-ventilation ratio
   a. 30:2 for single rescuer CPR
   b. 15:2 for dual rescuer CPR

G. AED

1. Child: use AED as soon as available for sudden collapse and in-hospital; use child pads or a child system for children ages 1 to 8, if available; if child pads or a child system are not available, use adult AED and pads

2. Infant: AED is not recommended for infants less than 1 year of age

TABLE IV-7
RENAL DISORDERS

	NEPHROTIC SYNDROME	ACUTE GLOMERULONEPHRITIS
Other names	Childhood nephrosis	Poststreptococcal glomerulonephritis
Etiology	Cause unknown; likely autoimmune	Antigen - antibody reaction secondary to infection elsewhere in the body; usually a Group A beta-hemolytic streptococcal infection of the upper respiratory tract
Incidence	Average age of onset about 2 1/2 years; more common in boys	2/3 of cases in children from 4 to 7 years; more common in boys
Pathology	Increased permeability of the glomerular membrane to protein	Inflammation of the kidneys; damage to the glomeruli allows excretion of RBCs
Clinical manifestations	Edema: appears insidiously; usually first noticed about the eyes and can advance to the legs, arms, back, peritoneal cavity and scrotum; massive proteinuria; anorexia; pallor	Periorbital edema: appears insidiously; tea-colored urine from hematuria; hypertension; oliguria
Blood pressure	Usually normal; transient elevation may occur early	Varying degrees of hypertension may be present; when blood pressure is elevated, cerebral manifestations may occur as a result of vasospasm; these may include headache, drowsiness, diplopia, vomiting, convulsions
Laboratory findings	Urine shows heavy albuminuria	Urine contains RBCs; has a high specific gravity
Blood	Involves reduction in protein (mainly albumin); gamma globulin is reduced; during the active stages of the disease, the sedimentation rate is greatly increased	BUN value is elevated; anemia (reduction in circulating RBCs, in Hgb or both) tends to develop rapidly
Course and prognosis	Characterized by remissions and relapses; with protection against infection and suppression of proteinuria by steroid therapy, most children can eventually expect a favorable outcome	Recovery from acute glomerulonephritis is to be expected in nearly all children; mild illnesses last as little as 2 to 3 weeks; in exceptional instances, the disease is progressive and takes on the characteristics of chronic nephritis
Treatments	1. Prednisone (Deltasone) 2. Furosemide (Lasix) 3. Salt-poor albumin	1. Antibiotics for strep infection 2. Antihypertensives and diuretics 3. Corticosteroids
Nursing interventions	Control edema; provide skin care; prevent infection; monitor nutrition: low sodium, high protein, high potassium; monitor urine for proteinuria; monitor for side effects from steroid therapy	Bed rest if hypertensive; restrict fluids; monitor neuro status; monitor blood pressure; provide low potassium diet, no added salt; prevent infection

TABLE IV-8
COMPARISON OF CYSTIC FIBROSIS AND CELIAC DISEASE

	CYSTIC FIBROSIS	CELIAC DISEASE
Onset	0 to 6 months	6 to 18 months
Characteristics	Production of abnormally viscid secretions of: pancreas, respiratory, salivary, and sweat glands	Intestinal malabsorption: malnutrition; fat and gluten intolerance; dietary intolerance: fat, gluten
Etiology	Autosomal recessive: 25% chance	Inborn error of metabolism
Manifestations	Meconium ileus in newborn; large, fatty foul-smelling stools in older child; chronic respiratory disease; digestive problems; sweat abnormalities	Diarrhea: large bulky stools; anemia; retarded growth; frequent infections; malabsorption of vitamin D
Diagnosis	Sweat test; pancreatic enzymes	Bowel biopsy; sweat test; gluten-free diet

Treatment	- Pulmonary: postural drainage, aerosol therapy, antibiotic
	- Nutrition: pancreatic, enzymes with meals, high calorie, vitamins A, D, E, K (fat soluble) twice normal dose, free use of salt
	- Lung transplantation (experimental)
		- Gluten free diet:
		   - meat, eggs, milk, fruit, vegetables, gluten-free bread, vitamins A, D, E, K (fat soluble)
		- Avoid:
		   - Barley, rye, oats, wheat (BROW)

Nursing interventions	- Avoid infection - Respiratory toilet - Frequent, small feedings - Pancreatic enzymes - Developmental issues - Anticipatory grieving	- Avoid infection. - Instruct how to implement diet. - Developmental issues
Prognosis	Short lifespan 20 to 25 years	Normal lifespan if follows gluten-free diet

TABLE IV-9
NURSING CARE OF THE CHILD WITH CANCER

MANAGE PROBLEMS RELATED TO CHEMOTHERAPY	PREPARE CHILD/FAMILY FOR RADIATION THERAPY	TERMINAL PHASE—PROVIDE COMFORT CARE

- Nausea and vomiting
  - Administer antiemetic prior to treatment and regularly administer PRN medications.
  - Teach guided imagery.
 	
- Anorexia: difficult to handle with children
 	
- Mucosal ulceration
  - Stomatitis: bland diet, soft tooth brush, oral hygiene
  - Rectal ulcers: sitz baths, stool softeners, no rectal temperatures
 	
- Neuropathy (vincristine related)
  - Note bowel movements,
  - Instruct parents concerning foot-drop, weakness, numbness, and jaw pain.
 	
- Hemorrhagic cystitis (cyclophosphamide related)
  - 1½ to 2 times normal fluid intake
  - Frequent voiding
  - Administer early in day to allow for sufficient oral intake.
	- Meticulous skin care: avoid exposure to sun; limit use of soap and lotions; do not wash off markings
	
	- Radiation to chest and abdomen frequently results in nausea and vomiting, weight loss, esophagitis
	
	- Malaise is most frequent report of adolescents and prevents peer involvement
	
	- Discuss effects radiation therapy has on puberty, fractures and spinal deformities
	- Could cause sterility
		- If poor prognosis, assist family in dealing with life-threatening illness
		
		- Perception of death
		  - Infant and toddler: different way of life (e g., "Mommy is sleeping"); major fear is separation
		
		- Preschooler: reversible, cannot separate life and death
		
		- School-age child and preadolescent: similar to preschooler's reaction until 9 to 10 years, then adult concept of death; magical thinking may still be evident
		
		- Adolescent: adult concept - of all age groups, has most difficulty dealing with death

TABLE IV-10
COMMUNICABLE DISEASES GUIDE

DISEASE	INFECTIOUS AGENTS	TRANSMISSION	INCUBATION	CLINICAL MANIFESTATIONS	TREATMENT AND NURSING INTERVENTIONS	PREVENTION
Chickenpox	Varicella zoster virus	Direct contact, droplet spread, and contaminated objects or contact with skin lesions	2 to 3 weeks (usually 10 to 14 days)	Prodromal stage: slight fever, malaise and anorexia, first 24 hr; pruritic rash; macule to papule to vesicle to pustule; rash occurs in all different stages; lesions crust over and usually heal without scarring; client is communicable	Do not use aspirin; control itching; prevent secondary infection; acyclovir may lessen severity of outbreak and promote faster healing; strict isolation if child hospitalized	Varicella zoster immunoglobin (Zovirax)
Derma-tophytosis (tinea capitis) (ringworm)	Microsporum audouinii	- Person to person - Animal to person	N/A	Red, scaly patches on scalp and skin that blister and drain	Keep skin clean and dry. Apply antifungal cream for 4 weeks.	Caution children about sharing hair items
Enterobiasis (pinworms)	Enterobius vermicularis	Ingested; inhaled; poor hygiene after toilet; reinfect self	Eggs hatch and mature in 2 to 4 weeks 7 to 18 days	Parasites that live in rectum causing intense perianal itching; diagnosed with tape test.	Sanitize bedding; tight diapers and pants; family precautions; mebendazole (Vermox) to prevent itching	Handwashing (especially after using toilet)
Fifth disease (erythema infectiosum)	Human parvovirus 19	Respiratory secretions, blood Highly infectious	N/A	Red rash on cheeks: gives face a "slapped cheeks" appearance; followed by "lace-like" rash on extremes that may fade and reappear	Symptomatic treatment only; monitor for anemia	None
Impetigo	Group A beta strep or staph aureus	Direct contact with skin lesion or articles soiled with discharge	3 days to 1 month	History of trauma or minor injury; honey-colored blisters that rupture and become crusted; lymphadenopathy; highly contagious	Soak lesions; topical ointment; communicability; prevent scratching; family precautions	Good hygiene; short fingernails
Lyme disease	Borrelia burgdorferi	- Transmitted by bite of deer tick - High risk areas: Michigan, New York, New Jersey, Minnesota, Connecticut, Pennsylvania, Massachusetts		Initially flu-like manifestations; red rash in bulls-eye pattern at bite site; later, joint pain, neurologic and cardiac involvement; may become chronic	Antibiotics; remove tick as soon as possible; symptomatic; analgesics; antipyretic	Avoid tick-infested areas; dress appropriately in woods (tuck socks into jeans and long sleeves)

TABLE IV-10
COMMUNICABLE DISEASES GUIDE (CONTINUED)

DISEASE	INFECTIOUS AGENTS	TRANSMISSION	INCUBATION	CLINICAL MANIFESTATIONS	TREATMENT AND NURSING INTERVENTIONS	PREVENTION
Meningitis	Viral or bacterial (H. Influenza: 3 months to 3 years; meningococcal meningitis)	Direct invasion via otitis media, upper respiratory infection, head injury	2 to 10 days	Onset abrupt with fever, headache, irritability, altered level of consciousness, nuchal rigidity, increased intracranial pressure; must do lumbar puncture to isolate organism	Isolate; reduce environmental stimuli; monitor hydration; seizure precautions; IV antibiotics	(Rifampin): given to contacts of client with meningococcal meningitis as prophylaxis
Mumps	Viral (paramyxovirus)	Saliva, direct contact or droplet	14 to 21 days	Prodromal stage: headache, malaise, anorexia, followed by earache; parotitis 3 days later with pain/tenderness	Symptomatic and supportive; analgesics; antipyretics; hydration	MMR
Pediculosis capitis (head lice)	Pediculus humanus capitis	Sharing of personal items, (e.g., hair ornaments, caps, hats)	Eggs hatch in 7 to 10 days	Intense itching; can visually see nits attached to base of hair shafts; differentiate from dandruff	Do not share personal items. Shampoo with anti-lice products, wash linens and clothing in hot water.	Caution children about sharing hair items
Pertussis (whooping cough)	Bordetella pertussis	Respiratory droplets and direct contact	7 to 21 days	Initially "cold" manifestations; progresses to spasms of paroxysmal coughing (whooping cough)	Antibiotics; corticosteroids; supportive care; isolation; stay with child during coughing spells	DTaP
Rabies	Viral	Contact with saliva of infected animal	1 to 3 months or as short as 10 days	Prodromal: malaise, sore throat followed by hypersensitivity, excitation, convulsions, paralysis; high mortality	Irrigate wound; psychologic follow up	Avoid contact with wild animals; rabies shot (given after exposure)
Reye syndrome	Viral	Unknown: proceeded by viral infection and associated with use of aspirin	N/A	Prodromal: malaise cough, upper respiratory infection; 1 to 3 days after: fever, decreased level of consciousness, hepatic and cerebral dysfunction; high mortality	Monitor liver function; peak age 4 to 11 years; neuro assessments; intracranial pressure monitoring	Avoid use of aspirin in adolescents and children.
Rheumatic fever	Group A beta-hemolytic strep	Nasopharyngeal secretions; direct contact with infected person or droplet spread	1 to 3 weeks after acute infection, develops inflammatory disease	Carditis, arthritis, chorea (involuntary ataxic movements), subcutaneous nodules, erythema marginatum (rash)	Bed rest in acute phase to decrease cardiac workload; full course of antibiotics (penicillin/ erythromycin); high dose aspirin therapy (monitor for toxicity, tinnitus)	Adequate, prompt treatment of strep infection (must finish entire course of therapy)

TABLE IV-10
COMMUNICABLE DISEASES GUIDE (CONTINUED)

DISEASE	INFECTIOUS AGENTS	TRANSMISSION	INCUBATION	CLINICAL MANIFESTATIONS	TREATMENT AND NURSING INTERVENTIONS	PREVENTION
Roseola (exanthem subitum)	Viral (human herpes virus type 6)	Unknown (limited to children 6 months to 2 years of age)	Unknown	Persistent high fever for 3 to 4 days; precipitous drop in fever with appearance of rash (rose-pink maculopapule on trunk, then spreading to neck, face and extremities); lasts 1 to 2 days	Antipyretics to control temperature and prevent febrile seizures; hydrate	None
Rubella (German measles)	Viral (rubella virus)	Nasopharyngeal secretions: direct contact, indirect via freshly contaminated nasopharyngeal secretions or urine	14 to 21 days	Prodromal phase; absent in children, present in adults; rash; first face and rapidly spreads downward to neck, arms, trunk, and legs; teratogenic to fetus	No treatment necessary; isolate child from pregnant women; women of childbearing years should have rubella titer drawn	MMR
Rubeola (measles)	Viral	Respiratory-droplets	10 to 21 days	Prodromal stage: fever and malaise, coryza, conjunctivitis, Koplik spots (spots with blue/white center on buccal mucosa opposite molars); rash: starts on face, spreads downward, may desquamate (peel)	Antipyretics to control temperature and prevent seizures; dim lights if photophobia; respiratory precautions	MMR
Scarlet fever	Group A beta-hemolytic strep	Nasopharyngeal secretions, direct contact with infected person or droplet spread	2 to 4 days	Prodromal stage: abrupt high fever, pulse increased, vomiting, chills, malaise, abdominal pain; enanthema: tonsils enlarged, edematous reddened, covered with patches of exudate; strawberry tongue; exanthema: rash appears 12 hr after prodromal signs	Full course of antibiotics (penicillin/erythromycin); isolate; monitor for rheumatic fever, glomerulonephritis; hydrate	Adequate, prompt treatment of strep infection (must finish entire course of therapy)
Tetanus	Clostridium tetany	Deep puncture, not contagious, "anaerobic"	7 to 14 days	Gradual stiffening of voluntary muscles until rigid (i.e., lockjaw, rigid abdomen); sensitive to stimuli; clear sensorium	Eliminate stimuli; monitor respirations, blood gases; muscle relaxants; monitor hydration	DTaP, Td

UNIT FIVE

NURSING MANAGEMENT

UNIT CONTENT

SYMBOLS

 Key Points

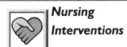 Nursing Interventions

 Points to Remember

SECTION I

MANAGEMENT

A. Concepts of Management

1. Leadership
   a. Definition: A way of behaving that influences others to respond, not because they have to, but because they want to; leaders help others to identify and focus on goals and the achievement of them; think of leadership as a personal interaction that focuses on the personal development of the members of the group
   b. Essential components of leadership
      1) Knowledge
      2) Self-awareness
      3) Communication
      4) Energy
      5) Goals
      6) Action
    c. **NURSING INTERVENTIONS:** All nurses will need leadership skills to manage other nurses, assistive personnel, and clients. It is essential to the nursing role to identify and implement effective leadership practices.
2. Management
   a. Definition: A problem-oriented process with a focus on the activities needed to achieve a goal; supplying the structure, resources, and direction for the activities of the group; management involves personal interaction, but the focus is on the group's process; the most effective managers are also effective leaders
   b. Essential components of management
      1) Planning/organization
      2) Direction
      3) Monitoring
      4) Recognition and reward
      5) Development of staff
      6) Representation
   c. Management styles
      1) Autocratic
      2) Laissez-faire
      3) Democratic
    d. **NURSING INTERVENTIONS:** All nurses need to learn management skills and identify their own personal leadership style. Additionally, nurses need to know the differences between being an autocratic and democratic leader. The most effective management style in a health care environment is the democratic leader who uses an interdisciplinary approach that encourages open communication and collaboration and promotes individual autonomy and accountability.

3. Communication
   a. Definition: Communication involves sending, receiving, and interpreting both verbal and nonverbal information between at least two people
   b. Components of communication
   c. Basic elements of effective communication
   d. Assertive communication
    e. **NURSING INTERVENTIONS:** Effective communication requires commitment, effort, focus, and cooperation, especially when dealing with complex clinical issues and people with diverse backgrounds and perspectives; it is essential to understand and use effective communication skills to successfully manage others
4. Conflict
   a. Definition: Conflict arises when there are two opposing views, feelings, expectations, or many other issues; it can occur within an individual, between individuals, or between groups and organizations; conflict can be managed
   b. Sources of conflict
   c. Conflict resolution
      1) Avoidance
      2) Accommodation
      3) Compromise
      4) Competition
      5) Collaboration
   d. Process of negotiation
   e. Sexual harassment
    f. **NURSING INTERVENTIONS:** A nurse manager's role is to identify the source of conflict, understand the issues that have developed, and work toward conflict resolution while maintaining positive regard for each individual. It is essential to address the person with whom you have conflict before going to his superiors (use the chain of command). Remember, the most important conflict strategy involves collaboration that results in a win-win solution for everyone.

B. Power vs. Influence

1. Definition
   a. Power: the ability, strength, and capacity to do something
   b. Influence: control over people and their actions
2. Types of power
   a. Reward: power based on the ability to control resources
   b. Coercive: power based on the ability to inflict aversive outcomes or punishment
   c. Legitimate: power based on one's position

d.   Referent: power based on attractive characteristics

e.   Expert: power based on expertise or knowledge

3.   Influence Tactics

a.   Ingratiation: the ability to manipulate others through flattery and style

b.   Conformity pressure: the pressure to conform to the group; this pressure increases as group size increases to greater than six, or as familiarity with the topic decreases

c.   Foot-in-the-door: a small request followed by a larger request

d.   Door-in-the-face: a large request that is intended to be denied, followed by a smaller request that is intended to be granted

e.   Guilt: the practice of inducing guilt before making a request; granting the request reduces the feeling of guilt

 4.   **NURSING INTERVENTION:** the power of influence is aimed at accomplishing well-defined goals, preferably as a cohesive team

C. Team Building

1.   Definition: Activities or efforts intended to unify people into a team to more effectively accomplish the overall objectives and mission of the organization

2.   Components of team building

a.   Clear expectations: Expectations should be clearly defined and communicated to members of the team.

b.   Context: Team members should understand why they are participating in the team.

c.   Commitment: Members should feel valuable, excited, and challenged, and be committed to the success of the team.

d.   Competence: Team should feel like it has the resources, strategies, and support it needs to meet its goals.

e.   Collaboration: Rules of conduct should be followed for conflict resolution and cooperative decision-making.

f.   Communication: There should be a clear, honest, respectful dialogue between team members.

g.   Creativity: New, innovative ideas should be encouraged and welcomed.

h.   Consequences: Contributions and success should be recognized and rewarded.

 3.   **NURSING INTERVENTIONS**

a.   Foster a teamwork culture that values collaboration and cooperation.

b.   Communicate that teamwork is expected.

c.   Publicly celebrate team success.

d.   Bring a sense of play and fun to the team.

D. Continuity of Care

1.   Definition: Continuity of care focuses on the experience of the client as the client moves through the health care system; guiding the client through this experience requires coordination, integration, and facilitation of all the events along the continuum.

2.   Nursing role

3.   Factors impacting the continuum of care

E. Quality Improvement

1.   Definition: A planned process to evaluate the delivery of care and to develop ways to address any problems or difficulties.

2.   Continuous vs. Total Quality Improvement

3.   Types of quality indicators

a.   Structure

b.   Process

c.   Outcome

4.   Data collection

F. Variance/Incidence/Occurrence Reports

1.   Definition: A variance or incident is an event that occurs outside the usual expected "normal" events or activities of the client's stay, unit functioning, or organizational processes.

2.   Purpose

3.   Documentation standards

 4.   **NURSING INTERVENTIONS:** Incidence or variance reports are not intended to point blame, just document the facts; the purpose is to identify situations or system issues that contributed to the occurrence and to engage strategies to prevent reoccurrence or to correct the situation.

G. Resource Management

1.   Health care delivery

a.   Retrospective vs. prospective payment

b.   Health-maintenance organizations

2.   Budgeting

a.   Types of budgets

b.   The budget process

1)   Planning

2)   Preparation

3)   Modification and approval

4)   Monitoring

3.   Nurse's role in resource management

 4.   **NURSING INTERVENTIONS:** A nurse manager must also be aware of economic issues in health care. Budgetary terms are fundamental to understanding financial management of institutions. Remember, the more information available to the nurse, the better the decisions and input into long-range planning for the institute.

H. Case Management
1. Definition: Case management involves the development of a partnership with the client, with a goal of managing declines in health and/or function that are due to serious, acute, or chronic and persistent illness and disability
2. Types of case management
   a. Independent
   b. Hospital based
   c. Provider based
   d. Insurance based
3. **NURSING INTERVENTIONS:** A nurse's role in case management is aimed at arranging services to respond to the hierarchy of client needs. This system provides care that minimizes fragmentation and maximizes holistic individualized client care.

I. Consultation and Referral
1. Definitions
   a. Consultation: To ask for help in solving a problem or meeting a need of an individual or group; this help is then applied and monitored by the nurse; often, it is a request for information from someone with specialized knowledge, including peers
   b. Referral: A request for assistance from someone with specialized knowledge or skills to help in the management of the client's problems; most often, it is a request for intervention from another professional who has the needed skills and knowledge; the intervention becomes that specialist's responsibility, but the nurse continues to be responsible for the monitoring of the client's response and progress
2. Common nursing consultation and referral situations
3. Appropriate use of consultation and referral
4. **NURSING INTERVENTIONS:** The processes of consultation and referral are integral for effective use of services along the continuum. The nurse supports the client and families with appropriate consultation and referral to contacts in the community.

SECTION II

DELEGATION

A. Delegation/Supervision
1. Definitions
   a. Delegation: The act of asking another to do some aspect of care, assignment, or work that needs to be accomplished; Delegation can be horizontal to peers, upwardly vertical to management, or downwardly vertical to subordinate

   b. Supervision: Monitoring the progress toward completion of delegated tasks; the amount of supervision required depends on the direction of the delegation, the abilities of the person being delegated to, and the location of the ultimate responsibility for outcomes
2. Accountability
3. Five rights of delegation
   a. Right person
   b. Right task
   c. Right supervision
   d. Right circumstance
   e. Right instruction
4. **NURSING INTERVENTIONS:** It is very important for a nurse manager to understand legal responsibilities when managing and delegating nursing care to a wide variety of health care workers. The nurse manager must delegate activities thoughtfully, taking into account individual job descriptions, knowledge base, and demonstrated skills. Remember, the professional nurse is accountable to determine the extent and complexity of client needs and to assign work that is consistent with the individual's position, description, and duties.

B. Roles and Responsibilities of Levels of Staff
1. Assistive Personnel (AP)
   a. Also referred to nursing assistant or patient-service technician.
   b. Training is often on the job
   c. AP may complete a certification program - Certified Nursing Assistant
   d. Function under the direction of the licensed practical nurse (LPN) or RN
   e. Skills:
      1) Basic hygiene care and grooming
      2) Communication
      3) Assistance with ADLs such as nutrition, elimination, and mobility
      4) Emphasis is on maintaining a safe environment and recognizing situations to report to their immediate superior
2. LPN
   a. May also be called a licensed vocational nurse (LVN)
   b. Education is approximately 12 to 18 months in a formal program
   c. LPNs must complete and pass the NCLEX®-PN exam for licensure
   d. Function under direction of the RN or primary care provider
   e. Advanced clinical skills in caring for clients who are chronic and stable. Scope of practice determined by Nurse Practice Act, which varies from state to state. Requirements to maintain active license determined by each state.

1) Meeting health needs of clients
2) Caring for clients whose condition is considered to be stable

3. RN
   a. May be diploma, associate degree, baccalaureate degree (or higher)
   b. Education ranges from 2 to 4 (or more) years
   c. RNs must complete and pass the NCLEX®-RN exam for licensure
   d. Function under direction of the primary care provider
   e. Advanced clinical skills in caring for client who is acute and critical. Scope of practice determined by Nurse Practice Act, which varies from state to state. Requirements to maintain active license determined by each state.

4. Advance practice nurses
   a. May be nondegree or master's degree (or higher)
   b. Education ranges from 18 months to 4 (or more) years (in addition to basic RN program)
   c. Must complete and pass a certification exam (in addition to the NCLEX®-RN exam) applicable to the specialty and practice (e.g., adult nurse practitioner, diabetic educator)
   d. Functions vary according to the state practice act which may be either autonomously or under the direct or indirect supervision of a provider
   e. Skills: vary according to the state practice act, may include ability to prescribe, diagnose, and treat

5. Primary care provider
   a. May be a provider, provider's assistant, or nurse practitioner
   b. In general, only an attending provider has admitting privileges to an institution, although another care provider in the practice may direct the care given to the client

SECTION III

ETHICAL ISSUES

A. Ethical Practice
1. Basic ethical principles
   a. Nonmaleficence: the obligation not to harm other people (e.g., Hippocrates statement, "First do no harm.")
   b. Beneficence: the obligation to do good for other people
   c. Autonomy/self-determination: the right to make one's own decisions
   d. Fidelity: the obligation to be faithful to the agreements and responsibilities one has undertaken

   e. Justice: obligation to be fair to all people (e.g., when allocating limited resources)
2. The American Nurses Association's (ANA): guidelines to use when giving client care, which outline the nurse's responsibility to the client, the profession of nursing, and assist the nurse in ethical decision making
3. Ethical dilemmas: an ethical issue for which two opposing viewpoints can each be supported by sound ethical principle
4. Ethical decision making: a process in which the nurse, the client, the client's family, and the health care team make decisions, taking into consideration personal and philosophical viewpoints, the ANA code for nurses, and ethical principles

B. Organ Donation
1. Determination of death
2. Nursing role
3. Family needs
4. Criteria for donation
 5. **NURSING INTERVENTIONS:** Today's nurses have an ethical responsibility to participate in the donation process by presenting the option of organ donation to all suitable clients and families. Remember, families in this situation may be receptive to organ donation because they want something positive to come from their loss. The nurse needs to be comfortable when discussing and providing information about organ donation.

C. Advance Directives
1. Definition: A document in which a competent client is able to express his or her wishes regarding future acceptable health care (including the desire for extraordinary lifesaving measures including resuscitation, intubation, and artificial hydration and nutrition) and/or designate another person to make decisions for the client if the client is physically or mentally unable
2. Legislative action
3. Living will
   a. Definition: Declaration of what the client finds acceptable or would refuse under identified situations that may occur in the future
   b. Legal standing
   c. Content
4. Durable power of attorney
   a. Definition: Designation of another person to make decisions (often financial) for the client when the client becomes unable to make decisions independently
   b. Legal issues
   c. Purpose

5. **NURSING INTERVENTIONS:** It is important for a nurse to identify clients who do not have advance directives, to inform them of their rights, and to ensure that clients with advance directives have copies placed in their charts.

SECTION IV

LEGAL ISSUES

A. Informed Consent
1. Definition: Consent given by the client that is based on adequate information to consider the risks and benefits of the offered service
2. Elements of informed consent
3. Nursing roles and responsibilities

B. Client Rights
1. Client Bill of Rights
2. Americans with Disabilities Act
3. Confidentiality
   a. Definition: The right to privacy with respect to one's personal medical information
   b. Legislation: Health Insurance Portability and Accountability Act (HIPAA) of 1996
      1) A uniform, federal (national) floor of privacy protection for health consumers
      2) State laws that may provide additional protections to consumers are not affected by HIPAA
      3) Guarantees clients access to their medical records
      4) Provides clients with control over how their personal health information is used and disclosed
      5) HIPAA outlines limited circumstances in which a client's personal health information can be disclosed without first obtaining consent of the client or client's family including:
         a) Suspicion of child abuse
         b) When otherwise required by law (such as suspicion of criminal activity due to gunshot wounds)
         c) Incidences of state or other health department; reportable communicable disease
4. Nursing role, responsibilities
5. Legal implications

C. Legal Responsibilities
1. Types of law
2. Nurse Practice Act
3. Good Samaritan Law
4. Mandatory Reporter of Abuse
5. Malpractice
6. Negligence
7. Torts
8. Breach of duty
9. Standard of professional practice

D. Advocacy
1. Definition: A process by which the nurse assists the client to grow and develop toward self-actualization
2. Nursing role as advocate

E. NURSING INTERVENTIONS: An astute professional
 nurse who recognizes rights and responsibilities in legal matters is better able to protect himself against liability or loss of licensure.

POINTS TO REMEMBER:

Remember, the nurse has a duty to intervene when the safety or well being of a client or another person is obviously at risk.

SECTION V

INFORMATION SYSTEMS AND TECHNOLOGY

A. Impact of Technology on Nursing Profession
1. Allows candidate testing for nursing licensure (NCLEX®) with rapid results
2. Permits verification of licensure online for nurses and other health care professionals
3. Improves communication within and between departments through the use of e-mail, Intranet, and the Internet
4. Eases the retrieval of medical histories to optimize decision making
5. Automates medication delivery systems to help prevent error
6. Automates distribution of client care supplies, including sterile materials, medical equipment, and hygiene care supplies
7. Facilitates client-centered care with portable and wireless terminals, workstations, and laptops
8. Improves and facilitates client education through the use of multimedia software, including graphics, photographs, videos, and 3-D visuals
9. Supports continuing education with distance learning
   a. Videoconferencing via satellite
   b. Online degrees and certification programs
   c. Computer-mediated instruction
10. Increases client monitoring capabilities
11. Decreases deviation from standards of practice
12. Allows electronic documentation
    a. Bedside charting
    b. Computerized charting

B. Potential Future Impact of Technology
1. Federally mandated electronic transferable medical records
2. Virtual and augmented reality allowing for simulated client teaching activities

C. Data Security
1. Passwords are necessary to prevent improper access to computers and medication systems
2. Only people with a professional relationship with a client may access the client's personal health information, per HIPAA regulations
3. Computer terminals must be logged off and locked when not in immediate use
4. Monitor screens must be shielded or situated so that unauthorized persons cannot see the information on the monitor

POINTS TO REMEMBER:

NEVER share your computer passwords with another person, including coworkers and family members.

NOTES

COMMUNITY HEALTH

UNIT CONTENT

SYMBOLS

 Key Points

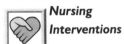 **Nursing Interventions**

 Points to Remember

SECTION I

RELIGIOUS COMPETENT CARE

A. Buddhism

1. Many forms of Buddhism; some sects are based on the country of origin
2. Spiritual beliefs
   a. Important figure: Buddha Siddhartha
   b. Spiritual leaders: priests, monks
   c. Central focus is enlightenment and the attainment of a clear, calm state of mind
   d. Illness is a result of karma (cause and effect) and a consequence of actions in this, or a previous, life
3. Practices associated with life transitions
   a. Birth
      1) Belief in reincarnation
      2) Contraception that prevents conception is acceptable
   b. Death
      1) State of mind at time of death believed to influence rebirth; therefore nurse should ensure a calm, peaceful environment for the client who is dying
      2) Organ donation is encouraged as an act of mercy
      3) Cremation is common
4. Dietary restrictions
   a. Vegetarian diet practiced by many
5. Healing practices
   a. A quiet and peaceful atmosphere is important to allow the client to rest better, as well as to practice meditation and prayer

B. Catholicism

1. Form of Christianity; also known as "Roman Catholic"
2. Spiritual beliefs
   a. Important figures: Savior Jesus Christ, born to the Virgin Mary
   b. Spiritual leaders: priests, nuns, deacons
   c. God has revealed himself to humanity as Father to Jesus; the Holy Trinity is the Father, the Son, and the Holy Spirit
   d. Illness may be God's punishment for sinful thinking or behavior
3. Practices associated with life transitions
   a. Birth
      1) Contraception, abortion, and sterilization are prohibited
      2) Infant baptism is required if prognosis is grave. If death of a newborn is imminent, a nurse (of any religion) can baptize the infant by pouring a small amount of warmed water on the infant's head and saying, "I baptize thee in the name of the Father, and of the Son, and of the Holy Spirit."
   b. Death
      1) If death is imminent a priest should be called to administer the Sacrament of the Sick, otherwise known as the "last rites"
      2) Organ donation is acceptable
      3) Suicide may prevent burial in a Catholic cemetery
4. Dietary restrictions
   a. Some Catholics may abstain from eating meat on Ash Wednesday and on Fridays during Lent, which is a 40-day period between Ash Wednesday and Easter
5. Healing practices
   a. Most observant Catholic clients will want to see a priest when hospitalized
   b. Client may request the Eucharist (communion) and/or the Sacrament of Reconciliation (confession) to aide in healing
   c. Client may wear a cross, medal (symbol of a saint), or scapular (small piece of cloth on a string worn around the neck)
   d. Client may display a statue of Jesus, Mary, or a saint at bedside, and make use of a rosary (string of prayer beads)

C. Christian Scientist

1. Form of Christianity also known as the Church of Christ, Scientist
2. Spiritual beliefs
   a. Founder: Mary Baker Eddy
   b. No clergy
   c. Central beliefs: God is divine love; God's infinite goodness heals
   d. Illness is viewed as a manifestation of human imperfections that can be healed through prayer and spiritual regeneration; no disease is beyond the power of God to heal
3. Practices associated with life transitions
   a. Birth
      1) Contraception is an individual decision
      2) Abortion is prohibited
      3) May choose to give birth at home aided by a midwife, or to minimize hospitalization by going home the same day of the delivery
   b. Death
      1) Unlikely to seek medical help to prolong life
      2) Organ donation discouraged
4. Dietary restrictions
   a. No requirements, but most abstain from alcohol

5. Healing practices
    a. Most practitioners rely on spiritual healing, but are not completely opposed to medical providers; individuals are free to make their own decisions in each situation
    b. May avoid diagnostic testing to avoid unwanted medical treatment in violation of spiritual beliefs
    c. Medications and blood products are avoided; immunizations are accepted only to comply with the law
    d. Full-time healing ministers (Christian Science Practitioners) practice spiritual healing and do not use medical or psychological techniques. The church also maintains a directory of Christian Science nurses available to provide medical care in a spiritual atmosphere

D. Hinduism
1. Many forms of Hinduism, each with its own practices and customs
2. Spiritual beliefs
    a. No single founder, universally accepted scripture, or religious hierarchy; may be monotheistic (one god), polytheistic (many gods), or atheistic (no god)
    b. Spiritual leaders: priests
    c. Central belief: spiritual well-being comes from leading a dedicated life based on nonviolence, love, good conduct, and selfless service
    d. Illness is a result of karma (cause and effect) and a consequence of actions in this, or a previous, life; illness, accident, or injury may be viewed as a form of purification
3. Practices associated with life transitions
    a. Birth
        1) Contraception is acceptable
        2) Abortion may be prohibited
        3) Noting the exact time of birth is crucial to determining the child's horoscope
        4) Males are not circumcised
        5) Traditionally, the child is not named until the 10th day of life
    b. Death
        1) Belief in reincarnation: the soul will reincarnate until its karma is exhausted
        2) Prolonging life artificially is up to the individual, but allowing a natural death is traditional
        3) Nurse should ensure a calm, peaceful environment for the client who is dying
        4) Organ donation is acceptable
        5) Prefer cremation and the casting of ashes in a river

4. Dietary restrictions
    a. Vegetarian diet encouraged and practiced by many; of those who eat meat, most abstain from beef and pork
    b. According to traditional dietary law, the right hand is used for eating and the left hand for toileting and hygiene
    c. There are several fasting days during a year which vary by sect
5. Healing Practices
    a. Personal hygiene is very important and the client may want to bathe daily
    b. Prayer for health is considered a low form of prayer, and therefore stoicism may be preferred
    c. Future lives are influenced by how one faces illness, disability, and death

E. Islam
1. Adherents to the Islamic belief are known as Muslims. Sunni Muslims form the worldwide majority and differ from Shi'a Muslims, a worldwide minority, in some matters of faith and practice
2. Spiritual beliefs
    a. Important figures: the Prophet Mohammed
    b. Spiritual leaders: Iman
    c. Central beliefs: one God, Allah; holy text, Qur'an; Judgement Day; Final Day of Resurrection
    d. Illness, pain, and suffering are manifestations of God's will and are necessary to remove sin
3. Practices associated with life transitions
    a. Birth
        1) Contraception acceptable
        2) After 130 days gestation (about 18 weeks) fetus is considered a full human being
        3) Abortion is permitted under certain circumstances (i.e., mother's life is in danger), but only if fetus has not attained personhood
        4) Circumcision of males is customary
    b. Death
        1) Any attempt to shorten life is prohibited, but prolonging death by means of futile medical interventions is also prohibited
        2) The client who is dying may wish to be placed facing Mecca (usually east)
        3) Organ donation is acceptable
        4) Autopsy is permitted for medical or legal reasons
        5) Rituals following death include traditional bathing and burial within 24 hr; cremation is prohibited
4. Dietary restrictions
    a. Food must be "halal"

b. Pork, alcohol, and some shellfish are prohibited
c. Ramadan: fasting occurs from sunrise to sundown during the ninth lunar month (dates vary year to year); children, pregnant women, and sick persons are exempted

5. Healing practices
a. Client may wish to pray five times a day (dawn, midday, mid-afternoon, sunset, and nightfall) facing Mecca, and may have a prayer rug and Qur'an at bedside for prayers
b. Privacy during prayer is important
c. Women are very modest and frequently wear clothes that cover their entire body; during treatment and care the women's modesty should be respected as much as possible

F. Jehovah's Witness
1. Form of Christianity; name is derived from the Hebrew name for God
2. Spiritual beliefs
a. Founded in the 1870s as the "Watchtower Society"
b. Spiritual leaders: older adults
c. Central beliefs: Bible is the literal word of God and is historically accurate; all other religions are "false teachings"; conversion of others is important
d. Suffering and illness is permitted by God and results from Satan's influence on the world
3. Practices associated with life transitions
a. Birth
1) Contraception is an individual choice
2) Abortion is prohibited
3) No infant baptism
b. Death
1) Organ donation is permitted
2) Autopsy permitted if legally required
4. Dietary restrictions
a. Moderate use of alcohol is permitted, but drunkenness is a sin
5. Healing practices
a. Strongly opposed to blood products for transfusion and will refuse even if refusal means certain death
1) Volume expanders permitted if not derived from blood
2) Organ transplantation is permitted if all of the blood is drained from the organ or tissue before being transplanted
3) Advocate "bloodless surgery"
4) Courts have ordered transfusions for very young children; in other cases they have respected the declared choice of an underage minor who is able to defend his beliefs to the court in a manner that reflects a mature understanding without undue influence from the parents

b. Reading scriptures believed to comfort the client and leads to mental and spiritual healing

G. Judaism
1. Predates Christianity; several major divisions with different customs and practices
2. Spiritual beliefs
a. Spiritual leader: rabbi
b. Central beliefs: one God; holy text is the Torah (the Old Testament of the Bible); the Messiah has yet to come
c. Illness and suffering are not judgements from God, since everyone is mortal
3. Practices associated with life transitions
a. Birth
1) Contraception is considered an individual choice
2) Abortion is permitted under certain circumstances
3) Ritual circumcision of males, "Bris," performed on the eighth day of life
b. Death
1) Autopsy is discouraged, but not prohibited
2) Organ donation is permitted
3) Rituals following death include traditional bathing and burial within 24 hr; cremation is prohibited
4) Bereavement does not begin until after burial
4. Dietary restrictions
a. Orthodox and observant Jews will observe dietary laws requiring food to be "kosher" (properly prepared) and may request a kosher food tray
1) Complex rules regarding food preparation, including blessing when meat is slaughtered
2) Milk and meat cannot be served at the same meal
3) Pork and shellfish are prohibited
b. Fasting is required on Yom Kippur, the Day of Atonement (in fall, exact date is determined by the Jewish calendar); children, pregnant women, and sick persons are exempted
c. Lactose intolerance is common among Jews of European descent
5. Healing practices
a. Jewish law places the life of the person above all else
1) Saving a life overrides nearly all religious obligations
2) It is considered to be one of the highest commandments to tend to the sick or dying
3) In case of illness, medical care is obligated and health care providers are seen as instruments of God

b. Prayers for the well-being of the sick may be said

c. Anything that can be done to ease the client's suffering is encouraged

d. Males who strictly practice their religion will wear a yarmulke (skull cap) at all times; very observant females may dress modestly and cover their heads at all times

H. Church of Jesus Christ of Latter-Day Saints

1. Members refer to selves as belonging to The Church or Mormon faith
2. Spiritual beliefs
   a. Founded by the Prophet Joseph Smith
   b. Spiritual leaders: priests, older adults
   c. Central beliefs: God has revealed himself to humanity as Father to Jesus; Holy Trinity is the Father, the Son, and the Holy Spirit; the holy text is the Book of Mormon
   d. The body is a gift from God; to help keep bodies and minds healthy and strong God gave a law of health; illness, trials, and adversity are a part of life
3. Practices associated with life transitions
   a. Birth
      1) Contraception and abortion are forbidden
      2) No infant baptism
   b. Death
      1) Organ donation is permitted
      2) Autopsy permitted
      3) Life continues beyond death
4. Dietary restrictions
   a. Alcohol, coffee, and tea prohibited (some may drink caffeinated soft drinks or herbal teas)
   b. Fasting is required once per month; children, pregnant women, and sick persons are exempted
5. Healing practices
   a. Medical intervention is God's way of using humans to heal
   b. May want to use herbal remedies in addition to medical care
   c. Blessing of the sick: anointing with oil by two older adults

I. Seventh Day Adventist

1. Form of Christianity also known as Adventist
2. Spiritual beliefs
   a. Central belief: Bible is the literal word of God
   b. Religious leaders: pastors, older adults
   c. Body is the temple of the Holy Spirit (God) and must be kept healthy
3. Practices associated with life transitions
   a. Birth
      1) Contraception is an individual choice
      2) Abortion is acceptable in cases of rape, incest, or threat to the life of the mother

3) Opposed to infant baptism; adults are baptized by total immersion
   b. Death
      1) Autopsy is acceptable
      2) Organ donation is acceptable
4. Dietary restrictions
   a. Vegetarian diet is encouraged
   b. Alcohol, coffee, and tea are prohibited
5. Healing practices
   a. Healing can be accomplished both through medical intervention and divine healing
   b. Prayer and anointing with oil may be performed for the sick person

J. Nursing Process for Spiritually Sensitive Care

1. Assessment
   a. What is the client's religion?
   b. What is its importance in the client's daily life?
   c. What dietary prohibitions does the client follow?
   d. Are there rituals or customs that the client may wish to keep, particularly as related to transitions such as birth and death?
   e. Is there a spiritual leader that the client wishes to have involved in his or her care?
   f. Is the client using herbal or other traditional remedies?
   g. Are there any practices which the client may find provide comfort or support?

 2. **NURSING INTERVENTIONS**
   a. Remain sensitive to the client's spiritual beliefs, even if they are in opposition to the nurse's own beliefs.
   b. Provide a diet consistent with the client's customs.
   c. Provide the client privacy, as desired, for prayer and other rituals.
   d. Allow visits by clergy or supportive members of the member's congregation.
   e. Provide the client with an atmosphere conducive to religious practices that provide comfort or support.
   f. Check that herbal or alternative remedies do not interact poorly with medications the hospital is providing.

SECTION II

CULTURALLY COMPETENT CARE

A. African American

1. African Americans comprise a very diverse population that varies considerably by geographic region, age, and socioeconomic status.
2. Spiritual beliefs
   a. Church and religious life are typically very important
   b. Primary religious/spiritual affiliation: most are Christian, primarily Baptist; from other Protestant sects; or Muslim
   c. Illness may have both natural and supernatural causes
      1) Mental illness may be viewed as a lack of spiritual balance
      2) Some chronic or congenital illnesses may be considered "God's will"
3. Practices associated with life transitions
   a. Birth
      1) May give child a name of African origin, or one that is unique
   b. Death
      1) The deceased is highly respected
      2) Cremation is avoided
      3) Organ donation is unusual except in the case of an immediate family member
4. Dietary preferences
   a. May prefer cooked and fried foods
   b. Traditional "southern" cooking may include cooked greens (collard, mustard, turnip) or yams
5. Cultural variations
   a. Language: English with traditional dialects spoken in Louisiana (Creole) and many parts of the south; "Black" English is often spoken in urban areas, primarily inner cities, and is a distinct, expressive dialect with its own rules of grammar and slang
   b. Eye contact: viewed as a sign of respect and trust
   c. Time orientation: primarily present oriented with flexible time frame
   d. Personal space: affection is shown by touching, hugging, and being close
   e. Family: nuclear, extended, frequently matriarchal (women head the household); grandparents often involved in the care and raising of children
   f. Sick role: attention from family and relatives is expected

6. Healing practices
   a. Home and folk remedies often used first; usually it is the role of the mother or wife to obtain the remedy from a "knowing person"
   b. Prayer and a visit from minister may be important
   c. There may be some mistrust of the medical establishment
7. Health Risks
   a. Hypertension
   b. Coronary artery disease
   c. Sickle-cell anemia
   d. Diabetes mellitus
   e. Prostate, breast, colorectal cancer
   f. Renal disease

B. Asian American

1. Asian Americans comprise a very diverse population including ethnic groups of Pacific Islanders, Southeast Asians, Chinese, Japanese, Koreans, and others, each of which have their own customs and practices.
2. Spiritual beliefs
   a. Primary religious or spiritual affiliations: Buddhism, Christianity, and Hindu
   b. View of illness:
      1) Chinese traditionally believe that illnesses are caused by imbalances in the yin and yang
      2) External influences block the circulation of vital energy, or "chi"
3. Practices associated with life transitions
   a. Birth
      1) May want female kin at bedside during labor
      2) Breastfeeding is the norm
      3) Genetic defects may be blamed on something the mother did during pregnancy
      4) A new mother may be expected to eat a special diet and remain at home to recuperate for several weeks
      5) Circumcision is a decision which depends on religious and ethnic practice
   b. Death
      1) Organ donation is uncommon
      2) Autopsy is discouraged
4. Dietary preferences
   a. Depending on the individual ethnic group, food may be considered important in maintaining a healthy balance, and the client may believe that certain foods are "hot" or "cold"
   b. Chinese traditionally believe that food is critical to maintaining the balance of yin (cold) and yang (hot) in the body

5. Cultural variation
   a. Language: Many different dialects exist for most major Asian languages, and English competence varies considerably; use a trained, bilingual interpreter if client has limited English skills
   b. Eye contact: avoided with authority figures as a sign of respect
   c. Time orientation: present oriented; punctuality is not a traditional value, except in Japanese culture where promptness is important
   d. Personal space: clients may be very modest and public display of affection (physical touching) is not typical; the head may be considered to be sacred, and therefore touching someone on the head may be disrespectful
   e. Family: patriarchal, extended families common; wife may become a part of husband's family; filial piety (duty and obedience to one's parents) is expected
   f. Sick role: sick persons usually assume a passive role; client may not ask questions as this is seen as disrespectful, but may nod politely at everything that is said; client may be stoic in regards to pain
6. Healing practices
   a. May want to use traditional and herbal remedies in addition to medical care
   b. Older adult immigrants may have a strong belief in traditional folk medicine, while second-generation Asian Americans are often more oriented toward Western medicine
   c. Chinese traditionally believe that health is achieved by restoring balance between yin and yang
   d. Other specific health practices may depend on religion or ethnic group
7. Health Risks
   a. Hypertension
   b. Stomach, cervical, liver cancer
   c. Osteoporosis
   d. Thalassemia anemia
   e. Tuberculosis

C. **Hispanic**
1. Also known as Latino; comprised of a very diverse population including individuals of Mexican, Cuban, Central-American, South-American, Spanish, and Puerto-Rican heritage
2. Spiritual beliefs
   a. Latinos are traditionally very religious
   b. Primary religious/spiritual affiliation: Catholic, Christian
   c. Traditional belief is that health is controlled by fate, environment, and the will of God
3. Practices associated with life transitions

   a. Birth
      1) May want female kin present for labor
      2) Most breastfeed
      3) New mother may be expected to eat a special diet and remain at home to recuperate for several weeks
      4) Circumcision is not the traditional practice
   b. Death
      1) Extended family may want to attend to the sick and dying
      2) Body extremely respected and organ donation discouraged
      3) Autopsy discouraged
      4) Pregnant women may be excluded from attending funeral
4. Dietary preferences
   a. Traditional diet contains fresh ingredients; processed foods may be distrusted
5. Cultural variation
   a. Language: majority are bilingual Spanish/English, although English competence varies significantly; use trained, bilingual interpreter if limited English skills; considered respectful to address individuals formally until a rapport has been established
   b. Eye contact: direct eye contact is avoided with authority figures
   c. Time orientation: primarily present oriented with flexible time frame
   d. Personal space: handshaking is considered polite, but other touching by a stranger is generally considered inappropriate; embracing is common among family and friends
   e. Family: family is believed to come first, and members are supposed to have a strong sense of family loyalty; most live in nuclear families with extended families and godparents
   f. Sick role: clients will often assume a passive role, and may be stoic with regard to pain
6. Healing practices
   a. Soup and herbal teas may be thought to speed healing process
   b. Siesta is a traditional period of rest after the midday meal thought to be important for maintaining health
   c. May seek medical care for severe symptoms while using traditional folk healing measures for chronic or "folk" illnesses
7. Health Risks
   a. Diabetes mellitus
   b. Childhood obesity
   c. Hypertension
   d. B12 deficiency anemia

D. Native American

1. There are 300 or more different Native American tribal groups, each with its own culture, beliefs, and practices
2. Spiritual beliefs
    a. Belief in the Creator; sacred myths and legends provide spiritual guidance
    b. Primary religious/spiritual affiliation: specific tribes follow rituals referred to in a general way by the tribal name; for example, the Navajo Indians follow "The Navajo Way"
    c. Illness results from not living in harmony, or being out of balance with nature
3. Practices associated with life transitions
    a. Birth
        1) May wish female kin to be present at birth
        2) No circumcision
    b. Death
        1) Organ donation usually not desired
        2) Autopsy usually not desired
        3) Some tribes avoid contact with dying person (hospital is preferable to home)
4. Dietary preference
    a. May vary with tribal affiliation, although most are assimilated to United-States style diet
5. Cultural variation
    a. Language: most speak English
    b. Eye contact: respect is communicated by avoiding eye contact
    c. Time orientation: primarily present oriented with flexible time frame; rushing a client is considered rude and disrespectful
    d. Personal space: keep a respectful distance
    e. Family: some tribes are matrilineal, meaning they trace ancestral descent through the mother's line instead of the father's line; mother may be head of the family or clan
    f. Sick role: usually quiet and stoic
6. Healing practices
    a. Ill person may seek both modern medical attention and the services of a traditional Medicine Man or Woman
    b. Home and herbal remedies may be used
    c. Medicine bag: leather pouch worn around the neck, the contents of which are considered sacred.; it is improper to ask about the contents of the bag, and every effort should be made not to remove it
    d. Health practices are intertwined with religious and cultural beliefs
7. Health Risks
    a. Alcoholism
    b. Gall bladder disease
    c. Diabetes mellitus
    d. Coronary artery disease
    e. Tuberculosis
    f. Maternal-infant mortality
    g. Obesity
    h. Hypertension

E. Nursing Process for Culturally Sensitive Care:

1. Assessment
    a. What is the client's ethnic affiliation?
    b. What is its importance in the client's daily life?
    c. How well does the client speak, write, read, and understand English?
    d. What dietary preferences or prohibitions does the client follow?
    e. Are there rituals or customs that the client wishes to keep related to transitions such as birth and death?
    f. Does the client want or need to have family involved in his or her care?
    g. Is the client using herbal or other traditional remedies?
2. **NURSING INTERVENTIONS**
    a. Remain sensitive to the client's cultural beliefs, even if they are in opposition to the nurse's beliefs.
    b. Provide a trained, bilingual interpreter if necessary.
    c. Provide a diet consistent with the client's customs.
    d. Allow family to be involved in the client's care, if desired.
    e. Be respectful of the client's cultural preferences for personal space.
    f. Be aware of the meaning of eye contact in the client's culture.
    g. Check for interactions between herbal or traditional remedies and the medicines and treatments the hospital is providing.

SECTION III

DISASTER PLANNING

A. Disaster: A disaster is a serious disruption of the functioning of a community, causing widespread human, material, economic, or environmental losses that exceed the ability of the affected community or society to cope with using its own resources.

1. Internal disasters are events in the health care facility that threaten to disrupt the care environment
    a. Structural (fire, loss of power)
    b. Personnel related (strike, high absenteeism)
2. External disasters may be man-made or natural
    a. Man-made disasters
        1) Transportation related incidents, including car, train, plane, and subway crashes

2) Terrorist attacks
   a) Bombs, including suicide bombs and dirty bombs
   b) Bioterrorism
3) Industrial accidents
4) Chemical spills or toxic gas leaks
5) Structural fires
b. Natural disasters
   1) Extreme weather conditions, including blizzards, ice storms, hurricanes, tornadoes, and floods
   2) Ecological disasters, including earthquakes, landslides, tsunamis, volcanoes, and forest fires
   3) Microbial disasters such as epidemics and pandemics
3. A combined internal/external disaster situation can arise when an external disaster, such as a severe weather condition, both causes mass casualties and prevents health care providers from getting to the facility, perhaps due to traffic or road conditions

B. Disaster Planning

1. Interagency cooperation within the community is essential in a disaster and requires:
   a. Community-wide planning for emergencies and/or hazards that may affect the local area
   b. Coordination between community emergency system and health care facilities
   c. Developing a local emergency communications plan and/or network
   d. Identification of potential emergency public shelters
2. Role of Nurse
   a. In the health care facility
      1) Joint Commission on Accreditation of Healthcare Organizations (JCAHO) mandates specific standards for hospital preparedness
         a) Disaster plan
         b) Disaster drills
   b. In the community
      1) Education about disaster planning for families
         a) Family disaster plan should include:
            (1) What to do in an evacuation
            (2) Plans for family pets
            (3) Where to meet in case of emergency
         b) Family disaster kit should include:
            (1) Flashlight with extra batteries
            (2) Battery powered radio
            (3) Nonperishable food that requires no cooking (along with a non-electric can opener)

(4) One gallon of water per person
(5) Basic first aid supplies

C. Disaster Management

1. Emergency Management System
   a. Provides public access to immediate health care (911)
   b. Dispatch communication center
   c. Trained first responders: Emergency Medical Technicians
   d. Transportation to medical resources: ground (ambulance), air (helicopter)
2. Declaration of a disaster
   a. Disaster area: local officials request that the governor of the state take appropriate action under state law and the state's emergency plan and declare a disaster area
   b. Federal disaster area: governor of the affected state requests declaration of a disaster area by the president to qualify the affected area for federal disaster relief
   c. Internal disaster: nursing or administrative supervisor may declare an internal disaster in case of a facility-related issue
3. Disaster relief organizations
   a. Federal Emergency Management Agency (FEMA)
      1) FEMA is part of the U.S. Department of Homeland Security
      2) Manages federal response and recovery efforts
   b. American Red Cross
      1) Not a government agency, but authorized by the government to provide disaster relief
      2) Provides:
         a) Shelter and food to address basic human needs
         b) Health and mental services
         c) Food to emergency and relief workers
         d) Blood and blood products to disaster victims
      3) Handles inquiries from concerned family members outside the disaster area
   c. Hazardous Material Response Team (HAZMAT)
      1) Hazardous materials may be radioactive, flammable, explosive, toxic, corrosive, biohazardous, or may have other characteristics that make them hazardous in specific circumstances
      2) HAZMAT team members are specially trained to respond to these situations and wear protective equipment
      3) In a toxic exposure disaster, HAZMAT will coordinate the decontamination effort

4. Role of Nurse
   a. Triage: process of prioritizing which clients must receive care first
     1) Nonmass casualty situation: nurse prioritizes so that clients with conditions of the highest acuity are evaluated and treated first
     2) Mass casualty triage: three levels; emergency services are stressed by a large number of casualties, but still functional and able to provide care to victims on all levels
       a) Slightly injured - also called "nonurgent"
       b) Seriously injured - also called "urgent"
       c) Critically injured - also called "emergent"
     3) Disaster triage: four levels; emergency services are overwhelmed by the number of casualties and/or ground conditions and cannot treat everyone; must provide the "greatest good for the greatest number"
       a) Black Tag - allowed to die, prepare for morgue
       b) Red Tag - critically injured, do not delay treatment
       c) Yellow Tag - seriously injured, can delay treatment for 1 to 2 hr
       d) Green Tag - slightly injured, can delay treatment for 2 to 4 hr
   b. Health care facility disaster plan
     1) Nursing or administrative supervisor may implement the disaster plan due to extreme weather conditions or anticipated mass casualties
     2) May include plans for:
       a) Establishment of an "incident command center"
       b) Premature discharge of stable clients from facility
       c) Transfer of stable clients from ICU
       d) Postponement of scheduled admissions and elective operations
       e) Mobilization of personnel (call in off-duty persons)
       f) Protection of personnel and visitors
       g) Evacuation plan
     3) Role of the charge nurse during a disaster
       a) Preparation of a "discharge list" of clients who can safely and quickly be discharged
       b) Personnel sent to the command center, if required
       c) Off-duty personnel called in, if requested

       d) Disaster victims are prepared for admittance

D. Psychosocial Aftermath of a Disaster
  1. Crisis intervention (See also page 88.)
   a. Mental health response team, which employs advanced crisis intervention techniques to help victims, survivors, and their families better handle the powerful emotional reactions associated with crises and disasters
   b. Goals:
     1) Reduce the intensity of an individual's emotional reaction.
     2) Assist the individual in recovering from the crisis.
     3) Help to prevent serious long-term problems from developing.
  2. Post-traumatic stress disorder (PTSD)
   a. Mental health condition that can develop following any traumatic, catastrophic life experience (see also page 93)
   b. PTSD symptoms can develop in survivors of a disaster weeks, months, or even years following the catastrophic event
  3. Critical Incident Stress Debriefing
   a. Health care providers who respond to a highly stressful event that is extremely traumatic or overwhelming may experience significant stress reactions
   b. The Critical Incident Stress Debriefing process is designed to prevent the development of post-traumatic stress among first responders and health care professionals
     1) Defusing: discussion of feelings shortly after the disaster/critical incident (such as at the end of shift)
     2) Formal debriefing: discussion some hours or days after the disaster/critical incident, in a large group setting, with mental health teams of peer support personnel as leaders

SECTION IV

ALTERNATIVE AND COMPLEMENTARY THERAPIES

A. Herbal Medications and Supplements
  1. Safety and efficacy
   a. The Dietary Supplement Health and Education Act (DSHEA) limits the Food and Drug Administration's (FDA) control over dietary supplements.

b. Many herbal drug companies make claims, based on their own studies, indicating health benefits from herbal drugs
   1) These studies are not approved by the FDA
   2) Labels on the herbal medications must include a disclaimer stating the FDA has not approved the product for safety and effectiveness
c. Herbal medications may interact with other medicines and can have serious side effects

2. Common supplements
   a. Saw Palmetto (*Serenoa repens*)
      1) Purported use: treatment and prevention of benign prostatic hypertrophy (BPH)
      2) Side effects: prolonged bleeding time, altered platelet function
      3) Herb/medication interactions: additive effect with anticoagulants
      4) Studies: several well-conducted studies support the use of saw palmetto for reducing symptoms of BPH
      5) Nursing considerations
         a) Allow 4 to 6 weeks to see effects
         b) Discontinue prior to surgery
   b. Valerian root
      1) Purported uses: insomnia, migraines, menstrual cramps
      2) Side effects: drowsiness, anxiety, hepatotoxicity (long-term use)
      3) Herb/medication interactions: additive effect with barbiturates and benzodiazepines
      4) Studies: several studies support the use of valerian for mild to moderate sleep disorders and mild anxiety
      5) Nursing considerations
         a) Advise client against driving or operating machinery
         b) Advise client against long-term use
         c) Discontinue valerian at least one week prior to surgery
   c. St. John's wort (*Hypericum perforatum*)
      1) Purported uses: depression, seasonal affective disorder, anxiety
      2) Side effects: headache, sleep disturbances, hepatotoxicity (long-term use), constipation
      3) Herb/medication interactions: may reduce the effects of many medications
         a) Theophylline (*Theo-Dur*)
         b) HIV protease inhibitors and non-nucleoside reverse transcriptase inhibitors
         c) Cyclosporine (*Neoral*)
         d) Diltiazem (*Cardizem*) and nifedipine (*Procardia*)
      4) Studies: several well-conducted studies support the use of St. John's Wort for mild to moderate depression
      5) Nursing considerations
         a) St. John's wort has many medication interactions and should not be taken with other medications.
         b) St. John's wort should not be used to treat severe depression.
         c) St. John's wort should only be used with medical guidance.
   d. Echinacea (*Echinacea purpurea*)
      1) Purported uses
         a) Prevent and treat common cold
         b) Stimulate the immune system
         c) Promote wound healing
      2) Side effects: headache, epigastric pain, constipation
      3) Herb/medication interactions:
         a) May reduce the effects of immunosuppressants
         b) May increase serum levels of alprazolam (*Xanax*), calcium-channel blockers, and protease inhibitors
      4) Studies: well-conducted studies have conflicted as to the effectiveness of echinacea in the treatment of the common cold
      5) Nursing considerations
         a) Long-term use may cause immunosuppression
   e. Ginkgo (*Gingko biloba*)
      1) Purported uses: improve cerebral circulation to treat dementia and memory loss
      2) Side effects: dizziness, palpitations
      3) Herb/medication interactions:
         a) May increase the effects of MAOIs, anticoagulants, and antiplatelet aggregates
         b) May reduce the effectiveness of insulin
      4) Studies: studies conflict as to the effectiveness of gingko in all purported uses
      5) Nursing considerations
         a) Discontinue 2 weeks prior to surgery.
         b) Keep out of reach of children, may cause seizures with overdose.
   f. Ginseng (*Panax Quinquefolius*)
      1) Purported uses
         a) Improve strength and stamina
         b) Prevent and treat cancer and diabetes mellitus
      2) Side effects: insomnia, nervousness

3) Herb/medication interactions
    a) May decrease the effectiveness of anticoagulants and antiplatelet aggregates
    b) May increase the effectiveness of antidiabetic agents and insulin
4) Studies: conflict as to the effectiveness of ginseng in all purported uses
5) Nursing considerations
    a) Contraindicated for pregnant and lactating women.

g. Glucosamine (2-Amino-2-deoxyglucose)
1) Purported uses
    a) Osteoarthritis
    b) Promote joint health
2) Side effects: itching, edema, and headache
3) Herb/medication interactions: may increase resistance to antidiabetic agents and insulin
4) Studies: several studies support the use of glucosamine in reducing the symptoms of osteoarthritis in the knee
5) Nursing considerations
    a) Use with caution in clients with a shellfish allergy.
    b) Monitor glucose frequently in clients who are diabetics.
    c) Allow extended time to see effects.
    d) Use often in combination with chondroitin.

h. Chondroitin Sulfate
1) Purported uses: osteoarthritis
2) Side effects: headache, hives, photosensitivity, hypertension, constipation
3) Herb/medication interactions: may increase the effects of anticoagulants
4) Studies: several studies support the use of chondroitin in reducing the symptoms of osteoarthritis in the knee
5) Nursing considerations
    a) Do not give to women who are pregnant or breastfeeding.
    b) Often used in combination with glucosamine.
    c) Allow extended time to see effects.

i. Omega-3 fatty acids
1) Purported uses:
    a) Hypertriglyceridemia
    b) Maintaining cardiac health
2) Side effects: nausea, diarrhea, hypotension
3) Herb/medication interactions: may increase the risk of vitamin A or D overdose

4) Studies: Several well-conducted studies support the use of omega-3 fatty acids in reducing blood triglyceride levels, preventing cardiovascular disease in clients with a history of a heart attack, and slightly reducing blood pressure.
5) Nursing considerations
    a) Omega-3 fatty acids are found in fish oils, nuts, and vegetable oils.
    b) Some fish contain methylmercury and polychlorinated biphenyls (PCBs) that can be harmful in large amounts, especially in women who are pregnant or nursing.

3. Nursing assessments for herbal medications
  a. It is important for the nurse to ask the client specifically about herbal medications, vitamins, or other supplements during the client interview.
    1) Over-the-counter medications are often not considered medications by the client.

 4. **NURSING INTERVENTIONS**
  a. Instruct the client that herbal medications and supplements are not regulated by the FDA, often interact with other medications, and may cause serious side effects.
  b. Instruct the client that it is important for him to use herbal medications and supplements cautiously and with medical supervision.

B. Alternative and Complementary Therapies
1. Nonbiomedical therapy
  a. Covers a wide range of healing practices and philosophies that mainstream "Western medicine" (biomedical model) does not commonly use, study, or advocate
  b. While some scientific evidence exists regarding some of these therapies, for most, there are key questions that are yet to be answered through well-designed scientific studies, such as whether they are safe and whether they work for the diseases or medical conditions for which they are used
  c. Studies show that up to 50% of Americans include alternative and complementary therapies in maintaining their health
  d. Nonbiomedical therapies are usually not covered by health insurance
  e. Practitioners may not be licensed or regulated
2. Common alternative therapies
  a. Mind-body medicine uses a variety of techniques designed to enhance the mind's capacity to affect bodily function and symptoms
    1) Prayer
    2) Meditation: focusing the mind upon a sound, phrase, object, or visualized image to promote relaxation

3) Yoga: a form of exercise that emphasizes specific postures in combination with controlled breathing

4) Biofeedback: A method of treatment that uses monitors to feed back to clients physiological information of which they are normally unaware; by watching a monitor, clients can learn by trial and error to adjust their mental processes to control "involuntary" bodily processes such as heart rate

b. Biologically based therapies use substances such as herbs, foods, vitamins, and other "natural," but as yet unproven, substances
   1) Aromatherapy
      a) Ancient therapy that uses plant and essential oils
      b) May be inhaled, placed in compresses, or applied to the skin
   2) Special diets: macrobiotic, vegan
   3) Herbal supplements

c. Manipulative methods use manipulation and/or movement of one or more parts of the body
   1) Chiropractic: manipulation of the vertebrae to relieve pressure on the nerves and return the body to balance
   2) Therapeutic massage: a range of therapeutic approaches involving the practice of kneading or manipulating a person's muscles and soft tissues
   3) Hydrotherapy: practice of physiotherapy in a pool (typically heated)
   4) Tai Chi: ancient Chinese practice designed to exercise body, mind, and spirit, improving the flow of "chi," the vital life energy that sustains health and calms the mind
      a) Described as "meditation in motion," participants perform a defined series of postures or movements in a slow, graceful manner
      b) Scientific studies have shown that Tai Chi:
         (1) Improves muscle flexibility and builds muscle strength
         (2) Reduces falls in older adults and those with balance disorders

d. Energy therapies involve the use of energy fields, the existence of which has not yet been scientifically proven
   1) Reiki: Japanese technique for stress reduction and relaxation
      a) Administered by "laying on hands"
      b) Based on the idea that an unseen "life-force energy" flows through us and is what causes us to be alive
   2) Therapeutic touch

3) Electromagnetic fields

e. Traditional or folk medicine
   1) Traditional Chinese therapies
      a) Acupressure: placing physical pressure by hand or elbow onto certain points of the body (acupoints) to stimulate the flow of "chi," the vital life energy
      b) Acupuncture: placing very thin needles into certain points of the body (acupoints) to stimulate the flow of "chi," the vital life energy; often used to eliminate or reduce pain
      c) Herbs (ginger, green tea)
   2) Native-American therapies
   3) Various cultural folk remedies

3. Nursing assessments
   a. Ask the client about the use of alternative, complementary, or folk remedies.

 4. **NURSING INTERVENTIONS**
   a. Assist the client with appropriate use of therapy.
   b. Provide client teaching; safety, contraindication of complimentary choice.
   c. Refrain from endorsing products.

NOTES

ALTERNATE
TEST ITEM FORMATS

UNIT CONTENT

SYMBOLS

 Key Points   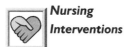 **Nursing Interventions**   **Points to Remember**

SECTION I

OVERVIEW

A. NCLEX® Item Types

1. Standard Multiple Choice Question
(See Introduction p. 5 to 7.)
    a. Traditionally the format of NCLEX® questions
    b. Still the most commonly seen type of question on the NCLEX®
    c. Has four options, only one of which is correct ("one best option")
    d. Mastering this format is critical to success on the NCLEX®
    e. The average standard question takes 60 to 70 seconds to answer
2. As of April 2003, the NCLEX® started including items other than standard multiple choice questions. These items are known as Alternate Test Item Formats.
    a. Supply answer
    b. Drag and drop
    c. Multiple response
    d. Hot spot
    e. Chart exhibit

POINTS TO REMEMBER:

 Students should allow a slightly longer time for answering alternate test items.

SECTION II

SUPPLY ANSWER

A. Overview

1. Definition: Supply answer items are a type of alternate item that will be primarily numerical. This type of question typically involves solving a math problem. Read the question carefully. If the question is asking for the answer in a specific unit amount, it is not necessary to put units in the answer.
2. Method of answer: To answer these questions, a number will need to be typed into the answer box on the screen.

POINTS TO REMEMBER:

1. Write the equation down on scrap paper.
2. Be certain to solve for the correct unit value.
3. Show calculations on test material provided.
4. Bring up the drop-down calculator.
5. Double-check work.

EXAMPLE VII-1
SUPPLY-ANSWER ITEM

> There are thirteen clients being seen in the emergency department and five clients in the waiting room. What is the total number of clients?

> Type your answer in the box below.

> 18

SECTION III

DRAG AND DROP

A. Overview

1. Definition: Drag-and-drop items are one of the newer types of alternate test questions. In this type of question every option will be used, placing each item in the correct sequence as indicated by the prompt.
2. Method of answer: To answer these questions, drag options in left-hand column into the appropriate order of performance in the right-hand column.
3. There is only one correct sequence to maintain the client's safety at each step in the care continuum.
4. Avoid including actions that would properly be done both prior to and after an intervention (i.e. handwashing).

EXAMPLE VII-2
DRAG-AND-DROP ITEM

A nurse is caring for a client who is to receive an indwelling urinary catheter. In what order should the nurse proceed with this procedure? (Move the steps of catheter insertion into the box on the right, placing them in the selected order of performance. All steps must be used.)

Unordered Options   Ordered Response

Don sterile gloves.	
Insert the catheter into the urethra.	
Drape the client exposing only genitalia.	
Instill saline into the balloon of the catheter.	
Cleanse the meatus with bactericidal solution.	

SECTION IV

MULTIPLE SELECT

A. Overview

1. Definition: Multiple-select items are a type of alternate item that requires test takers to choose more than one answer from up to six options. Any number of the options may be correct.
2. Method of answer: To answer these questions, click on all the answers that apply.
3. On the NCLEX®, credit will only be given for completely correct answers; there is no "partial credit" given for these item types

POINTS TO REMEMBER:

Consider each response as a true-false question - Is that a true or false statement about the question? Click on all that are true.

EXAMPLE VII-3
MULTIPLE-RESPONSE ITEM

Which of the following are types of vegetables?

Select all that apply.

☑ 1. Broccoli
☑ 2. Cucumber
☐ 3. Peach
☐ 4. Orange
☐ 5. Grape

SECTION V

HOT SPOT

A. Overview

1. Definition: Hot spot items are a type of alternate item that will be a "point and click" exercise. Hot spot items will usually require identification of an anatomical location on a figure.
2. Method of answer: To answer these questions, point at an area on the screen with the cursor and click on the correct spot. Move the mouse around the screen until an arrow appears. Once a spot is selected, click, and the arrow will change into a circle with an "X" in it.
3. Read the question carefully, then analyze the image.
4. The NCLEX® will allow reclicking as many times as necessary.

POINTS TO REMEMBER:

It is very important to remember that the screen is NOT a mirror image! If the question is asking for an answer on the right or left side of the body, make sure to click on the correct side.

EXAMPLE VII-4
HOT SPOT ITEM

A nurse is performing a cardiac assessment. Identify where the nurse will place the stethoscope to best auscultate the apical pulse. (Selectable areas, or "Hot Spots," can be found by moving your cursor over the artwork until the cursor changes appearance, usually into a hand. Click only on the Hot Spot that corresponds to your answer.)

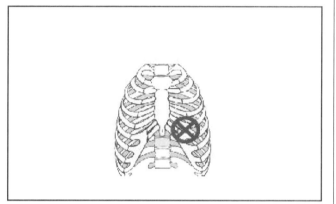

SECTION VI

CHART EXHIBIT

A. Overview

1. Any of the NCLEX® standard multiple choice questions may also include chart exhibits that must be analyzed and understood to correctly answer the question. In this alternative item format, the question cannot be answered without obtaining further information; this is where the chart format of the question comes in to play. On-screen tabs, similar to the tabs in either a client's paper or computerized medical record, will allow the testtaker to select various client documents. For example, one tab may say "Medication Administration Record," another may be labeled "Vital Signs," or "Laboratory Results." These documents will contain the information that the testtaker must analyze to correctly answer the question.

2. It is important to read the question carefully first, then analyze the three charts. The testtaker must use the mouse to click on each tab to open the pertinent document. When the tab is clicked, a separate window will open to display the data contained in the selected section of the "client's chart." Analysis of the data in each of these documents will provide the testtaker with all of the information necessary to answer the question.

EXAMPLE VII-5
CHART-EXHIBIT ITEM

A nurse in an antepartum clinic is collecting data from a pregnant client in her second trimester. Based on the review of the client's chart, the nurse should instruct the client to do which of the following? (Click on the "Exhibit" button below for additional client information. There are three tabs that contain separate categories of data.)

A. Rest for 8 hr.
B. Walk 1 hr a day.
C. Increase protein intake.
D. Consume applesauce daily.

Exhibit

History and Physical
Gravida 1, Para 0
Weight gain of 3 lb in 1 week

Vital Signs
Blood pressure 135/70 mm Hg
Respirations 20/min

Laboratory Findings
Hct 32%
Hgb 12 g/dL

APPENDICES

UNIT CONTENT

SYMBOLS

 Key Points

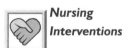 Nursing Interventions

 Points to Remember

APPENDIX A

REVIEW OF CALCULATIONS AND CONVERSIONS

A. Metric System

```
1 kg = 1,000 gm
1 gm = 1,000 mg
1 mg = 1,000 mcg
1 L = 1,000 mL
1 mL = 1 cc = 1 gm
1 cm = 10 mm
```

B. Apothecary System (rarely used today)

```
1 dram = 60 grains
1 oz = 8 drams
1 dram = 60 minims
1 fluid oz = 8 fluid drams
```

C. Household System

```
1 lb = 16 oz
1 tbsp = 3 tsp
1 oz = 2 tbsp
1 cup = 8 oz
1 pint = 16 oz
1 quart = 2 pints
1 gallon = 4 quarts
```

D. Conversions Between Systems

```
1 grain = 60 mg
1 gm = 15 grains
1 tsp = 5 mL
1 tbsp = 15 to 16 mL
2 tbsp = 1 oz = 30 to 32 mL
1 cup = 8 oz = 240 mL
8 oz = 240 to 250 mL
2 cups = 1 pint = 500 mL
1 inch = 2.54 cm
1 kg = 2.2 lb
1 lb = 454 gm
1 minim = 1 drop
1 mL = 15 minims = 15 drops
```

E. Temperature Conversions

```
37.0° C = 98.6° F
C = (F - 32) x 5/9
F = (C x 9/5) + 32
```

F. Calculations for IV Administration

1. $\# \text{ of hours} = \dfrac{\text{total volume}}{\text{mL/hour}}$

2. $\text{gtts per min} = \dfrac{\text{total volume x gtts/mL in administration set}}{\text{total number of minutes}}$

G. Calculations for Dosage

$$\dfrac{\text{Dosage on hand (H)}}{\text{mL}} = \dfrac{\text{Dosage desired (D)}}{\text{xmL}}$$

Fill-in-the-Blank question format is an NCLEX® Alternate Test Item Format. Place your answer in the box below the question.

Test Questions

1. A client has the following served for lunch: one cup of tea, one cup of coffee, and 240 mL of milk. The client drinks all of the tea and coffee and half of the milk. The total intake for lunch is

2. A client has a prescription for 0.25 mg of lanoxin (Digoxin). There are 0.5 mg tablets of lanoxin on hand. How many tablets should the client receive?

3. A client's IV infusion rate is 75 mL/hr. How many hours will a 500 mL bag of IV fluid last?

4. When the IV rate is 100 mL/hr and the administration set is 15 drops/mL, how many drops per minute should the IV run?

5. A 4-year-old child is prescribed 5 mL of ampicillin (Polycillin Pediatric) for otitis media every 6 hr. When preparing for the child's discharge, the nurse should tell the child's mother to give how much ampicillin every 6 hr at home?

6. A client has a prescription for heparin (Heparin Sodium) 7,000 units IV. The vial contains 10,000 units/mL. How many milliliters of heparin should be administered?

7. A nurse is preparing 300,000 units of procaine penicillin (*Wycillin*). The vial contains 1,500,000 units per 2 mL. How many milliliters should the nurse administer?

[ ]

8. A client weighs 180 lb and has a prescription for 0.5 mL of medication per kilogram of body weight. How many milliliters of medication should the client receive?

[ ]

9. A client is receiving D_5W at 50 mL/hr in one IV and D_5NS 75 mL/hr in another IV. The client also receives IV piggyback medication every 8 hr prepared in 100 mL of fluid. How much IV fluid will the client receive in 8 hr?

[ ]

10. When the IV administration set delivers 10 drops/mL, the rate of flow in drops/min for 1,000 mL D_5NS to infuse in 8 hr is

[ ]

11. While measuring a client's output, the nurse has measured 300 mL urine at 0800, 450 mL liquid stool at 1130, 225 mL urine at 1300, and 35 mL emesis at 1430. What is the client's total output for this shift?

[ ]

12. A client receiving an IV infusion has a prescription for 1,000 mL in 12 hr. Using a micro-drip system that delivers 60 micro drops/mL, the nurse should adjust the infusion for how many drops per minute?
   a. 45 drops
   b. 68 drops
   c. 83 drops
   d. 96 drops

[ ]

13. A client's temperature is 100° F. What is this temperature in degrees centigrade?

[ ]

14. A nurse has available meperidine (Demerol) 50 mg per mL. The provider order is to administer meperidine 35 mg. How many milliliters should the nurse safely administer?

[ ]

15. A client with fluid restriction may have 800 mL in 8 hr. The IV is running at 50 mL/hr. How much fluid may the client have by mouth?

[ ]

Test Answers

1.	600	9.	1,100
2.	0.5	10.	21
3.	7	11.	1,010
4.	25	12.	83
5.	1	13.	37.7
6.	0.7	14.	0.7
7.	0.4	15.	400
8.	41		

NUTRITION

Therapeutic Diets

A. Adult Nutritional Requirements

1. Protein: 0.8 to 1.0 g/kg daily
2. Fat: < 30% of total kcal
3. Carbohydrates: 45 to 65% of daily caloric intake
4. Calcium: 1,000 mg/daily
   a. Postmenopausal: 1,500 mg/day
5. Potassium: 2,300 mg/day
6. Iron:
   a. Men (19 and older) 8 mg/day
   b. Women (19 to 50) 18 mg/day
   c. Women (> 51) 8 mg/day
7. Daily fluid requirement in mL = Body weight in lb x 15
8. Fiber: 30 to 38 g/day

B. Nutrient Modification

1. Low-protein diet
   a. Indicated for renal impairment, hepatic coma, and advanced cirrhosis
   b. Controls end products of protein metabolism by limiting protein intake
   c. Encourage high-carbohydrate foods.
   d. Limit foods high in protein such as eggs, meat, milk, and milk products.
2. High-protein diet
   a. Used for tissue building, burns, correction of malabsorption syndromes, mild to moderate liver disease, undernutrition, and pregnancy
   b. Corrects protein loss and/or maintains and rebuilds tissues
   c. Encourage high-protein foods such as fish, fowl, organ and meat sources, and dairy products.
   d. May include protein supplements
3. Abnormalities in amino acid metabolism
   a. Use for phenylketonuria (PKU), galactosemia, and lactose intolerance.
   b. Reduce or eliminate the offending enzyme.
   c. Avoid milk and milk products for all three diets.
   d. Use milk substitutes.
4. Low-cholesterol diet
   a. Indicated for cardiovascular diseases, diabetes mellitus, and high-serum cholesterol levels
   b. Controls cholesterol levels by limiting cholesterol intake
   c. Limit foods high in low-density lipoproteins, saturated fats, and trans-fatty acids such as animal products (egg yolks, organ meats, bacon, fatty meats, and butter).
   d. Encourage low-cholesterol foods, foods containing high-density lipoproteins, and unsaturated fats, including omega-3 fatty acids, such as fatty fish; shellfish; walnuts; flaxseed oil; and raw or cooked vegetables, fruits; lean meats; and skinless fowl.
5. Modified-fat diet
   a. Indicated for malabsorption syndromes, cystic fibrosis, gallbladder disease, obstructive jaundice and liver disease, and obesity
   b. Fat content in the diet is lowered
      1) To stop contractions of the diseased organs
      2) When there is inadequate absorption of fat
      3) To decrease fat storage in the body
   c. To reduce fat intake, avoid gravies, fatty meat and fish, cream, fried foods, rich pastries, whole milk products, cream soups, salad and cooking oils, nuts, and chocolate; allow two to three eggs per week, lean meat, and butter and margarine.
   d. For a fat-free diet, restrict all fatty meats and fat; allow vegetables, fruits, lean meats, fowl, fish, bread, and cereal.
6. High-polyunsaturated fat diet
   a. Indicated for cardiovascular diseases
   b. Reduce saturated fats and trans-fatty acids by avoiding foods from animal sources, whole-milk products, egg yolks, organ meats, bacon, fatty meats, tropical oils, and partially hydrogenated vegetable oils.
   c. Increase polyunsaturated fats by including vegetable sources, corn/soybean/safflower oils, foods high in omega-3 fatty acids such as fatty fish and walnuts.
7. Carbohydrate modification (diabetic diet or American Diabetes Association diet)
   a. Principles of diabetic diet management
      1) Attain or maintain ideal body weight.
      2) Ensure normal growth.
      3) Maintain plasma glucose levels as close to normal as possible.
      4) Provide 30 calories/kg of ideal body weight.
      5) Provide 25% of calories at each meal and 25% for snacks.
      6) Provide 20% of calories as protein, 55 to 60% as carbohydrates, and 20 to 30% as fats.
      7) Include unsaturated fats, high fiber, and complex carbohydrates.
   b. Develop meal plans designed for individual needs using exchange lists.
      1) Milk exchanges
      2) Vegetable exchanges
      3) Fruit exchanges
      4) Bread exchanges
      5) Fat exchanges

C. Mineral Alterations

1. Potassium-modified diets
   a. Increase potassium intake for diabetic acidosis, thiazide diuretics, 48 hr after burns, vomiting, and/or fevers.
   b. Reduce potassium intake for kidney failure.
   c. Foods high in potassium include: fruits and fruit juices, (e.g., orange, grapefruit, banana, apple); avocados, prunes, dried apricots; dried beans, soy beans, lima beans, kidney beans, squash, baked potatoes, milk, and broiled meats.
   d. Foods low in potassium include breads, cereals, sugar, fats, and cranberry and grape juice.

2. Sodium-restricted diets
   a. Sodium is restricted in hypertension, heart failure, myocardial infarction, hepatitis, adrenal cortical diseases, kidney disease, lithium carbonate therapy, cystic fibrosis, and conditions such as cirrhosis of the liver and pre-eclampsia, which cause persistent edema.
   b. Mild restriction is 2 to 3 g of sodium
   c. Moderate restriction is 1,000 mg of sodium
   d. Strict restriction is 500 mg of sodium
   e. Severe restriction is 250 mg of sodium
   f. Limit foods high in sodium, such as potato chips and other salted snack foods; canned soups and vegetables; baked goods that contain baking powder or soda; cereals; seafood; beef; processed meats such as bologna, ham, and bacon; dairy products, especially cheese; pickles; olives; and condiments such as soy sauce, steak sauce, Worcestershire sauce; and salad dressings.
   g. Encourage low-sodium foods such as fresh fruits and vegetables, chicken, salt substitutes, and low-sodium products.

3. Iron alterations
   a. Increased iron intake is indicated for correction or prevention of iron deficiency anemia, which is most likely to occur in infants, toddlers, adolescents, and pregnant women.
   b. Food sources high in iron include fish, meats (particularly organ meats), green leafy vegetables, enriched breads, cereals and macaroni products, whole grain products, dried fruits such as raisins and apricots, and egg yolks
   c. Vitamin C enhances absorption of iron from the gastrointestinal tract.
   d. Administration of iron supplements
      1) Oral administration with a straw
      2) Maximum absorption occurs when administered between meals
      3) Fewer gastrointestinal side effects occur when administered with meals
      4) Injectable iron administered deep IM with Z track

4. Calcium alterations
   a. Increased calcium intake is indicated for growing children and adolescents, pregnant and lactating women, and postmenopausal women (prevents osteoporosis).
   b. Decreased calcium intake is indicated for kidney stones composed of calcium.
   c. Food sources high in calcium include milk and milk products like yogurt and cheese; dark green vegetables, such as collard greens, kale, broccoli; dried beans and peas; and shellfish and canned salmon.
   d. Some antacids contain calcium.
   e. Vitamin D enhances absorption of calcium from the gastrointestinal tract.

D. Consistency Modifications

1. Clear-liquid diet
   a. Indicated for resting the gastrointestinal tract, maintaining fluid balance; immediately postoperative; for diarrhea, nausea, and vomiting
   b. Includes water, tea, broth, gelatin, apple juice
   c. Not nutritionally adequate

2. Full-liquid diet
   a. When clear liquids are tolerated well, progress to full liquids
   b. Include clear liquids plus milk and milk products, such as custard, pudding, creamed soups, ice cream, sherbet, fruit juices
   c. Can be nutritionally adequate

3. Soft diet
   a. Include full liquids plus pureed vegetables, eggs that are not fried, tender meats, potatoes, cooked fruit

4. Bland diet
   a. Used to promote healing of gastric mucosa by eliminating chemically and mechanically irritating food sources
   b. Indicated for gastric and duodenal ulcers and postoperative stomach surgery
   c. Given in small, frequent feedings to assist in diluting or neutralizing stomach acid; protein foods are good at neutralizing; fat has some ability to inhibit the secretion of acid and delays stomach emptying
   d. Foods usually introduced in stages with gradual addition of foods
   e. Foods allowed include milk, butter, eggs that are not fried, custard, vanilla ice cream, cottage cheese, cooked refined or strained cereal, enriched white bread, gelatin, homemade creamed/pureed soups, baked or broiled potatoes

APPENDIX C

POSITIONING CLIENTS

TABLE APP-1

POSITION	DESCRIPTION	INDICATIONS
Semi-Fowler's	Head of bed elevated to 30°	Head injury, postoperative cranial surgery, respiratory diseases with dyspnea, postoperative cataract removal, increased intracranial pressure
Fowler's	Head of bed elevated to 45°	Head injury, postoperative cranial surgery, postoperative abdominal surgery, respiratory diseases with dyspnea, cardiac problems with dyspnea, bleeding esophageal varices, postoperative thyroidectomy, postoperative cataract removal, increased intracranial pressure
High-Fowler's	Head of bed elevated to 90°	Respiratory diseases with dyspnea: emphysema, status asthmaticus, pneumothorax, cardiac problems with dyspnea, feeding, meal times, hiatal hernia, during and after meals
Supine (dorsal recumbent)	Lying on back, head, and shoulders; usually slightly elevated with a small pillow	Spinal cord injury (no pillow), urinary catheterization
Prone	Lying on abdomen, legs extended, and head turned to the side	Immobilized client, amputation of lower extremity, unconscious client, post-lumbar puncture 6 to 12 hr, post myelogram 12 to 24 hr (oil-based dye), postoperative tonsillectomy and adenoidectomy
Lateral (side lying)	Lying on side with most of body weight borne by the lateral aspect of the lower ilium	Post abdominal surgery, unconscious client, seizures (head to side), postoperative tonsillectomy and adenoidectomy, postoperative pyloric stenosis of lower scapula and the lateral (right side), post-liver biopsy (right side), rectal irrigations
Sims' (semi-prone)	Lying on left side with most of body weight borne by the anterior aspect of the ilium, humerus, and clavicle	Unconscious client, rectal irrigations
Lithotomy	Lying on back with hips and knees flexed at right angles and feet in stirrups	Perineal procedures, rectal procedures, vaginal procedures
Trendelenburg	Head and body are lowered while feet are elevated	Shock
Reverse Trendelenburg	Head elevated while feet are lowered	Cervical traction
Elevate one or more extremities	Elevate legs/feet or arms/hands by adjusting bed or supporting with pillows	Thrombophlebitis, application of cast, edema, postoperative surgical procedure on extremity

APPENDIX D

ERGONOMIC GUIDELINES

A. General Guidelines to Prevent Injury
1. Use assistive devices such as slides and mechanical lifts whenever possible.
2. Use other staff members to help and instruct client on what to do.
3. Use correct body mechanics:
    a. Face the object being moved.
    b. Bend at your legs, instead of your back.
    c. Work using your legs, not your back.
    d. Turn pivoting your body. Do not twist.
    e. Have the object you are moving close to you and at waist level.
    f. Move the object toward, not away from you. Push instead of pull.
    g. Have a wide base of support; feet should be a shoulder width apart.
    h. Move object using smooth, even motion.
    i. Keep beds or objects at waist level and close to you.
    j. Do not lift, if you can slide.
    k. Do not bend, reach, or twist.

B. Transferring Clients from Bed to Chair or Chair to Bed
1. Lower the bed to lowest setting.
2. Position bed or chair so that the client is moving toward his/her strong side.
3. Position bed or chair so that the client can stand, then pivot.

C. Repositioning Clients in Bed
1. Raise bed to waist level.
2. Lower side rails.
3. Use slide boards or draw sheets.
4. Kneel on the bed if needed to maintain good body mechanics.
5. Use other staff members for help.

D. Working at a Computer
1. Body should be in a neutral aligned position.
2. Hands, wrists, and forearms parallel to the ground.
3. Head should be level.
4. Bend elbows 90 to 120° and close to the body.
5. Back should be supported.
6. Knees should be at hip level.
7. Adjust position at least every 15 min.

E. Assisting During Surgery
1. Raise table to waist level.
2. Prevent reaching by standing on stools.
3. Adjust position at least every 15 min.
4. Position trays at a level between the waist and shoulders.
5. Elevate one foot when standing.

APPENDIX E

PHARMACOLOGY

Antianxiety Agents (Minor Tranquilizers)
ANXIOLYTICS

MEDICATION: GENERIC/TRADE
- buspirone (BuSpar)

ACTION
- Serotonin reuptake inhibition and agonist effects on dopamine receptors of the brain

ADVERSE EFFECTS
- Depression, stimulation, insomnia
- Tremors
- Hypotension
- Tachycardia, palpitations

INDICATIONS
- Relief of short-term anxiety

 NURSING INTERVENTIONS
- Teach 3 to 4 week lag time before therapeutic effect achieved.
- Monitor blood pressure, and pulse.

OTHER INFORMATION
- This medication has no sedative/hypnotic properties or muscle relaxation properties
- Do not use with MAOIs.
- Avoid use of alcohol while taking this medication.

BENZODIAZEPINE COMPOUNDS

MEDICATION: GENERIC/TRADE
- chlordiazepoxide (*Librium*)
- diazepam (*Valium*)
- oxazepam (*Serax*)
- clonazepam (*Klonopin*)
- clorazepate (*Tranxene*)
- lorazepam (*Ativan*)
- alprazolam (*Xanax*)

ACTION
- CNS depression
- Muscle relaxation
- Anticonvulsant

ADVERSE EFFECTS
- Drowsiness, sedation

LONG-TERM ADVERSE EFFECTS
- Tolerance
- Dependency
- Rebound insomnia/anxiety

INDICATIONS
- Anxiety disorder
- Detoxification alcohol dependence disorder
- Skeletal muscle relaxation
- Premedication operative procedures
- Seizures

NURSING INTERVENTIONS
- Teach client to avoid activities that require alertness, such as driving.
- Caution to avoid falls.
- Discourage social isolation.
- Carefully observe client and offer support.
- Medication use is short-term only.
- Avoid alcohol or other CNS depressant.
- Discontinue by slowly tapering off.
- Use with caution in clients with a history of depression, suicide attempts, or drug abuse.
- Monitor for CNS depression.

OTHER INFORMATION
- Avoid during pregnancy and lactation.
- Older adults are more vulnerable to side effects.

BETA-BLOCKERS

MEDICATION: GENERIC/TRADE
- propranolol (Inderal)
- clonidine (Catapres)

ACTION
- Nonselective B-blocker

ADVERSE EFFECTS
- Dizziness, confusion
- Hypotension, bradycardia
- Dry mouth
- Drowsiness, sedation

INDICATIONS
- Anxiety disorders
- Narcotic withdrawal
- Convulsions

NURSING INTERVENTIONS
- Observe client carefully.
- Monitor client when out of bed.
- Monitor blood pressure, and pulse.
- Increase the client's fluids.

SEDATING ANTIHISTAMINES

MEDICATION: GENERIC/TRADE
- hydroxyzine (Vistaril, Atarax)

ACTION
- CNS depressant (subcortical levels)

ADVERSE EFFECTS
- Convulsions
- Tremors, fatigue
- Dizziness, confusion, depression
- Headache
- Dry mouth

INDICATIONS
- Preoperative medication
- Anxiety disorders

NURSING INTERVENTIONS
- Observe client closely; may lower seizure threshold.
- Teach client to avoid activities that require alertness.

SEDATIVE HYPNOTICS

MEDICATION: GENERIC/TRADE
- flurazepam (Dalmane)
- temazepam (Restoril)
- triazolam (Halcion)

ACTION
- Produces CNS depression and sedation

ADVERSE EFFECTS
- Drowsiness
- Dizziness, lightheadedness

OVERDOSE
- Somnolence
- Confusion
- Impaired coordination
- Coma

INDICATIONS
- Sleep disturbance of anxiety
- Short-term use only

NURSING INTERVENTIONS
- Carefully observe the client.
- Have client use caution when out of bed.
- Complete a suicide assessment.
- Obtain emergency medical treatment for the client.

Antidepressant Agents
TETRACYCLIC ANTIDEPRESSANTS

MEDICATION: GENERIC/TRADE
- amoxapine (Asendin)
- maprotiline (Ludiomil)

ACTION
- Blocks reuptake of norepinephrine and serotonin into nerve endings

ADVERSE EFFECTS
- Agranulocytosis
- Hypotension
- Paralytic ileus

INDICATIONS
- Depression

NURSING INTERVENTIONS
- Monitor the client's CBC.
- Caution the client to stand up slowly.
- Observe the client for nausea and vomiting.
- Use with caution in children under 18 years of age. Suicidal tendencies have been seen in children/adolescents taking antidepressants, primarily at the onset of treatment or when the dosage is changed. Instruct family to monitor closely for changes in behavior or signs of suicidal ideas.

TRICYCLIC ANTIDEPRESSANTS

MEDICATION: GENERIC/TRADE
- imipramine (Tofranil)
- desipramine (Norpramin)
- amitriptyline (Elavil)
- nortriptyline (Aventyl, Pamelor)
- clomipramine (Anafranil)
- doxepin (Sinequan)
- protriptyline (Vivactil)
- trimipramine (Surmontil)

ACTION
- Blocks reuptake of norepinephrine and serotonin into nerve endings

ADVERSE EFFECTS
- Agranulocytosis
- Hypotension

- Paralytic ileus
- Cardiovascular

INDICATIONS
- Major depressive disorders
- Agoraphobia
- Panic disorders
- Obsessive-compulsive disorder
- Psychogenic pain disorder

 NURSING INTERVENTIONS
- Monitor the client's CBC.
- Caution the client to stand up slowly.
- Observe the client for nausea and vomiting.
- Use cautiously in clients with known heart disease.
- Use with caution in children under 18 years of age. Suicidal tendencies have been seen in children/adolescents taking antidepressants, primarily at the onset of treatment or when the dosage is changed. Instruct family to monitor closely for changes in behavior or signs of suicidal ideas.

MONOAMINE OXIDASE INHIBITORS (MAOIs)

MEDICATION: GENERIC/TRADE
- isocarboxazid (Marplan)
- phenelzine (Nardil)
- tranylcypromine (Parnate)

ACTION
- Acts on CNS by increasing concentration of epinephrine, serotonin, and dopamine, thereby reducing depression effective

ADVERSE EFFECTS
- Excessive perspiration
- Erection/orgasm difficulty
- Anxiety, restlessness
- Hypertensive crisis
- Anticholinergic manifestations
- CNS effects: drowsiness, fatigue, headache, restlessness, insomnia, constipation
- Orthostatic hypotension
- Insomnia (Parnate)
- Weight gain

INDICATIONS
- Because of dietary restrictions, use as second-line antidepressant if other antidepressants are not effective

 NURSING INTERVENTIONS
- Observe, report, and provide comfort measures.
- Lower dose or switch to a less anticholinergic preparation.
- Teach the client to avoid foods with high tyramine content such as aged cheese, fava or Italian green beans, fermented foods, liver, yeast extracts, bologna, beer, and Chianti and red wines; limit sour cream and yogurt.
- Teach the client to avoid over-the-counter cold preparations.
- (See antipsychotic medications.)
- Medication can produce some side effects for short period.
- Treat symptoms medically if not severe.
- Monitor blood pressure, both sitting and standing.
- Give single morning dose.
- Use with caution in children under 18 years. Suicidal tendencies have been seen in children/adolescents taking antidepressants, primarily at the onset of treatment or when the dosage is changed. Instruct family to monitor closely for changes in behavior or signs of suicidal ideas.

OTHER INFORMATION
- Medication Interactions:
  - Tricyclic antidepressants cause hypertensive crisis.
  - Cocaine and amphetamines potentiate the action.

- Asthma inhalants
- Narcotics, especially meperidine (Demerol), which can cause cardiovascular collapse
- Local anesthetics with epinephrine
- Sinus and nasal decongestants

SELECTIVE SEROTONIN REUPTAKE INHIBITORS (SSRIs)

MEDICATION: GENERIC/TRADE
- trazodone (Desyrel)
- sertraline (Zoloft)
- fluoxetine (Prozac)
- paroxetine (Paxil)
- bupropion (Wellbutrin)
- Venlafaxine hydrochloride (Effexor)

ACTION
- Inhibits serotonin and potentiates behavioral changes

ADVERSE EFFECTS
- Anticholinergic effects
- Dry mouth
  - Constipation
  - Urinary retention
  - Blurred vision
  - Aggravates glaucoma
- Cardiovascular effects
  - Postural hypotension
  - Tachycardia, arrhythmias
- Allergic reactions
  - Rashes
  - Photosensitivity
  - Tremors
- CNS
  - Insomnia
  - Stimulation
  - Sedation
  - Delirium
  - Myoclonic twitches
  - Seizures (especially high doses)
  - Sexual side effects such as impaired libido

INDICATIONS
- Depression
- Anxiety disorders

 NURSING INTERVENTIONS
- Increase the client's fluids.
- Encourage good oral hygiene.
- Consume bulk diet, exercise, and use stool softeners.
- Monitor I&O, lower dose.
- Provide corrective lenses, large print, and/or change to another antidepressant.
- Provide ophthalmic consult.
- Take blood pressure regularly, both sitting and standing.
- Use smaller divided doses in conduction defects for clients with known heart disease.
- Avoid giving to clients with conduction defects or recent myocardial infarction.
- Conduct pretreatment ECG.
- Provide sunscreen, protective clothing.
- Carefully observe client.
- Advise client to avoid caffeine.
- Observe and report; may have to discontinue.
- Start at a low dose and gradually increase (maprotiline and bupropion) to monitor weight gain.
- Use with caution in children under 18 years of age. Suicidal tendencies have been seen in children/adolescents taking antidepressants, primarily at the onset of treatment or when the dosage is changed. Instruct family to monitor closely for changes in behavior or signs of suicidal ideas.

OTHER INFORMATION
- Response rate varies, but often takes 3 to 4 weeks for therapeutic effect.
- Allow 14-day waiting period before changing from antidepressant to MAOI and vice versa.
- Tricyclics can be fatal with overdose; do suicide assessment.
- Medication Interactions:
  - Antihypertensives (unable to control blood pressure)
  - Antacids inhibit absorption
  - Antipsychotics
  - Antiarrhythmics

Antimicrobial Agents
AMINOGLYCOSIDES

MEDICATION: GENERIC/TRADE
- gentamicin sulfate (Garamycin)
- neomycin sulfate (Mycifradin Sulfate)
- streptomycin sulfate
- tobramycin sulfate (Nebcin)
- vancomycin hydrochloride (Vancocin)
- amikacin (Amikin)

ACTION
- Bacteriostatic or bacteriocidal
- Inhibits protein synthesis

ADVERSE EFFECTS
- Nephrotoxicity
- Ototoxicity (tinnitus, vertigo, hearing loss)

INDICATIONS
- Serious bacterial infections
- Promote bowel sterility prior to gastrointestinal surgical procedures

NURSING INTERVENTIONS
- Weigh client and obtain baseline renal function studies prior to therapy.
- Monitor output for specific gravity, urinalysis, BUN, creatinine, and creatinine clearance.
- Monitor peak and trough therapeutic levels for duration of therapy.
- Encourage fluids.
- Evaluate client's hearing before and during hearing loss therapy.

ANTIFUNGALS

MEDICATION: GENERIC/TRADE
- amphotericin B (Fungizone)
- fluconazole (Diflucan)

ACTION
- Alters fungal cell permeability

ADVERSE EFFECTS
- Fever, chills, nausea, vomiting, and headache
- Thrombophlebitis
- Hypokalemia
- Diarrhea, rash, pruritus

INDICATIONS
- Systemic fungal infections

NURSING INTERVENTIONS
- Instruct the client to take this medication for the full course of therapy.
- Administer acetaminophen (Tylenol) and diphenhydramine (Benadryl) 1 hr before infusion.

- Add hydrocortisone to infusion.
- Observe for signs of hypokalemia.
- Large doses of potassium may be needed with systemic medications.
- Care with IV administration can harm tissue.

ANTIFUNGALS

MEDICATION: GENERIC/TRADE
- Nystatin (Mycostatin)

ACTION
- Alters fungal cell permeability

ADVERSE EFFECTS
- Rash, urticaria, stinging, burning

INDICATIONS
- Infections due to Candida in the mouth, gastrointestinal tract, or vagina

NURSING INTERVENTIONS
- Wash hands before and after application.

ANTIRETROVIRALS

MEDICATION: GENERIC/TRADE
- didanosine (Videx)
- lamivudine (Epivir)
- lamivudine and zidovudine (Combivir)
- nevirapine (Viramune)
- stavudine (Viramune)
- zalcitabine (Hivid)
- zidovudine (Retrovir)

ACTION
- Reverse transcriptase inhibitors stop the action of reverse transcriptase, preventing HIV viral replication in its early stage.

ADVERSE EFFECTS
- Nausea
- Seizures
- Thrombocytopenia
- Pancreatitis
- Fatigue
- Dizziness
- Insomnia
- Fever
- Rash
- Headache

INDICATIONS
- Treat HIV infections

NURSING INTERVENTIONS
- Stress the importance of medication compliance to avoid medication resistance and provide optimum effect.
- Monitor CBC and platelet counts.
- Advise client to take precautions to prevent the spread of HIV.

ANTIRETROVIRALS

MEDICATION: GENERIC/TRADE
- nelfinavir (Viracept)
- ritonavir (Norvir)
- saquinavir (Fortovase)

ACTION
- Protease inhibitors act by inhibiting the enzyme protease and preventing HIV viral maturation.

ADVERSE EFFECTS
• Nausea
• Adipogenic effects
• Thrombocytopenia
• Pancreatitis
• Fatigue
• Dizziness
• Insomnia

INDICATIONS
• Treat HIV infection

 NURSING INTERVENTIONS
• Stress the importance of medication compliance to avoid medication resistance and provide optimum effect.
• Give with a light meal or snack.
• Monitor the client's CBC and platelet counts.
• Advise the client to take precautions to prevent the spread of HIV.

ANTITUBERCULARS

MEDICATION: GENERIC/TRADE
• ethambutol (Myambutol)

ACTION
• Impairs RNA synthesis

ADVERSE EFFECTS
• Vision loss and loss of color discrimination

INDICATIONS
• Pulmonary tuberculosis

 NURSING INTERVENTIONS
• Evaluate the client's visual acuity and color discrimination before and during therapy.

ANTITUBERCULARS

MEDICATION: GENERIC/TRADE
• rifampin (Rifadin)

ACTION
• Impairs RNA synthesis

ADVERSE EFFECTS
• Hepatotoxicity
• Red-orange color to urine and feces
• Drowsiness
• Acute renal failure

INDICATIONS
• Pulmonary tuberculosis

 NURSING INTERVENTIONS
• Monitor liver function studies.
• Teach the client about color changes of body secretions.
• Teach the client to avoid activities that require alertness.
• For PO administration, give 1 hr before meals, or 2 hr after.

OTHER INFORMATION
• May require increased doses of warfarin, corticosteroids, and oral hypoglycemics

ANTITUBERCULARS

MEDICATION: GENERIC/TRADE
•isoniazid (INH)

ACTION
•Interferes with DNA synthesis

ADVERSE EFFECTS
•Hepatotoxicity
•Peripheral neuropathy

INDICATIONS
• Infection due to tubercle bacilli

 NURSING INTERVENTIONS
• Monitor liver function studies.
• Teach the client to notify the provider for loss of appetite, fatigue, malaise, jaundice, and/or dark urine.
• Teach the client to avoid alcohol.
• Administer pyridoxine (Vitamin B₆) (Beesix) to prevent peripheral neuropathy.

ANTITUBERCULARS

MEDICATION: GENERIC/TRADE
• para-aminosalicylic acid (PAS)

ACTION
• Inhibits folic acid synthesis

ADVERSE EFFECTS
• Hepatotoxicity
• Gastrointestinal symptoms: nausea, vomiting

INDICATIONS
• Tuberculosis

 NURSING INTERVENTIONS
• Monitor the client's liver function studies.
• Teach the client to notify provider of loss of appetite fatigue, malaise, jaundice, and/or dark urine.
• Administer with meals or antacid.

ANTIVIRALS

MEDICATION: GENERIC/TRADE
• amantadine (Symmetrel)
• oseltamivir (Tamiflu)
• rimantadine (Flumadine)
• zanamivir (Relenza)

ACTION
• Interrupts viral replication and reduces flu symptoms

ADVERSE EFFECTS
• Insomnia
• Bronchitis
• Cough

INDICATIONS
• Treat or prevent the flu

NURSING INTERVENTIONS
• Reduce dosage in clients with renal disease.
• Instruct client to take within 2 days of symptoms or within 10 days after exposure of the virus.

ANTIVIRALS

MEDICATION: GENERIC/TRADE
• ribavirin (Rebetol)

ACTION
• Interrupts viral replication and slows respiratory syncytial virus action

ADVERSE EFFECTS
• Conjunctivitis
• Rhinitis

- Skin rash
- Bronchospasms
- Anemia

INDICATIONS
- Treat severe respiratory syncytial virus

NURSING INTERVENTIONS
- Use Small Particle Aerosol Generator Model-2 (SPAG-2) for aerosol delivery.
- Use sterile USP water for reconstitution.
- Monitor the client for anemia.
- Avoid exposure to self or others with the aerosol (especially persons with asthma).
- Pregnant women and caregivers must not enter room where ribavirin is administered.

ANTIVIRALS

MEDICATION: GENERIC/TRADE
- acyclovir (Zovirax)
- foscarnet (Foscavir)
- ganciclovir (Cytovene)
- valacyclovir (Valtrex)

ACTION
- Interrupts viral replication, but does not completely eliminate the virus

ADVERSE EFFECTS
- Seizures
- Thrombocytopenia
- Leukopenia
- Fever

INDICATIONS
- Treat herpes simplex, herpes zoster, varicella zoster, cytomegalovirus and Epstein Barr virus

NURSING INTERVENTIONS
- Reduce dosage in clients with renal insufficiency.
- Use an infusion pump for IV infusions.
- Instruct client to take at the first sign of herpes infection.
- Instruct client to take measures to prevent the spread of infection to others.

CEPHALOSPORINS

MEDICATION: GENERIC/TRADE
- First generation
  - cefazolin sodium (Ancef, Kefzol)
  - cephalexin monohydrate (Keflex)
  - cephalothin sodium (Keflin)
- Second generation
  - cefaclor (Ceclor)
  - cefuroxime (Zinacef)
  - loracarbef (Lorabid)
- Third generation
  - cefixime (Suprax)
  - cefotaxime (Claforan)
  - ceftriaxone (Rocephin)

ACTION
- Bacteriocidal or bacteriostatic
- Inhibits cell wall synthesis

ADVERSE EFFECTS
- Hypersensitivity
- Local irritation at injection site
- Anaphylaxis
- Diarrhea
- Do not breastfeed while taking this medication.

INDICATIONS
- Infections due to gram-positive cocci and some gram-negative cocci
- Prophylactically before certain operative procedures

NURSING INTERVENTIONS
- Obtain client history
- Change IV sites after 3 days
- Use with caution in clients with renal impairment
- Use with caution on clients with penicillin allergy

OTHER INFORMATION
- Structurally related to penicillin
- May cause false positive urine glucose test
- Excreted unchanged in urine

PENICILLINS

MEDICATION: GENERIC/TRADE
- amoxicillin (Polymox)
- ampicillin (D-Amp)
- cloxacillin (Cloxapen)
- dicloxacillin (Dycill)
- nafcillin (Unipen)
- penicillin G (Bicillin L-A)
- penicillin V (Beepen-VK)

ACTION
- Bacteriocidal against microbes by inhibiting cell wall synthesis during cell division

ADVERSE EFFECTS
- Hypersensitivity: rash, urticaria, anaphylaxis

INDICATIONS
- Infections due to gram-positive cocci and some gram-negative cocci

NURSING INTERVENTIONS
- Observe for hypersensitivity.
- Teach client to call provider if a rash, fever, or chills develop.
- Teach client to take medications as prescribed until entire amount taken.
- Administer 1 to 2 hr before meals or 2 to 3 hr after meals for best absorption.
- Do not breastfeed while taking this medication.

OTHER INFORMATION
- Resistant strains of bacteria may develop.

SULFONAMIDES

MEDICATION: GENERIC/TRADE
- sulfamethoxazole-trimethoprim (Bactrim, Septra)
- sulfisoxazole (Gantrisin)

ACTION
- Broad spectrum bacteriostatic

ADVERSE EFFECTS
- Hypersensitivity
- Blood dyscrasia-agranulocytosis, aplastic anemia
- Toxic to kidney when output is low
- Gastrointestinal manifestations: nausea, vomiting, diarrhea

INDICATIONS
- Urinary tract infections
- Otitis media
- Sinusitis

NURSING INTERVENTIONS
- Obtain client history.

- Monitor CBC routinely.
- Teach client to report skin rash, sore throat, fever, or mouth sores.
- Increase fluid intake to maintain output of 3,000 to 4,000 mL.
- Administer 1 hr before or 2 hr after meals for best absorption.

Antipsychotic Agents
ANTIPSYCHOTICS

MEDICATION: GENERIC/TRADE
- chlorpromazine *(Thorazine)*
- mesoridazine *(Serentil)*
- perphenazine *(Trilafon)*
- haloperidol *(Haldol)*
- loxapine *(Loxitane)*
- risperidone *(Risperdal)*
- thioridazine *(Mellaril)*
- fluphenazine *(Prolixin)*
- trifluoperazine *(Stelazine)*
- thiothixene *(Navane)*
- molindone *(Moban)*
- clozapine *(Clozaril)*

ACTION
- Depresses cerebral cortex, which controls activity aggression

ADVERSE EFFECTS
- Sedation
- Extrapyramidal effects
  - Dystonia
  - Akathisia
  - Tardive dyskinesia
- Anticholinergic symptoms
  - Dry mouth
  - Constipation
  - Urinary retention
  - Blurred vision
  - Nasal congestion
  - Hypotension
- Photosensitivity
- Agranulocytosis (esp. *Clozaril*)
- Neuroleptic malignant syndrome
- Weight gain

INDICATIONS
- Schizophrenic disorders
- Bipolar disorder, manic phase
- Agitated organic disorders

NURSING INTERVENTIONS
- Ask provider if entire dose can be given at bedtime.
- Report parkinsonian manifestations, dystonia to provider.
  - Medication may be changed.
  - Antiparkinsonian medication may be given.
  - Discontinue at first sign.
- Provide laxatives or diet changes if constipation is a problem.
- Provide fluids, sugarless candies, and gum for dry mouth.
- Monitor I&O.
- Monitor blood pressure, both sitting and standing.
- Caution to stand up slowly.
- Caution client to use sunscreen, protective clothing for sun sensitivity.
- Observe and report signs of infection, discontinue if necessary.
- Observe and report signs: altered consciousness, unstable blood pressure and pulse, muscle rigidity, diaphoresis, tremors; discontinue medication of present.
- Monitor diet, increase physical exercise.

OTHER INFORMATION
- Medication Interactions: CNS depressants have additive effects; antacids inhibit absorption.
- Lowers seizure threshold
- Clozapine *(Clozaril)* requires weekly WBC.
- Use low doses only for older adults.
- Avoid thioridazine *(Mellaril)* in males who are sexually active.
- Risperidone *(Risperdal)* also effective on negative manifestation.

Autonomic Nervous System Medications
CHOLINERGIC BLOCKERS
(Not used as much today because of side effects)

MEDICATION: GENERIC/TRADE
- benztropine mesylate *(Cogentin)*
- procyclidine hydrochloride *(Kemadrin)*
- biperiden hydrochloride *(Akineton)*
- trihexyphenidyl hydrochloride *(Artane)*

ACTION
- Parasympatholytic

ADVERSE EFFECTS
- Anticholinergic
- Blurred vision
- Dry mouth
- Constipation
- Urinary retention
- Orthostatic hypotension
- Drowsiness

INDICATIONS
- Parkinson's disease
- Extra-pyramidal manifestations associated with antipsychotics

NURSING INTERVENTIONS
- Provide fluids, hard candy, ice chips.
- Increase dietary fiber, fluid intake, and exercise.
- Monitor I&O.
- Monitor blood pressure; teach client to stand up slowly.
- Teach client to avoid activities that require alertness.

OTHER INFORMATION
- Older adult clients are particularly sensitive to side effects.
- Euphoria and potential for abuse
- Amantadine *(Symmetrel)* is newer agent for treating Parkinson's disease; not a cholinergic blocker

DOPAMINERGIC THERAPY
(Used more often)

MEDICATION: GENERIC/TRADE
- levodopa *(Sinemet)*
- bromocriptine *(Parlodel)*
- amantadine *(Symmetrel)*

ACTION
- Increase dopamine

ADVERSE EFFECTS
* Impaired concentration
* Hypotension
* Gastrointestinal upsets
* Dizziness

INDICATIONS
* Parkinson's disease

NURSING INTERVENTIONS
* Change positions slowly.
* Minimize vitamin B$_6$ foods and vitamins (meat, eggs, poultry, sweet potatoes).
* Take with juice, low-protein snack.
* Abrupt discontinuation of therapy may precipitate a parkinsonian crisis.

Cardiovascular Medications
ANGIOTENSION-CONVERTING ENZYME INHIBITORS (ACE) - ANTIHYPERTENSIVE

MEDICATION: GENERIC/TRADE
* captopril *(Capoten)*
* enalapril *(Vasotec)*
* benazepril *(Lotensin)*

ACTION
* Prevents production of angiotensin II, causing systemic vasodilation

ADVERSE EFFECTS
* Dry cough
* Drop in blood pressure during first 1 to 3 hr following first dose
* Dizziness, orthostatic hypotension
* No reflux edema

INDICATIONS
* Hypertension
* Management of heart failure

NURSING INTERVENTIONS
* Advise client to change positions slowly.
* Monitor blood pressure, weight, signs of heart failure resolution.
* Avoid using in women who are pregnant or breastfeeding.

ANTIARRHYTHMICS

MEDICATION: GENERIC/TRADE
* lidocaine *(Xylocaine)*
* propranolol hydrochloride *(Inderal)*
* procainamide hydrochloride *(Pronestyl)*
* quinidine gluconate *(Dura-Tabs)*

ACTION
* Decreases cardiac conduction

ADVERSE EFFECTS
* Bradycardia
* Tachycardia - reflux
* Hypotension

INDICATIONS
* Prevention or treatment of atrial or ventricular arrhythmias including those secondary to myocardial infarction and digitalis toxicity

NURSING INTERVENTIONS
* Remain with client during infusion, tachycardia.
* Monitor ECG, blood pressure, and heart rate and rhythm.
* Stop immediately if ECG indicates excessive cardiac depression.

OTHER INFORMATION
* Narrow therapeutic index
* Do not confuse lidocaine with epinephrine used for local or topical anesthesia.
* IV dose of propranolol hydrochloride much smaller than by mouth dose
* Monitor blood levels.

ANTIARRHYTHMICS

MEDICATION: GENERIC/TRADE
* verapamil *(Calan, Isoptin)*

ACTION
* Calcium blocker
* Decrease cardiac conduction

ADVERSE EFFECTS
* Headache
* Constipation
* Dizziness
* Heart failure
* Reflux peripheral edema
* Bradycardia
* Hypotension

INDICATIONS
* Atrial arrhythmias
* Angina
* Hypertension
* Manage ventricular heart rate in clients receiving digoxin *(Lanoxin)*.

NURSING INTERVENTIONS
* Treat headache with acetaminophen *(Tylenol)*.
* Increase dietary fiber, fluid intake, and exercise.
* Monitor blood pressure and cardiac rhythm.

ANTIARRHYTHMICS

MEDICATION: GENERIC/TRADE
* amiodarone *(Cordarone)*
* bretylium *(Bretylate)*

ACTION
* Lengthens action potential and refractory period to reduce ventricular arrhythmias

ADVERSE EFFECTS
* Bradycardia
* Anorexia
* Heart failure
* Heart block
* Dizziness
* Nausea

INDICATIONS
* Ventricular arrhythmias
* Supraventricular rhythms

NURSING INTERVENTIONS
* Monitor ECG, blood pressure, and heart rate and rhythm.
* Monitor electrolytes.

ANTIHYPERTENSIVES

MEDICATION: GENERIC/TRADE
- hydralazine hydrochloride (*Apresoline*)
- prazosin hydrochloride (*Minipress*)
- nitroprusside (*Nipride*)

ACTION
- Relaxes smooth muscle

ADVERSE EFFECTS
- Tachycardia, palpitation
- Orthostatic hypotension
- Headache, dizziness
- Nausea, vomiting, diarrhea, anorexia
- Weight gain
- Administer diuretic if needed

INDICATIONS
- Hypertension, heart failure

 NURSING INTERVENTIONS
- Monitor heart rate and rhythm.
- Teach client to stand up and move around slowly.
- Treat headache with acetaminophen (*Tylenol*); teach client to lie down if dizzy.
- Administer with meals.
- Weigh daily.
- Administer diuretic if needed.

OTHER INFORMATION
- Compliance is biggest problem because side effects are worse than the disease - Not used very much today because of this.
- Side effects can be minimized by adjusting dose or changing medications.
- Giving medications daily rather than several times a day may increase compliance.

ANTILIPIDEMIC AGENTS

MEDICATION: GENERIC/TRADE
- lovastatin (*Mevacor*)
- atorvastatin (*Lipitor*)

ACTION
- Decreases level of cholesterol in the bloodstream
- Lowers low-density-lipoproteins and serum cholesterol HMG-COA reductase

ADVERSE EFFECTS
- HMG-COA reductase: gastrointestinal distress
- CNS: headaches, insomnia, fatigue, skin rashes
- Bile sequestrants: constipation, bloating, headache, tinnitus, orange color to urine

INDICATIONS
- Hypercholesterolemia

 NURSING INTERVENTIONS
- Fiber supplements, high-fiber diet
- HMG-COA reductase - take with meals. Change diet to include low fat and cholesterol.
- Have client take in the evening.
- Do not take with grapefruit juice.
- May increase digoxin (*Lanoxin*) levels by 20%; monitor care fully for toxicity.

CALCIUM CHANNEL BLOCKERS - ANTIANGINAL AND ANTIHYPERTENSIVE

MEDICATION: GENERIC/TRADE
- nifedipine (*Procardia*)
- diltiazem (*Cardizem*)

ACTION
- Decreases calcium in muscle so dilates coronary arteries and decreases heart rate

ADVERSE EFFECTS
- Bradycardia
- Peripheral swelling
- Coughing
- Hypotension
- Gastrointestinal upsets

INDICATIONS
- Hypertension
- Angina

 NURSING INTERVENTIONS
- Assess the client for bradycardia.
- Teach the client to be careful when using over-the-counter medications.
- Educate the client to change positions slowly.
- Monitor the client for swelling.

CARDIOTONIC GLYCOSIDES

MEDICATION: GENERIC/TRADE
- digitoxin (*Crystodigin*)
- digoxin (*Lanoxin*)
- dobutamine (*Dobutrex*)

ACTION
- Increases the force of cardiac contraction - positive inotropic
- Decreases heart rate - negative chronotropic

ADVERSE EFFECTS
- Bradycardia, arrhythmias
- Fatigue, muscle weakness, agitation
- Hallucinations
- Signs of toxicity: anorexia, nausea, yellow-green halos around visual images

INDICATIONS
- Heart failure
- Tachyarrhythmias

 NURSING INTERVENTIONS
- Take apical pulse for 1 full min; record and report significant changes in rate or rhythm. Hold if <60 or >120 in adult client.
- Monitor serum levels of potassium and medication, and monitor ECG.
- Teach how to take pulse and what signs to report.

OTHER INFORMATION
- Narrow range between therapeutic and toxic doses - (0.8 to 2.0 ng/mL); toxic level > 2 ng/mL
- Calcium salts are contraindicated

CORONARY VASODILATORS

MEDICATION: GENERIC/TRADE
- nitroglycerin (*Nitrostat*)

ACTION
- Dilate coronary arteries
- Decrease cardiac workload

ADVERSE EFFECTS
* Headache
* Flushing
* Orthostatic hypotension
* Palpitations
* Tachycardia

INDICATIONS
* Angina

NURSING INTERVENTIONS
* Treat headache with acetaminophen (*Tylenol*).
* Tolerance to medication usually develops.
* Monitor vital signs.
* Teach client to stand up, move slowly.
* Teach client to lie down if dizzy.

OTHER INFORMATION
* Protect this medication from light, moisture, and heat.
* Sublingual tablet taken at the first sign of anginal pain.
* Client should sit or lie down.
* May repeat tablet every 5 min times three if needed.
* Have client call provider if no relief.
* Topical medication measured on ruled application paper and applied to nonhairy area.

Central Nervous System Medications
ANTICONVULSANTS

MEDICATION: GENERIC/TRADE
* phenytoin sodium (*Dilantin*)
* carbamazepine (*Tegretol*)
* valproate (*Depakene*)

ACTION
* Inhibits spread of seizure activity

ADVERSE EFFECTS
* Ataxia
* Lethargy

INDICATIONS
* Tonic/clonic seizure disorder

NURSING INTERVENTIONS
* Determine if ataxia is a manifestation of the disease or a toxic effect of the medication.
* Teach client to avoid activities that require alertness.
* Use only NS solutions for infusion.
* Instruct client that good oral hygiene and regular dental care are required.
* Monitor therapeutic levels.
* Give IV medications slowly.

OTHER INFORMATION
* Do not mix with D_5W because precipitation will occur.

NARCOTIC ANALGESICS

MEDICATION: GENERIC/TRADE
* codeine sulfate
* meperidine hydrochloride (*Demerol*)
* morphine sulfate
* fentanyl (*Sublimaze*)

ACTION
* Alter perception of pain

ADVERSE EFFECTS
* Respiratory depression
* Hypotension, bradycardia
* Sedation, clouded sensorium, euphoria
* Nausea, vomiting, constipation
* Lethargy

INDICATIONS
* Moderate to severe pain

NURSING INTERVENTIONS
* Monitor respirations before and during treatment.
* Monitor blood pressure and pulse.
* Teach client to avoid activities that require alertness.
* Provide environment that enhances rest.
* Give IV medications slowly.
* Avoid alcohol or other CNS depressants. Dependence is a major unwanted effect.

OTHER INFORMATION
* Naloxone (Narcan) is used to reverse narcotic-induced respiratory depression.

NON-NARCOTIC ANALGESICS

MEDICATION: GENERIC/TRADE
* aspirin

ACTION
* Analgesic, antipyretic, anti-inflammatory

ADVERSE EFFECTS
* Prolonged bleeding time
* Nausea, vomiting, gastrointestinal distress

INDICATIONS
* Arthritis
* Mild pain, fever

NURSING INTERVENTIONS
* Teach client who takes large doses for a long time to watch for signs of bleeding.
* Administer with meals, milk, or antacids.

OTHER INFORMATION
* Contraindicated for children under 18 years old because use has been linked to Reye syndrome

NON-NARCOTIC ANALGESICS

MEDICATION: GENERIC/TRADE
* acetaminophen (*Tylenol*)

ACTION
* Analgesic antipyretic

ADVERSE EFFECTS
* Hepatotoxicity only with very large doses

INDICATIONS
* Mild pain, fever

NURSING INTERVENTIONS
* Teach client not to exceed recommended dosage.

NON-NARCOTIC ANALGESICS

MEDICATION: GENERIC/TRADE
* ibuprofen (*Motrin*)
* naproxen (*Naprosyn*)

ACTION
• Anti-inflammatory analgesic

ADVERSE EFFECTS
• Gastrointestinal distress, occult bleeding, allergy

INDICATIONS
• Arthritis, gout
• Pain from inflammation

NURSING INTERVENTIONS
• Administer with meals, milk, or antacids.
• Check stool for melena or occult blood.
• Treat gastrointestinal distress.
• Contraindicated in clients allergic to aspirin.

Eye Agents
MIOTICS

MEDICATION: GENERIC/TRADE
• pilocarpine hydrochloride (Carpine)

ACTION
• Decreases intraocular pressure and decreases production of aqueous humor

ADVERSE EFFECTS
• Myopia
• Blurred vision
• Retinal detachment
• Bronchospasm

INDICATIONS
• Glaucoma
• Surgical procedures on the eye

NURSING INTERVENTIONS
• Symptoms disappear after 10 to 14 days of treatment.
• Advise client to use caution when driving, especially at night.
• Advise client to use cautiously with bronchial asthma.
• Conjunctival irritation may subside in 10 to 14 days following treatment.

OTHER INFORMATION
• Press inner canthus for a minute or two to decrease systemic absorption.

MYDRIATICS

MEDICATION: GENERIC/TRADE
• atropine sulfate (Atropisol)

ACTION
• Pupillary dilatation, cycloplegia

ADVERSE EFFECTS
• Blurred vision
• Photophobia
• May cause cardiovascular changes such as hypotension, hypertension, and ventricular fibrillation.

INDICATIONS
• Acute inflammation of the eye
• Diagnostic procedure

NURSING INTERVENTIONS
• Warn client about temporary blurring of vision.
• Have client wear dark glasses.
• Teach client not to drive until vision is clear.

MYDRIATICS

MEDICATION: GENERIC/TRADE
• phenylephrine hydrochloride (Neo-Synephrine)

ACTION
• Pupillary dilatation

ADVERSE EFFECTS
• Hypertension
• Blurred vision

INDICATIONS
• Diagnostic procedure

NURSING INTERVENTIONS
• Monitor blood pressure.
• Avoid use in clients with hypertension.
• Teach client not to drive until vision is clear.

Fluid and Electrolyte Agents
ELECTROLYTE REPLACEMENT MEDICATIONS

MEDICATION: GENERIC/TRADE
• potassium chloride

ACTION
• Necessary for cardiac contraction, renal function, and transmission of nerve impulses

ADVERSE EFFECTS
• Cardiac arrhythmias, heart block, cardiac arrest
• Gastrointestinal distress

INDICATIONS
• Hypokalemia

NURSING INTERVENTIONS
• Administer IV infusions as dilute solution infuses slowly.
• Monitor ECG and serum potassium levels.
• Administer oral dose with meals and plenty of fluids.
• Monitor for signs of hyperkalemia.
• Potassium chloride is not given IV push. Infuse at rate not to exceed 10 mEq/hr.

LOOP DIURETICS

MEDICATION: GENERIC/TRADE
• furosemide (Lasix)
• ethacrynate sodium (Sodium Edecrin)
• ethacrynic acid (Edecrin)

ACTION
• Inhibit sodium and chloride reabsorption in the kidney
• Increase excretion of sodium and water

ADVERSE EFFECTS
• Fluid and electrolyte imbalances
• Hypocalcemia
• Hypokalemia
• Dehydration
• Hyponatremia
• Orthostatic hypotension
• Hypochloremia

INDICATIONS
• Edema
• Pulmonary edema

NURSING INTERVENTIONS
• Monitor I&O, weight, and serum electrolytes.

- Teach client to increase dietary potassium intake.
- Observe for signs of hypokalemia: muscle weakness, cramps, and metabolic alkalosis.
- Teach clients to stand up, take the stairs, and move around slowly.

OTHER INFORMATION
- Administer in the morning to prevent nocturia.
- High risk of digitalis toxicity due to potassium depletion

OSMOTIC DIURETICS

MEDICATION: GENERIC/TRADE
- mannitol *(Osmitrol)*

ACTION
- Increases osmotic pressure of glomerular filtrate
- Increases excretion of water and electrolytes

ADVERSE EFFECTS
- Fluid and electrolyte imbalances
- Transient plasma volume increase
- Pulmonary edema
- Cellular dehydration

INDICATIONS
- Oliguria
- Edema
- Increased intraocular pressure
- Increased intracranial pressure

 NURSING INTERVENTIONS
- Monitor vital signs hourly, including central venous pressure.
- Insert indwelling urinary catheter, record urine output hourly.
- Monitor weight, I&O, serum sodium, and potassium.
- A rebound increase in ICP may occur about 12 hr after medication administration; client may report headache or confusion.

OTHER INFORMATION
- IV solution may crystallize; dissolve before infusing by warming bottle and shaking.

POTASSIUM-SPARING DIURETICS

MEDICATION: GENERIC/TRADE
- spironolactone *(Aldactone)*
- triamterene *(Dyrenium)*

ACTION
- Increased excretion of sodium and water
- Reduces potassium excretion

ADVERSE EFFECTS
- Hyperkalemia

INDICATIONS
- Edema
- Hypertension

 NURSING INTERVENTIONS
- Monitor I&O, weight, blood pressure, and serum electrolytes.
- Teach client to avoid excessive dietary potassium.

OTHER INFORMATION
- Used in combination with potassium-depleting diuretics

THIAZIDES AND THIAZIDE-LIKE DIURETICS

MEDICATION: GENERIC/TRADE
- chlorothiazide *(Diuril)*
- hydrochlorothiazide *(Hydrodiuril)*
- chlorthalidone *(Hygroton)*
- quinethazone *(Hydromox)*

ACTION
- Inhibit sodium reabsorption in the kidney
- Increase excretion of sodium and water

ADVERSE EFFECTS
- Hypokalemia
- Altered glucose metabolism

INDICATIONS
- Hypertension
- Edema

 NURSING INTERVENTIONS
- Monitor I&O, weight, blood pressure, and potassium level.
- Teach client to increase dietary potassium intake.
- Observe for signs of hypokalemia: muscle weakness, cramps, and metabolic alkalosis.
- Monitor blood glucose.
- Observe for signs of hyperglycemia.

OTHER INFORMATION
- Administer in the morning to prevent nocturia.
- High risk of digitalis toxicity due to potassium depletion

Gastrointestinal Medications
ANTACIDS

MEDICATION: GENERIC/TRADE
- aluminum hydroxide *(Amphojel)*
- aluminum and magnesium hydroxide and simethicone *(Mylanta)*
- aluminum and magnesium hydroxide *(Maalox)*
- Aluminum magnesium complex *(Riopan)*
- calcium carbonate *(Tums)*

ACTION
- Reduce acid in gastrointestinal tract
- Decrease pepsin activity

ADVERSE EFFECTS
- Constipation
- Hypernatremia
- Hypermagnesemia
- Hypophosphatemia

INDICATIONS
- Gastritis
- Esophageal reflux
- Adjunct in treatment of gastric and duodenal ulcers

 NURSING INTERVENTIONS
- Record amount and consistency of stools.
- Teach client to increase phosphorous in diet when taking large doses for prolonged periods.
- Increase dietary fiber, fluid intake, and exercise.
- Use laxatives and stool softeners.
- For the client who needs salt restriction, administer aluminum magnesium complex, which has a very low sodium content.
- Do not give magnesium-containing antacids to a client with renal disease.
- When giving aluminum-containing antacids, observe for anorexia, malaise, and/or muscle weakness.

ANTIEMETICS

MEDICATION: GENERIC/TRADE
- prochlorperazine maleate (Compazine)
- trimethobenzamide hydrochloride (Tigan)
- ondansetron (Zofran)

ACTION
- Acts centrally by blocking chemoreceptor trigger zone, which acts on vomiting center

ADVERSE EFFECTS
- Drowsiness, dizziness - rare extrapyramidal reaction can occur
- Diarrhea

INDICATIONS
- Nausea and vomiting

NURSING INTERVENTIONS
- Teach client to avoid activities that require alertness.
- Headache is a common side effect requiring analgesic relief with ondansetron.

ANTIEMETICS

MEDICATION: GENERIC/TRADE
- dimenhydrinate (Dramamine)
- scopolamine (Transderm V)

ACTION
- Acts centrally by blocking chemoreceptor trigger zone, which acts on vomiting center

ADVERSE EFFECTS
- Drowsiness, dizziness
- Decreased respirations

INDICATIONS
- Prevention of nausea and vomiting associated with motion sickness

NURSING INTERVENTIONS
- Teach client to avoid activities that require alertness.
- Teach client to apply the night before an expected trip or anticipated motion. Wash hands carefully after handling.

ULCER MEDICATIONS

MEDICATION: GENERIC/TRADE
- cimetidine (Tagamet)
- sucralfate (Carafate)
- omeprazole (Prilosec)
- ranitidine (Zantac)

ACTION
- Ranitidine and cimetidine are gastrointestinal antihistamines; they act to reduce gastric acid secretion.
- Sucralfate coats and protects surface of ulcer.
- Omeprazole blocks acid production.

ADVERSE EFFECTS
- Abdominal cramps, diarrhea
- Agranulocytosis, increased protime

INDICATIONS
- Short-term treatment of duodenal and gastric ulcers, and GERD

NURSING INTERVENTIONS
- Administer with meals for prolonged medication effect.
- Avoid over-the-counter preparations such as aspirin and cough medications.
- Report bruising.
- Do not crush, chew, or open capsules (Prilosec).

OTHER INFORMATION
- Short-term treatment only
- Separate administration of these medications from administration of antacids by 1 hr.

Hematologic Agents
ANTICOAGULANTS

MEDICATION: GENERIC/TRADE
- heparin sodium (Hep-Lock, Hepalean)
- enoxaparin (Lovenox); low molecular weight heparin

ACTION
- Prevents conversion of fibrinogen to fibrin and prothrombin to thrombin

ADVERSE EFFECTS
- Hemorrhage
- Injection site reactions

INDICATIONS
- Thrombosis
- Pulmonary embolism
- Myocardial infarction

NURSING INTERVENTIONS
- Monitor platelet count.
- Monitor activated partial thromboplastin time (aPTT).
- Avoid salicylates.
- Observe for bleeding gums, bruises, nosebleeds, and petechiae.

OTHER INFORMATION
- IV absorption is more regular than subcutaneous injection.
- aPTT should be 1.5 to 2 times control value.
- Antagonist is protamine sulfate.

ANTICOAGULANTS

MEDICATION: GENERIC/TRADE
- warfarin (Coumadin)

ACTION
- Prevents prothrombin formations

ADVERSE EFFECTS
- Hemorrhage

INDICATIONS
- Pulmonary embolism
- Thrombosis, myocardial infarction, heart valve damage

NURSING INTERVENTIONS
- Monitor prothrombin time (PT).
- Avoid salicylates.
- Observe for bleeding gums, bruises, nosebleeds, and petechiae.
- Teach client to use soft toothbrush and electric razor.

OTHER INFORMATION
- Oral administration PT should be 1.5 to 2 times control value.
- Antagonist is vitamin K.

ANTINEOPLASTICS

MEDICATION: GENERIC/TRADE
- methotrexate *(Folex, Rheumatrex)*
- cisplatin *(Platinol)*
- bleomycin *(Blenoxane)*

ACTION
- Act by many different mechanisms, most affect DNA synthesis or function

ADVERSE EFFECTS
- Many cause bone marrow depression, thrombocytopenia, nausea, vomiting, and/or mouth ulcers

INDICATIONS
- Cancer
- Chemotherapy

NURSING INTERVENTIONS
- Assess client for signs of infection.
- Monitor platelet count.
- Monitor IV site carefully, ensure patency; follow protocols for infiltration to prevent tissue ulceration/necrosis.
- Wear gloves, masks, gowns while handling or preparing medication; discard equipment in designated containers.
- Give antimetics as prescribed.
- Monitor for ulcerative stomatitis and gingivitis (often the first signs of toxicity).

ANTIPLATELET AGGREGATE

MEDICATION: GENERIC/TRADE
- aspirin *(ASA)*
- clopidogrel bisulfate *(Plavix)*

ACTION
- Inhibits platelet aggregation and prevents clots from forming

ADVERSE EFFECTS
- Bleeding
- Liver disease
- Headache, dizziness
- Gastric ulcers
- Bruising
- Rash
- Nausea
- Additional adverse effects for aspirin (ASA):
  - Thrombocytopenia
  - Angioedema
  - Tinnitus
  - Reduced hearing
  - Reye syndrome

INDICATIONS
- Prevent clot formation in clients with atherosclerosis, unstable angina, or recent myocardial infarction

NURSING INTERVENTIONS
- Monitor for bruising or signs of gastricintestinal bleeding.
- Do not use in clients with a history of gastric ulcers or liver disease.
- Advise client bleeding from cuts may take longer than normal to stop.
- Advise client to notify the dentist that he is taking this medication prior to a dental procedure.
- Advise client to avoid over-the-counter products containing aspirin.
- Do not give aspirin to children or adolescents.
- Give aspirin with food.

COLONY-STIMULATING FACTORS

MEDICATION: GENERIC/TRADE
- erythropoietin *(Procrit)*

ACTION
- Corrects anemia by stimulating RBC production

ADVERSE EFFECTS
- Arthralgia
- Seizures
- Headache, fever, dizziness
- Hypertension
- Clotting of arteriovenous graft

INDICATIONS
- Anemia caused by end-stage renal disease, chemotherapy, rheumatic disease, or antiretrovirals.

NURSING INTERVENTIONS
- Monitor CBC and blood pressure.
- Monitor serum iron level.
- Advise the client that he may have pain in limbs and diaphoresis for up to 12 hr following treatment.
- Adjust heparin during dialysis to prevent clot formation.

COLONY-STIMULATING FACTORS

MEDICATION: GENERIC/TRADE
- filgrastim *(Neupogen)*

ACTION
- Increases WBCs by stimulating production of neutrophils.

ADVERSE EFFECTS
- Fever, fatigue
- Myocardial infarction
- Thrombocytopenia
- Bone pain
- Hair loss

INDICATIONS
- Prevent or correct neutropenia. Treat myelodysplasia.

NURSING INTERVENTIONS
- Monitor CBC and platelets.
- Provide relief for skeletal pain.
- Wait 24 hr after chemotherapy to give medications.

HEMATONICS

MEDICATION: GENERIC/TRADE
- ferrous sulfate *(Slow-Fe)*

ACTION
- Source of iron replacement

ADVERSE EFFECTS
- Nausea, constipation, black stool

INDICATIONS
- Iron deficiency anemia

NURSING INTERVENTIONS
- Ascorbic acid increases absorption; give with citrus juice (except the elixir).
- For gastrointestinal upset, give with meals or orange juice.
- Teach client to increase dietary fiber, fluid intake, and exercise.

Hormonal Agents
CORTICOSTEROIDS

MEDICATION: GENERIC/TRADE
- cortisone acetate (Cortone)
- dexamethasone (Decadron)
- prednisone (Meticorten)
- hydrocortisone (Solu-Cortef)

ACTION
- Anti-inflammatory

ADVERSE EFFECTS
- Euphoria, insomnia, psychotic behavior
- Hypokalemia
- Hyperglycemia and carbohydrate intolerance
- Peptic ulcer
- Cushingoid symptoms with long-term therapy
- Withdrawal symptoms

INDICATIONS
- Adrenal insufficiency
- Allergic inflammation, edema, immunosuppression

 NURSING INTERVENTIONS
- Assess the client's behavior, especially with high doses.
- A potassium supplement may be needed.
- Provide a high-protein diet that is also rich in potassium.
- A client who has diabetes mellitus may require higher doses of insulin.
- Administer medication with meals.
- Teach client manifestations.
- Reduce dose gradually, not abruptly.

INSULINS

MEDICATION: GENERIC/TRADE
- Humalog insulin (Lispro) (Rapid acting [NovoLog])
- Regular insulin (Humulin R, Novolin R) (Short acting)
- Lente NPH (Intermediate acting [Humulin N and Novolin N])
- Ultralente protamine (Long acting)
- Insulin glargine (Lantus) (Long acting)
- Combination insulin: 70/30 (70% NPH insulin and 30% Regular insulin)

ACTION
- Facilitates transport of glucose into cells
- Lowers serum glucose level

ADVERSE EFFECTS
- Hypoglycemia
- Hyperglycemia

INDICATIONS
- Insulin-dependent diabetes mellitus

 NURSING INTERVENTIONS
- Administer orange juice or candy for hypoglycemia.
- Follow hospital or medical protocols for hyperglycemia and hypoglycemia.
- Administer rapid-acting insulin for hyperglycemia.
- Monitor capillary blood glucose routinely.

OTHER INFORMATION
- Refrigeration is recommended for long-term storage.
- Do not inject cold insulin.

SULFONYLUREAS

MEDICATION: GENERIC/TRADE
- tolbutamide (Orinase)
- chlorpropamide (Diabinese)
- tolazamide (Tolinase)
- glyburide (Micronase, DiaBeta)
- glipizide (Glucotrol)

ACTION
- Increases insulin release from the pancreas

ADVERSE EFFECTS
- Hypoglycemia
- Hepatotoxicity

INDICATIONS
- Adult onset, noninsulin dependent
- Diabetes mellitus

 NURSING INTERVENTIONS
- Teach client to take medication in morning to avoid hypoglycemic reaction at night.
- Tell client to avoid over-the-counter medications and alcohol.
- Use with caution in clients with a history of cardiovascular disease. Cardiovascular mortality has been linked to oral hypoglycemic use.

Mood-Stabilizing Agents
MOOD STABILIZERS

MEDICATION: GENERIC/TRADE
- lithium carbonate (Eskalith, Lithonate, Lithotabs, Lithobid)

ACTION
- Alters Na, K, and ion transport in nerve; interferes with balance of epinephrine and serotonin in CNS, thereby affecting emotional responses

ADVERSE EFFECTS
- Fine tremor
- Transient nausea
- Drowsiness, lethargy
- Diarrhea, abdominal discomfort
- Polyuria
- Thirst
- Weight gain
- Signs of toxicity:
  - Vomiting
  - Diarrhea
  - Lethargy
  - Muscle twitching
  - Ataxia
  - Slurred speech
  - Coma
  - Seizure
  - Cardiac arrest

INDICATIONS
- Bipolar disorder, manic phase
- Major depression
- Aggressive conduct disorder

 NURSING INTERVENTIONS
- Teach client that side effects are short in duration.
- Observe client carefully for changes in manifestations.
- Monitor blood levels.
- Advise client to avoid caffeine.
- Keep side rails up.

- Teach client to avoid activities that require alertness.
- Administer medication with meals.
- Increase fluid intake.
- Restrict calories and increase physical exercise.
- Assess client for edema.
- Observe client carefully for manifestations, and monitor blood levels as sodium decreases and lithium levels increase.
- Hold next dose and report stat.
- Conduct pretreatment medical exam with thyroid and kidney function testing and ECG.
- Nonsteroidal anti-inflammatory drugs may lead to lithium toxicity.

OTHER INFORMATION
- Narrow therapeutic index
  - 0.8 mEq/L to 1.2 mEq/L; therapeutic
  - 1.5 mEq/L to 2.0 mEq/L; toxic
  - Above 2.0 mEq/L: can be lethal

MEDICATION INTERACTIONS
- Diuretics increase the risk of lithium toxicity.
- Antipsychotics may cause neurotoxicity, especially in older adults.
- Ingestion of excessive salt increases lithium excretion.
- Discontinue medication prior to elective surgery or electroconvulsive therapy.
- Do not take if pregnant.

MOOD STABILIZERS

MEDICATION: GENERIC/TRADE
- carbamazepine (Tegretol)

ACTION
- Affects mood by inhibiting nerve impulses, by limiting sodium exchange

ADVERSE EFFECTS
- Skin rash
- Sore throat, mucosal ulcerations
- Low-grade fever
- Drowsiness, ataxia, vertigo
- Diplopia, blurred vision
- Nausea and vomiting, hepatotoxicity

INDICATIONS
- Acute mania and prevention of manic episodes when lithium ineffective
- Temporal lobe epilepsy

 NURSING INTERVENTIONS
- Use cautiously with lithium and haloperidol (Haldol).

MOOD STABILIZERS

MEDICATION: GENERIC/TRADE
- valproic acid (Depakote)

ACTION
- Increases levels of gamma-aminobutyric acid in brain

ADVERSE EFFECTS
- Gastrointestinal reports
- Tremor, sedation, ataxia
- Increased appetite, weight gain
- Pancreatitis
- Severe hepatic dysfunction
- Thrombocytopenia

INDICATIONS
- Manic episodes when lithium ineffective (better tolerated)

 NURSING INTERVENTIONS
- Administer with food or milk.
- Use to manage seizures.
- Teach client to avoid activities that require alertness.
- Monitor liver function test and hematology levels.
- Monitor for therapeutic serum level of 50 to 100 mcg/mL.

Obstetrics-Setting Agents
ANTICONVULSANTS

MEDICATION: GENERIC/TRADE
- magnesium sulfate

ACTION
- Anticonvulsant

ADVERSE EFFECTS
- Respiratory depression
- Heart block
- Circulatory collapse
- Increased magnesium

INDICATIONS
- Pregnancy-induced hypertension; controls or prevents premature labor, seizures

 NURSING INTERVENTIONS
- Hold medication if respirations less than 12/min.
- Monitor client for arrhythmias.
- Monitor pulse and blood pressure.
- Monitor I&O.
- Observe for neuromuscular or respiratory depression.
- Give slowly through IV.

OTHER INFORMATION
- Antidote is calcium gluconate

ANTIDOTES

MEDICATION: GENERIC/TRADE
- calcium gluconate

ACTION
- Needed for nervous musculoskeletal enzyme reactions, cardiac contraction, blood coagulation, and endocrine and exocrine secretions

ADVERSE EFFECTS
- Bradycardia
- Arrhythmias
- Venous irritation

INDICATIONS
- Hypermagnesemia

 NURSING INTERVENTIONS
- Monitor the client's pulse.
- Monitor the client for arrhythmias during administration.
- Assess IV site.

OTHER INFORMATION
- Contraindicated in clients who are digitized

ANTI-INFLAMMATORY DRUGS

MEDICATION: GENERIC/TRADE
- betamethasone (Celestone)

ACTION
- Corticosteroid

ADVERSE EFFECTS
- Gastrointestinal distress, hemorrhage, and pancreatitis
- Poor wound healing
- CNS depression, flushing, and sweating
- Thrombocytopenia
- Hypertension, circulation collapse, and embolism

INDICATIONS
- Stimulate lung development in infant
- Strong immunosuppressant
- Anti-inflammatory

NURSING INTERVENTIONS
- Monitor the client's temperature.
- Monitor the client's blood pressure and reports of chest pain.

OTHER INFORMATION
- Do not discontinue abruptly; adrenal crisis may occur.

ESTROGENS

MEDICATION: GENERIC/TRADE
- estradiol (Estrace)

ACTION
- Hormone needed for adequate functioning of female reproductive system; inhibits ovulation
- Promotes calcium use in bone structure

ADVERSE EFFECTS
- Hypoglycemia
- Dizziness, hypotension
- Gastrointestinal: nausea, vomiting
- Appetite increase, weight gain
- Embolism
- May increase risk of endometrial and breast cancer

INDICATIONS
- Prevent postpartum breast engorgement

NURSING INTERVENTIONS
- Observe glucose in clients who have diabetes mellitus.
- Monitor the client's weight.
- Report client's reports of headache and/or chest pain.
- Monitor the client for signs of endometrial or breast cancer.
- Instruct the client on self breast exam.
- Instruct the client to report symptoms of abdominal pain, vaginal bleeding, and/or discharge.

NARCOTIC ANTAGONISTS

MEDICATION: GENERIC/TRADE
- naloxone (Narcan)

ACTION
- Interferes with narcotic absorption at narcotic receptor sites

ADVERSE EFFECTS
- Rapid pulse
- Drowsiness, nervousness
- Nausea, vomiting
- Pulmonary edema

INDICATIONS
- Treatment of narcotic-induced depression of neonate
- Respiratory depression caused by an opioid

NURSING INTERVENTION
- Monitor the neonate's respiratory rate and depth.

- Provide supplemental oxygen as needed.
- Monitor respirations and pulse oximetry.

OXYTOCICS

MEDICATION: GENERIC/TRADE
- oxytocin (Pitocin)

ACTION
- Stimulates contractions of the uterus

ADVERSE EFFECTS
- Hypotension
- Fetal bradycardia or tachycardia
- Tachycardia
- Decreased urine output

INDICATIONS
- Induction of labor

NURSING INTERVENTIONS
- Monitor uterine contractions, blood pressure, maternal heart rate, and fetal heart rate.
- Monitor I&O.

OTHER INFORMATION
- Use only when pelvis is adequate, vaginal delivery is indicted, fetus is mature, and fetal position is favorable.

OXYTOCICS

MEDICATION: GENERIC/TRADE
- methylergonovine maleate (Methergine)

ACTION
- Stimulates motor activity of the uterus

ADVERSE EFFECTS
- Headache
- Chest pain
- Nausea
- Palpitations

INDICATIONS
- Postpartum hemorrhage due to uterine atony

NURSING INTERVENTIONS
- Assess uterine contractions following administration.
- Monitor vital signs and vaginal bleeding.

OTHER INFORMATION
- Contraindicated prior to the fourth stage of labor

UTERINE RELAXANTS

MEDICATION: GENERIC/TRADE
- isoxsuprine hydrochloride (Vasodilan)

ACTION
- Vasodilator

ADVERSE EFFECTS
- Hypotension
- Tachycardia

INDICATIONS
- Premature labor
- Labor contractions too frequent or uncoordinated

NURSING INTERVENTIONS
- Monitor the client's blood pressure and pulse.

OTHER INFORMATION
- Contraindicated in immediate postpartum period

UTERINE RELAXANTS

MEDICATION: GENERIC/TRADE
- ritodrine hydrochloride *(Yutopar)*

ACTION
- Inhibits contraction of uterine smooth muscle

ADVERSE EFFECTS
- Hypotension
- Hypertension

INDICATIONS
- Premature labor

NURSING INTERVENTIONS
- Monitor the client's blood pressure; maternal heart and fetal heart rate.

UTERINE RELAXANTS

MEDICATION: GENERIC/TRADE
- terbutaline sulfate *(Brethine)*

ACTION
- Relaxes uterine smooth muscle

ADVERSE EFFECTS
- Nervousness
- Tremors
- Headache

INDICATIONS
- Premature labor

NURSING INTERVENTIONS
- Monitor the client's blood pressure and pulse.
- Monitor maternal heart rate and fetal heart rate.

OTHER INFORMATION
- Use cautiously in clients with diabetes mellitus, heart disease, and hypertension.

APPENDIX F

NCLEX® "NEED TO KNOW" LABORATORY VALUES*

A. Serum Electrolytes:
Sodium (Na$^+$) = 135 to 145 mEq/L
Potassium (K$^+$) = 3.5 to 5.0 mEq/L
Calcium (Ca^{++}) = 8.5 to 10 mg/dL
Magnesium (Mg^{++}) = 1.8 to 3.0 mg/dL
Phosphorus (PO4) = 2.5 to 4.5 mg/dL
Creatinine (Cr) = 0.5 to 1.0 mg/dL
BUN = 10 to 20 mg/dL
Glucose (fasting) = 70 to 110 mg/dL

B. ABGs:
pH = 7.35 to 7.45
PaCO$_2$ = 35 to 45 mm Hg
PO$_2$ = >80 mm Hg
HCO$_3^-$ (bicarbonate) = 22 to 26 mEq/L
SaO$_2$ = 90 to 100 %

C. CBC:
RBCs	Males 4.6 to 6.2 mm³
	Females 4.2 to 5.4 mm³
WBCs	4,800 to 10,800 mm³
Hgb	Males 13 to 18 g/dL
	Females 12 to 16 g/dL
HCT	Males 45 to 52%
	Females 37 to 48%

D. Other Hematologic Values:
Glycosylated hemoglobin (HgbA1c) 5% (up to 7% in clients with diabetes mellitus)
Erythrocyte sedimentation rate < 20 mm/hr

E. Coagulation Times:
Bleeding time = 4 to 7 min
Therapeutic INR = 2.0 to 3.0
Platelets = 150,000 to 450,000 cu/mm
Prothrombin time = 11 to 14 seconds
Activated partial thromboplastin time = < 40 seconds

F. Liver Function Tests:
Albumin = 3.8 to 5.0 g/dL
Ammonia = 35 to 65 mcg/dL
Total bilirubin = 0 to 1.5 mg/dL
Total protein = 6.0 to 8.0 gm/dL

G. Urinalysis:
Specific gravity = 1.010 to 1.025
pH = 4.5 to 7.5
Glucose = negative
RBCs = negative
WBCs = negative
Albumin = negative

H. Therapeutic Medication Monitoring:
Digoxin level = 0.8 to 2.0 ng/mL
Lithium level = 0.8 to 1.2 mEq/L

(Note: "Need to know values" are those listed in the 2007 Detailed Test Plan for the NCLEX-RN® examination under the heading of "Physiological Adaptation: Reduction of Risk Potential, Laboratory Values")

"Need to Know" laboratory values have been taken from the United States National Library of Medicine at the National Institutes for Health. Different institutions or laboratories may use slightly different normal laboratory values and ranges. NCLEX® exam questions addressing laboratory values will include easily identifiable high and low laboratory values.

INDEX

A

abortion, 136
abruptio placenta, 138
acid-base imbalance, 12
acidosis
    metabolic, 12, 14(t)
    respiratory, 12, 14(t)
acquired immune deficiency syndrome (AIDS), 79
acromegaly, 40
acyanotic heart defects, 160(t)
Addison's disease, 42
ADHD. *See* attention-deficit and hyperactivity disorder
adolescents
    activity/rest, 156
    developmental stages of, 157
    language development, 157
    motor skills, 156
    nutrition, 156
    physical development, 156
adrenal gland functions, 43(t)
advance directives, 192
African-American client, 201
agoraphobia, 93
AIDS. *See* acquired immune deficiency syndrome
alcohol abuse, 107
alcohol withdrawal delirium, 109
alcohol withdrawal syndrome, 109
aldosteronism, 43
alkalosis
    metabolic, 12
    respiratory, 14
alternate item formats
    chart review, 215
    drag and drop, 213
    supply, 213
    hot spot, 214
    multiple response item, 214
Alzheimer's disease, 111
amniocentesis, 130
amniotic fluid, 123
amputation, 39
amyotrophic lateral sclerosis (ALS), 74
ANA code for nurses, 192
anemia, 49
    hemolytic, 50
    hyperproliferation, 50
    iron deficiency, 50
        in children 150
    megaloblastic, 50

    sickle cell, 50
anesthetics
    general, 24
    local, 24
angina, 53
angiography
    cardiac, 52
    renal, 61
anorexia, 112
anxiety, 91
    generalized, 92
    levels of, 92, 92(t)
    social (social phobia), 93
    test-taking, 7
aortic aneurysm, 55
Apgar score, 138
appendicitis, 170
arterial blood gas interpretation, 14(t)
arteriogram
    cardiac, 52
    cerebral, 68
arteriosclerosis obliterans, 57
arthritis
    juvenile rheumatoid (JRA), 174
    rheumatoid, 37(t)
ASD. *See* atrial septal defect
Asian-American Client, 201
asthma, 16
    in children, 172
atrial septal defect (ASD), 160 (t)
attention-deficit and hyperactivity disorder (ADHD), 97
autonomic hyperreflexia, 72
autism, 96

B

barium
    enema, 27
    swallow, 26
behavior modification, 87
benign prostatic hyperplasia (BPH), 65
bilirubin, 29
biophysical profile, 130
biopsy
    liver, 28
    renal, 61
bipolar disorder, 101
blood transfusion, 49
bowel surgery, 33

K

Kaposi's sarcoma, 80
ketoacidosis
    diabetic, 48
kick counts, 129
kidney
    functions of, 60
    transplantation, 65
knee
    total replacement of, 40

L

labor, 128
    induction of, 134
    premature, 132
    signs of, 130
    stages of, 130(t)
laminectomy, 73
laryngotracheobronchitis, 168
leadership, 189
leukemia
    in child, 176
lice, head. *See* pediculosis
liver
    function tests, 28
    functions of, 34
lochia, 134
lumbar puncture (LP), 68
lungs
    functions of, 14
    subdivisions of, 15
Lyme disease, 182(t)

M

magnetic resonance imaging (MRI), 69
management styles, 189
mania, 101
Mantoux test, 15
Maslow Hierarchy of Needs, 87, 87(t)
measles, 184(t)
medications
    administration to child, 171
    analgesia for labor and delivery, 132(t)
    antianxiety, 94(t)
    anticonvulsants, 70, 104(t)
    antidepressants, 102(t)
    antidepressants MAOI, 103(t)
    antihypertensive, 56
    antimania, 104(t)
    antipsychotics, 98(t)

    bronchodilators, 23
    chemotherapy, 77
    contraceptives, 143
    diuretics
        potassium depleting, 56
        potassium sparing, 56
    insulin preparations, 48(t)
    nonsteroidal agents, inhaled, 23
    organic mental disorders, 110
    sleep agents, 106(t)
    steroids, inhaled, 23
    used in labor and delivery, 131(t)
Ménière's disease, 75
meningitis, 183(t)
menopause, 143
mental health continuum, 89
mental retardation, 113
metered-dose inhalers, 23
milieu therapy, 88
mind-body alternative therapies, 207
mitral valve replacement, 55
MRI. *See* magnetic resonance imaging
multiple sclerosis, 73
mumps, 183(t)
Münchausen syndrome by proxy, 171
myasthenia gravis, 74
myelogram, 68
myelomeningocele, 162
myocardial infarction, 53
myxedema, 44

N

Nägele's rule, 124
Native-American client, 203
NCLEX®, 3, 213
    alternate item formats, 213
    communication questions, 6
    computerized adaptive testing, 3
    exam day, 7
    exam structure, 4
    priority setting questions, 7
    screen design, 3
    study skills, 4
    test-taking strategies, 6
neonate
    assessment of, 138
    care of, 138
    initial care of, 138
    postmature, 141
    premature, 140
nephroblastoma, 178
nephrosis, 62

nephrotic syndrome, 176(t)
neuroblastoma, 176
nonstress test, 129

O

obsessive-compulsive disorder (OCD), 93
omega-3 fatty acids, 207
organ donation, 192
organic mental disorders, 110
osteoarthritis, 37(t)
osteoporosis, 39
otitis media, 167
oxygen toxicity, 17

P

pacemaker
    cardiac, 52
pain
    child's reaction to, 158
pancreas functions, 47(t)
pancreatitis, 36
panic disorder, 92
para, 124
paracentesis, 28
parathyroid gland functions, 46
Parkinson's disease, 73
patent ductus arteriosus (PDA), 160
pediculosis, 183(t)
PEG. See tube, percutaneous endoscopic gastrostomy
pelvic inflammatory disease (PID), 143
percutaneous transhepatic cholangiogram (PTCA), 28
percutaneous transthoracic cardiac angioplasty (PTCA), 58
peripheral vascular disease, 57
pernicious anemia, 28
personality
    antisocial, 107
    borderline, 107
    paranoid, 96
pertussis, 183(t)
pheochromocytoma, 43
phobia,
    school, 156
phobic disorders, 93
PID. See pelvic inflammatory disease
PIH. See pregnancy-induced hypertension
pinworms, 182(t)
pituitary gland functions, 41(t)
placenta
    functions of, 123
    previa, 138
pleural effusion, 22
pneumonia, 20

pneumothorax
    open, 18
    spontaneous, 18
    tension, 18
polyhydramnios, 136
postoperative care, 24
postoperative complications, 25(t)
postpartum
    assessment, 134
    hemorrhage, 135
post-traumatic stress disorder (PTSD), 93
postural drainage, 22
pre-eclampsia, 137
pregnancy
    ectopic, 137
    emotional adaptations, 128
    high risk, 135
    induced hypertension (PIH), 137
    molar, 137
    objective signs of, 124
    adaptations to pregnancy, 125(t)
    positive signs of, 124
    presumptive signs of, 124
premature rupture of membranes (PROM), 132
prenatal care, 128
preoperative care, 24
preschooler
    activity and rest, 153
    developmental stages, 154
    language development, 154
    motor skills, 154
    nutrition, 153
    physical development, 153
    play, 154
PROM. See premature rupture of membranes
psychosocial development, 85
PTCA. See percutaneous transhepatic cholangiogram
PTCA. See percutaneous transthoracic cardiac angioplasty
PTSD. See post-traumatic stress disorder
pulmonary edema, 54
pulmonary emphysema, 16
pulmonary toilet, 22
pyloric stenosis, 170

Q

quality improvement, 190

R

rabies, 183(t)
radiation therapy
    external, 79
    internal, 79
rape, 115
Raynaud's syndrome, 58
renal failure
    acute, 63
    chronic, 63
renal function tests, 60
renal transplantation, 65
resource management, 190
retina
    detached, 76
Reye syndrome, 183(t)
rheumatic fever, 174
    in child, 183(t)
ringworm, 182(t)
roseola, 184(t)
rubella, 184(t)
rubeola, 184(t)

S

saw palmetto, 206
scarlet fever, 184(t)
schizophrenia, 96
school-age child
    activity and rest, 155
    developmental stages, 155
    language development, 155
    motor skills, 155
    nutrition, 155
    physical development, 155
    play, 155
school phobia, 156
scoliosis, 174
scope of practice
    advance practice nurse, 191
    nursing assistant, 191
    practical nurse, 191
    primary care provider, 191
    registered nurse, 192
seizure
    disorder, 70
    febrile, 165
sensory assessment, 75
Seventh Day Adventists, 200
shock, 59
SIADH. *See* syndrome of inappropriate secretion of antidi-
    uretic hormone
SIDS. *See* sudden infant death syndrome

SLE. *See* systemic lupus erythematosus
spinal cord injury, 72
spiritually sensitive care, 200
sputum examination, 15
St. John's wort, 206
status asthmaticus, 17
    in child, 173
status epilepticus, 70
steroids
    replacement therapy, 43
stone, kidney. *See* urolithiasis
stool analysis, 27
substance abuse, 108(t), 109(t)
    and the neonate, 141
suctioning
    pulmonary, 23
sudden infant death syndrome (SIDS), 152
suicide, 101
syndrome of inappropriate secretion of antidiuretic
    hormone (SIADH), 42
systemic lupus erythematosus (SLE), 80

T

T.O.R.C.H., 127
Tai Chi, 208
team building, 190
teratogens, 124
terms, mental health, 117(t)
tetanus, 184(t)
tetralogy of Fallot, 161(t)
thoracentesis, 15
thrombophlebitis, 56
thyroid gland functions, 44(t)
thyroidectomy, 45
TIA. *See* transient ischemic attacks
toddlers
    activity and rest, 152
    developmental stages, 153
    language development, 153
    motor skills, 152
    nutrition, 152
    physical development, 152
    play, 153
toilet training, 153
tonsillectomy, 169
tooth eruption
    permanent, 155(t)
    primary, 149(t)
total parenteral nutrition (TPN), 29
traction, 38
traditional (folk) alternative therapies, 208
transfusion reaction, 49
transient ischemic attacks (TIA), 71

transposition of the great vessels, 161(t)
transurethral resection of the prostate (TURP), 65, 66(t)
triage
    in mass casualty situation, 205
    in non-mass casualty situation, 205
trichomoniasis, 142
tubal ligation, 144
tube
    chest, 18
    feeding, 29
    gastrostomy, 29
    Miller-Abbot, 29
    nasogastric, 29
    percutaneous endoscopic gastrostomy, 29
    Sengstaken-Blakemore, 29
tuberculosis, 19
TURP. *See* transurethral resection of the prostate

U

ulcer
    duodenal, 30, 31(t)
    gastric, 30, 31(t)
ulcerative colitis, 32, 32(t)
ultrasound
    fetal, 129
urinalysis, 60
urinary diversion, 65
urolithiasis, 62

V

valerian root, 206
valve disorders,
    cardiac, 55
varicose veins, 57
vasectomy, 144
ventricular septal defect (VSD), 160
ventriculoperitoneal shunt, 162
violence
    family, 114
    sexual assault, 115
vomiting
    in children, 166
VSD, *See* ventricular septal defect

W

Wernicke-Korsakoff's syndrome, 111
whooping cough, 183(t)

X

x-ray
    chest, 15
    flat plate, 28
    KUB, 60

Z

Zollinger-Ellison syndrome, 28